CONTENTS

Differential Diagnosis

Commissioning Editor: Laurence Hunter
Project Development Manager: Siân Jarman / Ailsa Laing
Project Manager: Frances Affleck
Designer: Erik Bigland

Differential Diagnosis

Andrew T. Raftery BSc MD Cl Biol MI Biol FRCS
Consultant Surgeon, Sheffield Kidney Institute,
Northern General Hospital NHS Trust, Sheffield,
UK; Member (formerly Chairman) of the Court
of Examiners, Royal College of Surgeons of
England; Member of Panel of Examiners,
Intercollegiate Speciality Board in General
Surgery; Honorary Senior Clinical Lecturer
in Surgery, University of Sheffield

Eric Lim MB ChB MRCS
Specialist Registrar in Cardiothoracic Surgery,
Papworth Hospital, Cambridge University
Teaching Hospitals
NHS Trust, Cambridge, UK

SECOND EDITION

ELSEVIER
CHURCHILL
LIVINGSTONE

EDINBURGH LONDON NEW YORK OXFORD
PHILADELPHIA ST LOUIS SYDNEY TORONTO 2005

ELSEVIER
CHURCHILL
LIVINGSTONE

First edition 2001
Second edition 2005

ISBN 0 443 10061 6
International Student Edition ISBN 0 443 10062 4

British Library Cataloguing in Publication Data
A catalogue record for this book is available from the British Library

Library of Congress Cataloging in Publication Data
A catalog record for this book is available from the Library of Congress

Note
Medical knowledge is constantly changing. Standard safety precautions must be
followed, but as new research and clinical experience broaden our knowledge,
changes in treatment and drug therapy may become necessary or appropriate.
Readers are advised to check the most current product information provided by
the manufacturer of each drug to be administered to verify the recommended
dose, the method and duration of administration, and contraindications. It is
the responsibility of the practitioner, relying on experience and knowledge of
the patient, to determine dosages and the best treatment for each individual
patient. Neither the Publisher nor the authors assume any liability for any injury
and/or damage to persons or property arising from this publication.
The Publisher

ELSEVIER your source for books,
journals and multimedia
in the health sciences
www.elsevierhealth.com

The
publisher's
policy is to use
**paper manufactured
from sustainable forests**

Printed in China

PREFACE

We are grateful to the publishers, Elsevier, for the invitation to produce a second edition of the *Pocketbook of Differential Diagnosis*. We are pleased with the way the first edition has sold and that, in these days of self-directed problem-based learning, medical students still see the need for a book offering a didactic approach. In this edition, several chapters have been revised, some extensively, and a new chapter on Palpitations added. We have welcomed comments from students who have suggested additions and corrections and these have been taken into account when revising the text. However, if any reader still feels that there are omissions or that the book can be further improved in any way, we would be pleased to hear from you. We hope this book will continue to help you on the wards and in the clinics – and in examinations.

Sheffield and Cambridge 2005

A.T.R.
E.L.

ACKNOWLEDGEMENTS

We wish to gratefully acknowledge the help, advice and criticisms of the following, who kindly read various sections of the book: Mr John Lund, Specialist Registrar in General Surgery, Northern General Hospital, Sheffield; Mr John Wright, Specialist Registrar in Orthopaedic Surgery, Northern General Hospital, Sheffield; Mr Neil Sheehan, General Dental Practitioner, Sheffield; Mr Aris Papageorghiou, Specialist Registrar in Obstetrics and Gynaecology, London.

Any errors that may have occurred, however, remain our responsibility and not theirs. We would particularly like to express our thanks to our junior staff and medical students who have suggested corrections, amendments and improvements to the book. We would also like to thank our wives for their patience and encouragement shown throughout the production of the second edition. Mr Raftery would also like to thank his secretary, Mrs Louise Rowan (formerly Miss Louise Griffiths – she has married since the first edition, although how she found the time I don't know!), for the hard work and long hours she has put into typing and retyping the manuscript (Mr Raftery cannot use a word processor!).

ABBREVIATIONS

ABC	airway, breathing and circulation
ABGs	arterial blood gases
AC	air conduction
ACE	angiotensin-converting enzyme
ACTH	adrenocorticotrophic hormone
ADH	antidiuretic hormone
AF	atrial fibrillation
AFP	alpha fetoprotein
ANA	antinuclear antibody
ANF	antinuclear factor
ANCA	antineutrophil cytoplasmic antibody
AP	anteroposterior
APTT	activated partial thromboplastin time
AXR	abdominal X-ray
BC	bone conduction
BCG	bacille Calmette–Guérin
BPPV	benign paroxysmal positional vertigo
CAPD	continuous ambulatory peritoneal dialysis
CCF	congestive cardiac failure
CDH	congenital dislocation of the hip
CK-MB	creatine kinase-myocardial type
CMV	cytomegalovirus
CNS	central nervous system
COPD	chronic obstructive pulmonary disease
CREST	calcinosis cutis–Raynaud phenomenon–oesophageal hypomobility–sclerodactyly–telangiectasia
CRP	C-reactive protein
C&S	culture and sensitivity
CSF	cerebrospinal fluid
CT	computerised tomography
CVA	cerebrovascular accident
CXR	chest X-ray
DDAVP	1-deamino-8-D-arginine vasopressin
DDH	developmental dysplasia of the hip
DHEA	dihydroepiandrosterone
DIC	disseminated intravascular coagulation
DIP	distal interphalangeal

DMSA	dimercaptosuccinic acid
DVT	deep venous thrombosis
EBV	Epstein–Barr virus
ECG	electrocardiogram
EEG	electroencephalogram
ELISA	enzyme-linked immunosorbent assay
EMG	electromyography
EMSU	early morning specimen of urine
ERCP	endoscopic retrograde cholangiopancreatography
ESR	erythrocyte sedimentation rate
FBC	full blood count
FEV1	forced expiratory volume (1 second)
FNAC	fine-needle aspiration cytology
FSH	follicle-stimulating hormone
FVC	forced vital capacity
GBM	antiglomerular basement membrane
GCS	Glasgow Coma Scale
GI	gastrointestinal
G6PD	glucose-6-phosphate dehydrogenase
GTN	glyceryl trinitrate
Hb	haemoglobin
βHCG	β human chorionic gonadotrophin
5HIAA	5-hydroxyindoleacetic acid
HIV	human immunodeficiency virus
IGF-1	insulin growth factor-1
IgG	immunoglobulin G
IP	interphalangeal
IVC	inferior vena cava
IVU	intravenous urography
JVP	jugular venous pressure
KUB	kidney ureter bladder (plain X-ray)
LDH	lactate dehydrogenase
LFTs	liver function tests
LH	luteinising hormone
MCH	mean corpuscular haemoglobin
MCP	metacarpophalangeal
MCV	mean corpuscular volume

MEN	multiple endocrine neoplasia
MRCP	magnetic resonance cholangiopancreatography
MRI	magnetic resonance imaging
MSU	midstream specimen of urine
MTP	metatarsophalangeal
NSAID	non-steroidal anti-inflammatory drug
NSTEMI	non ST elevation myocardial infarction
OGD	oesophago-gastro-dudenoscopy
PAS	periodic acid–Schiff
PCR	polymerase chain reaction
PCV	packed cell volume
PIP	proximal interphalangeal
PR	per rectum
PSA	prostate specific antigen
PT	prothrombin time
PTC	percutaneous transhepatic cholangiography
PTH	parathyroid hormone
PV	per vaginam
RAST	radioallergen sorbent test
RDW	red cell distribution width
RTA	road traffic accident
SLE	systemic lupus erythematosus
T$_3$	tri-iodothyronine
T$_4$	thyroxine
TB	tuberculosis
TFT	thyroid function test
TIA	transient ischaemic attack
TIBC	total iron-binding capacity
TPN	total parenteral nutrition
TSH	thyroid-stimulating hormone
TT	thrombin time
U&Es	urea and electrolytes
US	ultrasonography
UTI	urinary tract infection
V/Q	ventilation/perfusion ratio
VDRL	Veneral Disease Research Laboratory
WCC	white cell count

CONTENTS

ABStrongDOMINAL PAIN

Abdominal pain is an extremely common presenting symptom. The pain may be acute (sudden onset) or chronic (lasting for more than a few days or presenting intermittently). It is important to be able to distinguish causes of abdominal pain which need urgent surgery, e.g. ruptured aortic aneurysm, perforated diverticular disease, from those that do not, e.g. biliary colic, ureteric colic, acute pancreatitis. The causes of abdominal pain are legion and the list below contains some of the more common causes but is not intended to be comprehensive.

CAUSES

Gastrointestinal

Gut

Gastroduodenal
- Peptic ulcer
- Gastritis
- Gastric volvulus
- Malignancy

Intestinal
- Appendicitis
- Obstruction
- Diverticulitis
- Gastroenteritis
- Inflammatory bowel disease
- Mesenteric adenitis
- Strangulated hernia
- Intussusception
- Volvulus
- Tuberculosis

Hepatobiliary
- Acute cholecystitis
- Chronic cholecystitis
- Cholangitis
- Hepatitis

Pancreatic
- Acute pancreatitis
- Chronic pancreatitis
- Malignancy

Splenic
- Infarction
- Spontaneous rupture

Urinary tract
- Cystitis
- Acute retention of urine
- Acute pyelonephritis
- Ureteric colic
- Hydronephrosis
- Pyonephrosis
- Polycystic kidney
- Tumour

Gynaecological
- Ruptured ectopic pregnancy
- Torsion of ovarian cyst
- Ruptured ovarian cyst
- Salpingitis
- Severe dysmenorrhoea
- Mittelschmertz
- Endometriosis
- Red degeneration of a fibroid

Vascular
- Mesenteric angina (claudication)
- Aortic aneurysm
- Mesenteric embolus
- Mesenteric venous thrombosis
- Ischaemic colitis
- Acute aortic dissection

Peritoneum
- Primary peritonitis (rare)
- Secondary peritonitis

Abdominal wall
- Rectus sheath haematoma
- Cellulitis
- Strangulated hernia

Retroperitoneum
- Retroperitoneal haemorrhage, e.g. anticoagulants

Referred pain
- Herpes zoster
- Lobar pneumonia

- Thoracic spine disease, e.g. disc, tumour
- Pleurisy
- Myocardial infarction
- Pericarditis
- Testicular torsion

'Medical' causes
- Hypercalcaemia
- Uraemia
- Diabetic ketoacidosis
- Sickle cell disease
- Addison's disease
- Acute intermittent porphyria
- Henoch–Schönlein purpura
- Tabes dorsalis

HISTORY

Age
Certain conditions are more likely to occur in certain age groups, e.g. mesenteric adenitis in children, diverticular disease in the elderly.

Pain
- Time and mode of onset, e.g. sudden, gradual.
- Character, e.g. dull, vague, cramping, sharp, burning.
- Severity.
- Constancy, e.g. continuous (peritonitis); intermittent (pain of intestinal colic).
- Location: where did it start? Has it moved?
- Radiation, e.g. loin to groin in ureteric colic.
- Effect of respiration, movement, food, defecation, micturition and menstruation.
- Vomiting.
- Did vomiting precede the pain?
- Frequency.
- Character, e.g. bile, faeculent, blood, coffee grounds.

Defecation
- Constipation: absolute constipation with colicky abdominal pain, distension, vomiting, suggests intestinal obstruction.
- Diarrhoea: frequency, consistency of stools, blood, mucus, pus.

Fever
- Any rigors.

Past history

- Previous surgery, e.g. adhesions may cause intestinal obstruction.
- Recent trauma, e.g. delayed rupture of spleen.
- Menstrual history, e.g. ectopic pregnancy.

EXAMINATION

General

Is the patient lying comfortably? Is the patient lying still but in pain, e.g. peritonitis? Is the patient writhing in agony, e.g. ureteric or biliary colic? Is the patient flushed, suggesting pyrexia?

Pulse, temperature, respiration

Pulse and temperature are raised in inflammatory conditions. They may also be raised with impending infarction of bowel. An increased respiratory rate might suggest chest infection referring pain to the abdomen.

Cervical lymphadenopathy

Associated with mesenteric adenitis.

Chest

Referred pain from lobar pneumonia.

Abdomen

- Inspection. Does the abdomen move on respiration? Look for scars, distension, visible peristalsis (usually due to chronic obstruction in patient with very thin abdominal wall). Check the hernial orifices. Are there any obvious masses, e.g. visible, pulsatile mass to suggest aortic aneurysm?
- Palpation. The patient should be relaxed, lying flat, with arms by side. Be gentle and start as far from the painful site as possible. Check for guarding and rigidity. Check for masses, e.g. appendix mass, pulsatile expansile mass to suggest aortic aneurysm. Carefully examine the hernial orifices. Examine the testes to exclude torsion.
- Percussion, e.g. tympanitic note with distension with intestinal obstruction; dullness over bladder due to acute retention.
- Auscultation. Take your time (30–60 seconds); e.g. silent abdomen of peritonitis; high-pitched tinkling bowel sounds of intestinal obstruction.

Rectal examination

Always carry out a rectal examination.

Vaginal examination

There may be discharge or tenderness associated with pelvic inflammatory disease. Examine the uterus and adnexa, e.g. pregnancy, fibroids, ectopic pregnancy.

GENERAL INVESTIGATIONS

- **FBC, ESR**
  Hb ↓ peptic ulcer disease, malignancy. WCC ↑ infective/inflammatory disease, e.g. appendicitis, diverticulitis. ESR ↑ Crohn's disease, tuberculosis.
- **U&Es**
  Urea and creatinine ↑ uraemia. Electrolyte disturbances in vomiting and diarrhoea.
- **LFTs**
  Abnormal in cholangitis and hepatitis. Often abnormal in acute cholecystitis.
- **Serum amylase**
  Markedly raised in acute pancreatitis. Often moderately raised with perforated peptic ulcer or infarcted bowel.
- **MSU**
  Blood, protein, culture positive in pyelonephritis. Red cells in ureteric colic.
- **CXR**
  Gas under diaphragm (perforated viscus). Lower lobar pneumonia (referred pain).
- **AXR**
  Obstruction – dilated loops of bowel. Site of obstruction. Local ileus (sentinel loop) – pancreatitis, acute appendicitis. Toxic dilatation – dilated, featureless, oedematous colon in ulcerative colitis or Crohn's disease. Renal calculi. Calcified aortic aneurysm. Air in biliary tree (gallstone ileus). Gallstones (10% radio-opaque).
- **US**
  Localised abscesses, e.g. appendix abscess, paracolic abscess in diverticular disease. Free fluid – peritonitis, ascites. Aortic aneurysm. Ectopic pregnancy. Ovarian cyst. Gallstones. Empyema, mucocele of gall bladder. Kidney – cysts, tumour.

SPECIFIC INVESTIGATIONS

- **Blood glucose**
  Raised in diabetic ketoacidosis.

- **Serum calcium**
  Hypercalcaemia.
- **CRP**
  Crohn's disease.
- **VDRL**
  Syphilis (tabes dorsalis).
- **Sickling test**
  Sickle cell disease.
- **Urinary porphobilinogens**
  Acute intermittent porphyria.
- **ABGs**
  Metabolic acidosis, e.g. uraemia, infarcted bowel, sepsis, diabetic ketoacidosis.
- **βHCG**
  Pregnancy. Ectopic pregnancy.
- **ECG**
  Myocardial infarction (referred pain).
- **OGD**
  Peptic ulcer. Malignancy.
- **IVU**
  Stones. Obstruction.
- **Barium enema**
  Carcinoma. Volvulus. Intussusception.
- **Small bowel enema**
  Small bowel Crohn's disease. Lymphoma of small bowel. Carcinoma of small bowel.
- **Duplex Doppler**
  Superior mesenteric artery stenosis (mesenteric angina). Superior mesenteric artery thrombosis. Mesenteric venous thrombosis.
- **Angiography**
  Superior mesenteric embolus or thrombosis.
- **CT**
  Aneurysm. Pancreatitis. Tumour.

ABDOMINAL SWELLINGS

Abdominal swelling may be generalised or there may be a localised mass. Abdominal swellings are a common surgical problem. They are also frequently the subject of examination questions! Abdominal swellings may be divided into generalised and localised swellings. Generalised swellings are classically described as the 'five Fs', namely fat, faeces, flatus, fluid or fetus. For the purpose of description of localised swellings, the abdomen has been divided into seven areas, i.e. right upper quadrant, left upper quadrant, epigastrium, umbilical, right lower abdomen, left lower abdomen and suprapubic area. Hepatomegaly, splenomegaly and renal masses, although referred to in this section, are dealt with under the relevant heading in the appropriate section of the book.

RIGHT UPPER QUADRANT

CAUSES

Liver
See hepatomegaly, page 215.

Gall bladder
- Mucocele
- Empyema
- Carcinoma
- Secondary to carcinoma of the head of the pancreas

Right colon
- Carcinoma
- Faeces
- Diverticular mass
- Caecal volvulus
- Intussusception

Right kidney
- Polycystic kidney
- Hydronephrosis
- Pyonephrosis
- Perinephric abscess
- Carcinoma
- Tuberculosis

- Solitary cyst
- Wilms' tumour (nephroblastoma)

HISTORY

Liver

See hepatomegaly, page 215.

Gall bladder

Known history of gallstones. History of flatulent dyspepsia.
Jaundice. Dark urine. Pale stools. Pruritus. Recent weight loss may
suggest carcinoma of the head of the pancreas or carcinoma of the
gall bladder.

Right colon

Lassitude, weakness, lethargy suggesting anaemia from chronic
blood loss. Central abdominal colicky pain, vomiting and
constipation and change in bowel habit will suggest colonic
carcinoma. There may be a history of gross constipation to suggest
faecal loading. Known history of diverticular disease. History of
attacks of crying, abdominal pain and blood and mucus in the
stool ('redcurrant jelly' stool) will suggest intussusception in infants.

Right kidney

See kidney swellings, page 283.

EXAMINATION

Liver

See page 215.

Gall bladder

A mucocele is either non-tender or only mildly tender. It is large
and smooth and moves with respiration, projecting from under the
ninth costal cartilage at the lateral border of rectus abdominis.
Empyema presents with an acutely tender gall bladder, which is
difficult to define due to pain and tenderness. The patient may be
jaundiced due to Mirrizi syndrome (external pressure from a stone
impacted in Hartmann's pouch on the adjacent bile duct).
Carcinoma of the gall bladder may present as a hard, irregular
mass in the right hypochondrium, but normally presents as
obstructive jaundice due to secondary deposits in the nodes at the
porta hepatis causing external compression of the hepatic ducts.
A smooth enlarged gall bladder in the presence of jaundice may be

due to carcinoma of the head of the pancreas (Courvoisier's law: 'in the presence of obstructive jaundice, if the gall bladder is palpable the cause is unlikely to be due to gallstones').

Right colon

Faeces are usually soft and putty-like and can be indented but may also feel like a mass of rocks. Carcinoma is usually a firm to hard irregular mass, which may be mobile or fixed. A diverticular mass is usually tender and ill-defined unless there is a large paracolic abscess. With caecal volvulus there is a tympanitic mass which may be tender with impending infarction. With intussusception there will be a smooth, mobile tender sausage-shaped mass in the right hypochondrium. The mass may move as the intussusception progresses.

Right kidney

See kidney swellings, page 283.

GENERAL INVESTIGATIONS

- **FBC, ESR**
  Hb ↓ anaemia, e.g. carcinoma of the colon, haematuria with renal lesions. Hb ↑, e.g. hypernephroma (polycythaemia associated with hypernephroma). WCC ↑, e.g. empyema, diverticular mass. ESR ↑, malignancy.
- **U&Es**
  Vomiting and dehydration, e.g. gall bladder and bowel lesions. Ureteric obstruction with renal lesions leading to uraemia.
- **LFTs**
  Liver lesions. Secondary deposits in liver.
- **MSU**
  Renal lesions – red blood cells, pus cells, malignant cells. C&S.
- **AXR**
  Intestinal obstruction due to carcinoma of the large bowel. Gallstones (10% are radio-opaque). Caecal volvulus. Constipation. Calcification in renal lesions.
- **US**
  Liver lesions. Gallstones. Mucocele. Empyema. Bile duct dilatation.

SPECIFIC INVESTIGATIONS

- **Barium enema**
  Carcinoma of the colon. Diverticular disease. Intussusception.

- **Colonoscopy**

  Carcinoma of the colon. Diverticular disease.
- **CT**

  Liver lesions. Gall bladder lesions. Renal lesions.

LEFT UPPER QUADRANT

CAUSES

Spleen

See splenomegaly, page 396.

Stomach

- Carcinoma
- Gastric distension (acute dilatation, pyloric stenosis)

Pancreas

- Pseudocyst
- Carcinoma

Kidney

See right upper quadrant, page 7.

Colon

- Carcinoma of the splenic flexure
- Faeces
- Diverticular mass

HISTORY

Spleen

See splenomegaly, page 396.

Stomach

Vomiting will suggest pyloric stenosis, acute dilatation of the stomach and carcinoma. Vomiting food ingested several days previously suggests pyloric stenosis. Lethargy, loss of appetite and weight loss are seen in carcinoma of the stomach.

Pancreas

There may be a history of acute pancreatitis, which would suggest the development of a pseudocyst. Weight loss, backache and jaundice will suggest carcinoma of the pancreas. Recent onset of diabetes may occur with carcinoma of the pancreas.

Spleen (massive splenomegaly)
See splenomegaly, page 396.

Kidney
See kidney swellings, page 283.

Colon
Lower abdominal colicky pain and change in bowel habit may suggest carcinoma or diverticular disease. A long history of constipation may suggest faecal masses.

EXAMINATION

Stomach
Gastric distension may present with a vague fullness and a succussion splash. Carcinoma will present with a hard, craggy, immobile mass. Pancreatic tumours may be impalpable or present as a fixed mass, which does not move with respiration. Pancreatic pseudocysts are often large, smooth and may be tender.

Colon
See right upper quadrant, page 7.

GENERAL INVESTIGATIONS

- **FBC, ESR**
  Hb ↓ carcinoma. Hb ↑ hypernephroma (polycythaemia is associated with hypernephroma). WCC ↑ diverticular disease, renal infections.
- **U&Es**
  Vomiting, dehydration (with gastric and colonic lesions). Renal lesions.
- **LFTs**
  Liver lesions. Secondary deposits in liver.
- **Serum amylase**
  Acute pancreatitis.
- **US**
  Splenomegaly. Renal lesions. Paracolic abscess.

SPECIFIC INVESTIGATIONS

- **Blood glucose**
  May be raised in pancreatic carcinoma.

- **Barium enema**
  Carcinoma. Diverticular disease.
- **Colonoscopy**
  Carcinoma. Diverticular disease.
- **Gastroscopy**
  Carcinoma of the stomach. Pyloric stenosis.
- **CT**
  Carcinoma of the pancreas. Pancreatic pseudocyst. Liver secondaries. Splenomegaly. Paracolic abscess.

EPIGASTRIUM

Many of the swellings that occur here will have been described under swellings in other regions of the abdomen. Although a full list of epigastric swellings is given below; only those not referred to in other sections will be discussed in the history and examination sections.

CAUSES

Abdominal wall
- Lipoma
- Epigastric hernia
- Xiphisternum
- Metastatic deposits

Stomach
- Congenital hypertrophic pyloric stenosis
- Carcinoma
- Acute gastric volvulus

Pancreas
See left upper quadrant, page 10.

Transverse colon
- Carcinoma
- Faeces
- Diverticular mass

Liver
See hepatomegaly, page 215.

Retroperitoneum
- Aortic aneurysm
- Lymphadenopathy (lymphoma, secondaries from testicular carcinoma)

Omentum
- Omental secondaries, e.g. stomach and ovary

HISTORY

Abdominal wall

The patient may indicate a soft, subcutaneous swelling, which may be a lipoma or an epigastric hernia containing extraperitoneal fat. The latter always occurs in the midline through a defect in the linea alba. They may become strangulated, in which case they are tender, and occasionally the skin is red. Occasionally a patient may indicate a firm bony lump in the upper epigastrium, which is in fact a normal xiphisternum. This may have become apparent either due to a deliberate attempt to lose weight or sudden weight loss due to underlying disease. Metastatic deposits may present as single or multiple fixed lumps in the skin or subcutaneous tissue, e.g. from breast or bronchus.

Stomach

A baby may present with projectile vomiting. The infant thrives for the first 3–4 weeks of life and then develops projectile vomiting after feeds. The first-born male child in a family is most commonly affected. There may be a history of a familial tendency, especially on the maternal side.

Retroperitoneum

A history of backache may suggest an aortic aneurysm or the patient may complain of a pulsatile epigastric swelling. Backache may also be a presenting symptom of retroperitoneal lymphadenopathy.

EXAMINATION

Abdominal wall

A soft, lobulated mass suggests a lipoma. It will be mobile over the tensed abdominal musculature. A fatty, occasionally tender, non-mobile swelling in the midline will suggest an epigastric hernia. The majority of epigastric hernias are composed of extraperitoneal fat, although there may be a sac with bowel contents. A cough impulse will be palpable. The swelling may be reducible. Hard, irregular, fixed lumps in the abdominal wall suggest metastatic deposits, especially if there is a history of carcinoma of the breast or bronchus.

Retroperitoneum

An aneurysm presents as a pulsatile expansile mass. Check the distal circulation (emboli, associated peripheral ischaemia). Retroperitoneal lymph node metastases from testicular cancer may present as a large retroperitoneal mass. Check the testes for swellings. Check all other sites for lymphadenopathy (especially the left supraclavicular node). Lymphadenopathy may also result from lymphoma. Check for lymphadenopathy elsewhere and for splenomegaly. A hard, craggy, mobile mass, especially in the presence of ascites, suggests omental secondaries (ovary, stomach – check for Virchow's node, i.e. left supraclavicular node).

GENERAL INVESTIGATIONS

- **FBC, ESR**
  Hb ↓ carcinoma of the stomach, carcinoma of the colon, carcinomatosis. WCC ↑ diverticulitis.
- **U&Es**
  Vomiting and dehydration with gastric and colonic lesions.
- **LFTs**
  Liver lesions.
- **US**
  Aortic aneurysm. Lymphadenopathy. Pancreatic pseudocyst.

SPECIFIC INVESTIGATIONS

- **Blood glucose**
  May be abnormal with pancreatic carcinoma or previous pancreatitis.
- **CT**
  Pancreatic tumours. Pancreatic pseudocyst. Lymphadenopathy. Aortic aneurysm. Omental deposits. Guided biopsy/FNAC.
- **Barium enema**
  Carcinoma of the colon. Diverticular disease.
- **Colonoscopy**
  Carcinoma of the colon. Diverticular disease.
- **Gastroscopy**
  Carcinoma of the stomach.

- **Laparoscopy**
  Carcinoma of the ovaries. Omental secondaries. Carcinomatosis peritonei.
- **Biopsy**

UMBILICAL

Many of the swellings here will already have been described under swellings in other regions of the abdomen. Only those not referred to in those sections will be discussed in the history and examination sections.

CAUSES

Superficial
- Sister Joseph's nodule (malignant, rare)

Hernia
- Paraumbilical
- Umbilical

Stomach
- Carcinoma

Transverse colon
- Carcinoma
- Faeces
- Diverticular mass

Small bowel
- Crohn's disease
- Carcinoma (rare)
- Mesenteric cysts (rare)

Omentum
- Secondary deposits, e.g. stomach, ovary

Retroperitoneum
- Aortic aneurysm
- Lymph nodes, e.g. lymphoma, secondaries from testicular carcinoma

HISTORY

Superficial

Sister Joseph's nodule presents as hard lump at the umbilicus. It is due to secondary deposits of carcinoma of the stomach, colon, ovary or breast.

Hernia

An umbilical hernia presents in infancy as an umbilical swelling which is reducible, and will usually have been noted at birth. Paraumbilical hernias usually occur in obese adults, often female. The patient may have had a lump for a long time. It may present with incarceration or with a tender painful swelling, suggesting strangulation.

Small bowel

The patient may present with central abdominal colicky pain, vomiting and diarrhoea suggestive of Crohn's disease or more rarely a carcinoma of the small bowel.

EXAMINATION

Superficial

Sister Joseph's nodule presents as a hard lump or lumps at the umbilicus. Check for carcinoma of the stomach, colon, ovary or breast.

Hernia

In infants there may be an obvious large umbilical defect. The swelling is usually wide-necked and reducible. In adults there may be a reducible paraumbilical hernia. Occasionally it is soft, containing extraperitoneal fat. Frequently there is a sac containing omentum. Incarceration may occur. A tender red swelling suggests strangulation. A Richter's-type hernia may occur at this site.

Small bowel

Small bowel masses are usually very mobile, may be sausage-shaped, and may be tender.

GENERAL INVESTIGATIONS

- **FBC, ESR**

  Hb ↓ carcinoma. WCC ↑ diverticular disease.

- **U&Es**
  Vomiting. Dehydration, e.g. carcinoma of the stomach,
  carcinoma of the bowel, Crohn's disease.
- **LFTs**
  Alkaline phosphatase raised with liver secondaries.
- **US**
  Aortic aneurysm. Retroperitoneal lymphadenopathy.

SPECIFIC INVESTIGATIONS

- **CT**
  Aortic aneurysm. Retroperitoneal lymphadenopathy. Omental
  deposits. Guided biopsy/FNAC.
- **Barium enema**
  Carcinoma of the colon. Diverticular disease.
- **Colonoscopy**
  Carcinoma of the colon. Diverticular disease.
- **Gastroscopy**
  Carcinoma of the stomach.
- **Small bowel enema**
  Crohn's disease. Lymphoma. Carcinoma.
- **Laparoscopy**
  Carcinoma of the ovaries. Omental secondaries. Carcinomatosis
  peritonei.
- **Biopsy**
  Benign versus malignant.

RIGHT AND LEFT LOWER QUADRANTS

CAUSES

Abdominal wall
- Lipoma
- Spigelian hernia

Large bowel

Right lower quadrant
- Appendix mass/abscess
- Carcinoma of the caecum
- Carcinoma of the ascending colon

- Faeces
- Caecal volvulus
- Intussusception
- Crohn's disease

Left lower quadrant
- Carcinoma of the sigmoid colon
- Diverticular mass
- Faeces
- Sigmoid volvulus
- Crohn's disease

Small bowel
- Crohn's disease
- Carcinoma (rare)
- Lymphoma
- Ileo-caecal tuberculosis

Ovary/uterus/fallopian tube
- Ovarian cyst
- Ovarian neoplasm
- Ectopic pregnancy
- Tubo-ovarian abscess
- Uterine fibroid

Kidney
See kidney swellings, page 283.

Spleen (massive splenomegaly)
See splenomegaly, page 396.

Retroperitoneum
- Iliac artery aneurysm
- Lymphadenopathy
- Neoplasm of iliac bone, e.g. osteogenic sarcoma, Ewing's tumour (rare)

HISTORY

Anterior abdominal wall
The patient may have the development of a soft mass that is slow growing, suggestive of a lipoma. A spigelian hernia occurs just lateral to the rectus muscle, halfway between the umbilicus and symphysis pubis. It is usually reducible.

Large bowel
A short history of central abdominal, colicky pain followed by a sharply localised pain in the right iliac fossa will suggest the

diagnosis of acute appendicitis. After 48 hours, if there is not generalised peritonitis, an appendix mass will have formed and an abscess may subsequently form in the right iliac fossa. With carcinoma of the caecum the patient will either have noticed a mass or will present with alteration in bowel habit and the symptoms of anaemia, e.g. tiredness, lethargy. The same applies to carcinoma of the ascending colon. Faeces will be indentable and hard, rock-like masses will be felt around the colon. Caecal volvulus will present with central abdominal colicky pain and abdominal distension. Intussusception is more common in infants and usually presents with colicky abdominal pain and the classic 'redcurrant jelly' stool. Crohn's disease will present with malaise and diarrhoea with central abdominal colicky pain.

Carcinoma of the sigmoid colon will present with lower abdominal colicky pain, a change in bowel habit and bleeding PR. Diverticular disease may present with similar symptoms. Sigmoid volvulus will present with lower abdominal colicky pain and a tense, palpable mass in the left abdomen, which is tympanitic on percussion. Large bowel Crohn's disease will present with a sausage-like, palpable mass, which may be tender and is associated with diarrhoea.

Small bowel
If there is a mass palpable in the right iliac fossa the site of pathology is likely to be in the terminal ileum. This usually involves central abdominal colicky pain and a change in bowel habit. Ileo-caecal TB causes abdominal pain, diarrhoea which is associated with malaise and weight loss.

Spleen
With massive splenomegaly, the spleen may be palpable extending into the right lower quadrant.

Ovary/fallopian tube/uterus
The patient may feel a lump in the abdomen herself (ovarian cyst, fibroid) or notice generalised abdominal swelling, which may be associated with a massive ovarian cyst or ascites associated with ovarian cancer. Ectopic pregnancy will present with a missed period and abdominal pain, bleeding PV, and collapse with hypovolaemic shock if it ruptures. Salpingo-oophoritis will present with lower abdominal pain and tenderness and associated fever, and often a purulent vaginal discharge. Menorrhagia, lower abdominal pain and dyspareunia may suggest fibroids.

Retroperitoneum

The patient may present having noticed a pulsatile swelling in the iliac fossa. Pelvic lymphadenopathy may be suspected by history of removal of a malignant lesion from the lower limb, especially malignant melanoma. There may be an existing lesion present on the limb. A dull, boring pain may be suggestive of an iliac bone lesion. A palpable bony lesion suggests an osteogenic sarcoma or Ewing's tumour of bone.

EXAMINATION

The features of most of the lesions described above have been described in the other sections on abdominal swellings. Only those findings relavent to the ovary, uterus and fallopian tube will be described here. Examination may reveal a greatly distended abdomen which may be due to a huge ovarian cyst or ascites associated with an ovarian neoplasm. Huge ovarian cysts are often smooth and loculated. It is impossible to get below them as they arise out of the pelvis. Signs of ascites include shifting dullness and a fluid thrill. With ectopic pregnancy there may be a palpable mass in either iliac fossa. This may be associated with shock if rupture of the ectopic pregnancy has occurred. Shoulder-tip pain may occur from irritation of the undersurface of the diaphragm with blood. With tubo-ovarian abscess there may be a palpable mass arising out of the pelvis, or merely lower abdominal tenderness. Vaginal examination will reveal tenderness in the pouch of Douglas. Uterine fibroids may be extremely large and palpable as nodules on the underlying uterus.

GENERAL INVESTIGATIONS

- **FBC, ESR**
  Hb ↓ Crohn's disease, carcinoma. ESR ↑ carcinoma, Crohn's disease, ileo-caecal tuberculosis. WCC ↑ appendicitis, diverticulitis.
- **U&Es**
  Vomiting. Dehydration. Obstruction from carcinoma or Crohn's disease.
- **LFTs**
  Alkaline phosphatase ↑ with liver secondaries.
- **US**
  Ovarian lesions. Uterine lesions. Tubo-ovarian abscesses. Pregnancy. Ectopic pregnancy. Iliac artery aneurysms. Lymphadenopathy. Appendix mass. Crohn's mass.

- **AXR**
  Obstruction. Dilated loops of bowel. Ovarian teratoma (teeth, etc.). Erosion of iliac bone – bone tumours.

SPECIFIC INVESTIGATIONS

- **βHCG**
  Raised in pregnancy.
- **Mantoux test**
  Ileo-caecal TB.
- **CT**
  Ovarian lesions. Uterine lesions. Abscess. Ectopic pregnancy. Iliac artery aneurysm. Lymphadenopathy. Appendix mass. Bone tumours.
- **Barium enema**
  Carcinoma. Diverticular disease.
- **Small bowel enema**
  Crohn's disease. Carcinoma. Lymphoma.
- **Colonoscopy**
  Carcinoma (biopsy). Diverticular disease.
- **Laparoscopy**
  Carcinoma, Crohn's disease, ileo-caecal TB.
- **Bone scan**
  Bone tumour.

SUPRAPUBIC

CAUSES

Bladder
- Acute retention
- Chronic retention
- Carcinoma

Uterus
- Pregnancy
- Fibroids
- Carcinoma

Bowel
- Crohn's disease
- Carcinoma
- Diverticular mass

Other
- Urachal cyst (rare)

HISTORY

Bladder

Sudden onset of suprapubic pain with inability to pass urine suggests acute retention. There will usually be a past history of difficulty in starting and a poor stream. A history of dribbling may suggest acute renal failure associated with upper tract problems from chronic outflow obstruction. Haematuria, frequency, dysuria may suggest bladder carcinoma.

Uterus

Missed periods and early morning vomiting will suggest pregnancy. Menorrhagia and dyspareunia will suggest fibroids. Intermenstrual bleeding suggests carcinoma.

Urachus

Umbilical discharge may suggest a urachal cyst or abscess.

EXAMINATION

In acute retention there will be a smooth, tender swelling extending towards (but not above) the umbilicus. It is dull to percussion and it is impossible to get below it. Digital rectal examination will usually reveal benign prostatic hypertrophy or occasionally a hard, irregular prostate associated with carcinoma. With carcinoma of the bladder, a hard, irregular craggy mass may be felt arising out of the pelvis.

Uterus

A smooth, regular swelling arising out of the pelvis suggests a pregnant uterus. Later, as the uterus enlarges, fetal heart sounds may be heard. Fibroids are usually smooth and firm and may become very large. Uterine carcinoma is hard and craggy. Bimanual examination may confirm the diagnosis.

GENERAL INVESTIGATIONS

- **FBC, ESR**
  Hb ↓ tumour. WCC ↑ infection.
- **MSU**
  Red cells. White cells. Organisms, (infection precipitating) retention. Malignant cells with carcinoma.
- **US**
  Pregnancy. Fibroids. Bladder tumour. Urachal cyst.

SPECIFIC INVESTIGATIONS

- **βHCG**
  Pregnancy.
- **PSA**
  Carcinoma of the prostate.
- **Cystoscopy**
  Bladder tumour. Biopsy.
- **Barium enema**
  Colonic carcinoma. Diverticular disease. Crohn's disease.
- **Colonoscopy**
  Carcinoma. Diverticular disease.
- **CT**
  Ovarian lesions. Uterine lesions. Bladder lesions. Urachal cyst.

▶ ANAEMIA

Anaemia is defined as a haemoglobin concentration of less than 13.5 g/dl in adult males and 11.5 g/dl in adult females. Classification of anaemia according to red cell indices is useful because specific investigations can be tailored accordingly.

CAUSES

Microcytic (MCV <80 fl)
- Iron deficiency
- Anaemia of chronic disease
- Thalassaemia

Normocytic (MCV 80–95 fl)
- Acute blood loss
- Haemolytic anaemia
  - Hereditary spherocytosis
  - Sickle cell disease
  - G6PD deficiency
  - Autoimmune haemolytic anaemia
  - Malaria
  - Drugs (e.g. dapsone, quinine, sulphonamides)
  - Red cell trauma (burns, mechanical heart valves)
- Mixed deficiencies
- Secondary anaemia (liver and renal disease)
- Bone marrow failure
- Pregnancy

Macrocytic (MCV >95 fl)
- Megaloblastic anaemia
  - Pernicious anaemia
  - Vitamin B_{12} deficiency
  - Folate deficiency
- Alcoholism
- Liver disease
- Hypothyroidism
- Hyperthyroidism (Graves)
- Addison's disease
- Marrow infiltration
- Drugs
  - Azathioprine (dose-related)

HISTORY

Important aspects of the history are to enquire about symptoms suggestive of the diagnosis of anaemia, and to establish any underlying cause.

Symptoms of anaemia

The symptoms of anaemia are dependent on the degree of anaemia, speed of onset, age and the presence of coexisting disease. Mild to moderate chronic anaemia may be asymptomatic in young, fit individuals. Symptoms of anaemia include tiredness, lethargy and dyspnoea. Anaemia can precipitate or worsen angina and lower limb claudication.

History of the underlying disorder

Blood loss is a common cause of iron deficiency anaemia and frank bleeding can easily be established from the history. Occult bleeding from the gastrointestinal tract is an important cause of chronic blood loss. Patients may have melaena and may also experience upper abdominal pains from peptic ulceration, gastritis, gastro-oesophageal reflux or gastric carcinoma (page 1). The causes of lower gastrointestinal bleeding are detailed on page 372. The amount and frequency of blood loss with menstruation should be documented and the presence of haemoptysis and haematuria should be ascertained. Malabsorption can cause a deficiency of substrate or coenzyme requirements for the synthesis of haemoglobin. Gastrectomy or atrophic gastritis with pernicious anaemia may impair both iron and vitamin B_{12} absorption due to alterations in pH and effects on intrinsic factor, respectively. Impairment of vitamin B_{12} absorption may also result from extensive disease or resection involving the terminal ileum and predisposes to megaloblastic anaemia. A history of travel to areas where malaria and hookworm infections are endemic should be sought.

Dietary history

It is important to take a dietary history, as folate deficiency commonly results from poor dietary intake. This is in contrast to iron, as dietary deficiency of iron alone rarely results in anaemia unless accompanied by increased utilisation or blood loss. Due to intrinsic stores of vitamin B_{12}, dietary deficiencies may take up to 2 years before becoming clinically apparent. The amount of alcohol intake should also be noted because alcohol excess may result in a macrocytic anaemia.

Past medical and drug history

A number of chronic diseases can result in anaemia but it is important to exclude other concomitant causes before attributing anaemia to the effects of the primary illness. Diseases predisposing to macrocytic anaemia have been listed above. Aplasia of the marrow may occur as a complication of viral hepatitis or exposure to radiation and result in aplastic anaemia. Drugs such as chemotherapeutic agents, chloramphenicol and sulphonamides may also precipitate bone marrow failure. Respiratory tract infections with mycoplasma, infectious mononucleosis, lymphomas and connective tissue disease are associated with autoimmune haemolytic anaemia.

Family history

Haemoglobinopathies such as thalassaemia and sickle cell disease may be inherited. Alternatively, hereditary enzyme defects (G6PD) or red cell membrane defects (hereditary spherocytosis) may also result in intravascular haemolysis.

EXAMINATION

Classically, patients with anaemia have pallor of the palmar skin creases and conjunctivae; however, diagnosis based solely on these findings is unreliable. With iron deficiency, spoon-shaped nails (koilonychia) may be noted; these findings may be accompanied by angular cheilitis and glossitis. Jaundice can be a complication of haemolytic anaemia, or can result from chronic liver disease.

Subacute combined degeneration of the cord is a complication of severe vitamin B_{12} deficiency. Neurological examination reveals symmetrical loss of light touch, vibration and proprioception of the feet due to dorsal column involvement. In addition, Romberg's sign may be elicited. Less common features are peripheral neuropathy, optic atrophy and dementia.

With anaemia, examination of the cardiovascular system may reveal evidence of a hyperdynamic circulation with tachycardia, bounding pulse and a systolic flow murmur.

Splenomegaly is associated with hereditary spherocytosis and thalassaemia. Sickle cell disease.

SPECIFIC INVESTIGATIONS

Microcytic anaemia

- **FBC and blood film**
  Low haemoglobin concentration occurs with microcytosis (MCV <80 fl) and hypochromia (MCH <27 pg). The platelet count may be raised when anaemia is associated with acute bleeding. Microcytic, hypochromic red blood cells with accompanying pencil cells may also been seen on the blood film.
- **Serum iron and TIBC**
  Serum iron reduced and TIBC raised with iron deficiency. With chronic disease both are reduced, and with thalassaemia both are normal.
- **Serum ferritin**
  Concentration of serum ferritin, a protein–iron complex, will be reduced with iron deficiency. It is not affected by chronic disease or thalassaemia.
- **Faecal occult blood and faecal microscopy**
  Detects blood loss from the gastrointestinal tract. Hookworm ova can be identified on microscopy.
- **Free erythrocyte protoporphyrin**
  Iron is added to protoporphyrin to form haem; therefore, in the presence of iron deficiency, protoporphyrin levels will be raised. It is a sensitive indicator of iron deficiency and is unaffected by chronic disease or thalassaemia.
- **Hb electrophoresis**
  Allows the specific diagnosis and classification of thalassaemia and sickle cell disease.

Normocytic anaemia

- **FBC and film**
  Low haemoglobin levels are accompanied by normal red cell indices (MCV 80–95 fl, MCH >27 pg), which can also occur in the presence of coexisting microcytic and macrocytic anaemia (mixed deficiency), although this will usually be picked up on the blood film. Certain haematology laboratories report red cell distribution width (RDW), which is increased in the presence of differing red corpuscle sizes. The reticulocyte count will be increased with haemolytic anaemia and following acute blood loss, and the blood film may reveal evidence of damaged red cells or sideroblasts.

- **Tests for haemolysis**
  Unconjugated bilirubin, urine urobilinogen and faecal
  stercobilinogen are raised with all causes of haemolysis. Serum
  haptoglobins are absent. Plasma haemoglobin is raised
  specifically with intravascular haemolysis. Reference to
  haematology textbooks will be required for confirmatory tests for
  individual haemolytic disorders.
- **Urinalysis**
- **Haemosiderin and haemoglobin will be present in the urine
  specifically with intravascular haemolysis**
- **Bone marrow aspiration**
  Aspiration of the bone marrow will reveal erythroid hyperplasia
  with haemolytic anaemia; with aplastic anaemia, bone marrow
  hypoplasia with fat replacement results.

Macrocytic anaemia

- **FBC and film**
  Low haemoglobin is accompanied by macrocytosis (MCV >95 fl).
  The reticulocyte count is low and accompanying low platelet and
  white cell counts may indicate megaloblastic anaemia.
  Hypersegmented neutrophils may be seen on the blood film.
- **Serum vitamin B_{12} assay**
  Serum levels of vitamin B_{12} can be estimated and deficiency
  readily ascertained. If the aetiology of vitamin B_{12} deficiency is
  not apparent, a Schilling test can be performed to clarify if the
  problem lies within the stomach, terminal ileum, or is due to
  intrinsic factor.
- **Antiparietal cell antibodies and anti-intrinsic factor antibodies**
  Pernicious anaemia results from lack of intrinsic factor
  production or blocking antibodies.
- **Serum and red cell folate**
  Both of these tests are low with folate deficiency; however, in the
  presence of vitamin B_{12} deficiency the red cell folate may
  actually be increased.
- **Bone marrow aspiration**
  Megaloblasts are seen in marrow aspirates with vitamin B_{12} or
  folate deficiency.
- **Further tests**
  Further tests for individual diseases responsible for macrocytosis
  or secondary anaemia need to be tailored according to the
  clinical presentation.

ANORECTAL PAIN

Anorectal pain is a common problem. The majority of patients have an obvious cause, e.g. fissure-in-ano, perianal abscess or thrombosed haemorrhoids.

CAUSES

Acute
- Fissure-in-ano
- Perianal haematoma
- Thrombosed haemorrhoids
- Perianal abscess
- Intersphincteric abscess
- Ischiorectal abscess
- Trauma
- Anorectal gonorrhoea
- Herpes

Chronic
- Proctalgia fugax
- Fistula-in-ano
- Anorectal malignancy
- Solitary rectal ulcer
- Chronic perianal sepsis, e.g. Crohn's disease, TB
- Cauda equina lesions

HISTORY

Constipation with pain on defecation and blood (usually on the paper) will suggest fissure-in-ano. A sudden onset of pain with a tender lump in the perianal region will suggest perianal haematoma. A past history of prolapsing piles, with failure to reduce them, associated with pain and tenderness suggests thrombosed haemorrhoids. Gradual onset of pain and tenderness with swelling is suggestive of abscess formation. A careful history must be taken of trauma. A history of anal sexual exposure will suggest gonorrhoea or herpes. With gonorrhoea there may be irritation, itching, discharge and pain. With herpes there will be pain and irritation. Proctalgia fugax is diagnosed on the history of perineal pain, which is spasmodic, the spasms lasting up to

30 minutes. The pain often feels deep inside the rectum. The cause is unknown but may be related to paroxysmal contraction of levator ani. Anorectal malignancies will be suggested in alteration of bowel habit and bleeding on defecation. Pain will only be apparent if the tumour involves the anal canal below the dentate line, where sensation is of the somatic type. Solitary rectal ulcer may present with pain but more usually presents with bleeding PR, passage of mucus, and difficulty with defecation. Chronic perianal sepsis may be the presenting symptom of Crohn's disease or TB. These diseases may already be manifest at other sites of the body. Rarely lesions of the cauda equina may cause anal pain.

EXAMINATION

Inspection may reveal a chronic fissure-in-ano, perianal haematoma, thrombosed piles, or a tumour growing out of the anal canal. A tense, red, tender area may be present, representing a perianal abscess. A fullness in the buttock with redness may indicate a large ischiorectal abscess. A digital rectal examination should be carried out unless the diagnosis is obvious. With gonococcal proctitis, proctoscopy may reveal pus and blood in the rectal ampulla with oedematous and friable mucosa. The presence of vesicles in the anal area will suggest herpes. Solitary rectal ulcer is usually diagnosed on sigmoidoscopy when redness and oedema of the mucosa is seen, usually, but not always, in association with frank ulceration. If a cauda equina lesion is suspected a full neurological examination should be carried out. No abnormality is usually found with proctalgia fugax.

GENERAL INVESTIGATIONS

- **FBC, ESR**
  WCC ↑ infections, e.g. abscess. ESR ↑ Crohn's disease, TB and malignancy.
- **Blood glucose**
  Sepsis may be a presentation of diabetes mellitus.
- **Proctoscopy**
  Haemorrhoids. Anorectal malignancy. Anorectal gonorrhoea. Swab → Gram-negative intracellular diplococci.
- **Sigmoidoscopy**
  Anorectal malignancy.

SPECIFIC INVESTIGATIONS

- **Endo-anal ultrasound**
  This may demonstrate intersphincteric abscesses or fistulae-in-ano.
- **MRI**
  This will delineate complex fistula problems or may indicate a
  cauda equina lesion.
- **Antigen detection tests**
  Herpes.
- **Electron microscopy**
  Identification of virus in vesicle fluid.
- **PCR**
  For fast diagnosis of herpes.

▶ ARM PAIN

This section deals with pain in the upper limb unrelated to joint pains. The majority of causes of arm pain are related to either neurological or vascular lesions.

CAUSES

Cervical lesions
- Disc lesion
- Cervical spondylosis
- Syringomyelia
- Infection, e.g. osteitis, TB
- Tumours
  - Spinal cord
  - Meninges
  - Nerves
  - Vertebral bodies

Brachial plexus
- Cervical rib
- Malignant infiltration, e.g. Pancoast's tumour
- Thoracic inlet syndrome

Vascular lesions
- Subclavian artery stenosis
- Embolism
- Arterial thrombosis
- Axillary venous thrombosis
- Myocardial ischaemia (left arm)

Others
- Repetitive strain injury
- Peripheral neuropathy
- Carpal tunnel syndrome
- Bone tumours
- Compartment syndrome
  - Acute, e.g. crush injuries
  - Chronic, e.g. exertional

HISTORY

Symptoms of cervical lesions include: pain and stiffness in the neck; pain radiating down the arm. Cervical cord compression may occur. Cervical spondylosis represents 'wear and tear' of the cervical spine. It is common over the age of 60 years. Acute disc lesions usually occur in the younger patient. A careful history is needed to exclude trauma.

Brachial plexus lesions refer pain down the arm and may result from localised lesions, e.g. a cervical rib causing extrinsic compression will affect T1 and cause wasting of the small muscles of the hands and paraesthesia in the dermatomal distribution, i.e. the inner aspect of the upper arm.

Subclavian artery stenosis will result in 'claudication' in the arm, i.e. pain brought on by exercise, relieved by rest, due to inadequate blood flow. A history of cardiac problems, e.g. AF or widespread arterial disease, will suggest embolism or thrombosis. A sudden onset of a painful, swollen, cyanotic limb will suggest axillary vein thrombosis. Pain radiating into the left arm brought on by exercise and related to central chest pain and pain radiating into the neck suggests myocardial ischaemia. Pain associated with occupation, e.g. writing, word-processing (keyboard occupations), will suggest repetitive strain injury. A history of diabetes mellitus, renal failure, liver failure, alcohol abuse, vitamin B_{12} deficiency, drugs, e.g. phenytoin, vincristine, suggests peripheral neuropathy.

Pain, paraesthesia in the thumb, index and middle finger, which is worse in bed at night and relieved by hanging the arm out of bed, would suggest carpal tunnel syndrome. The latter may be associated with pregnancy, rheumatoid arthritis, myxoedema, anterior dislocation of the lunate, gout, acromegaly, amyloidosis, and arteriovenous fistula at the wrist created for haemodialysis.

Localised bone pain may be due to primary or secondary tumours. The latter are most common and may result from a primary in the breast, bronchus, thyroid, prostate or kidney. Pathological fractures may occur. With compartment syndrome there may be a history of crush injury, vascular injury or vascular surgery. Chronic compartment syndrome may result from unusual exertion, e.g. weight-lifting.

EXAMINATION

A full neurological examination should be carried out, looking for cervical lesions, brachial plexus lesions or carpal tunnel syndrome. There may be limitation in movements of the cervical spine. The limbs should be examined for swelling, e.g. axillary vein thrombosis, when there will be cyanosis and dilated veins. Examine for signs of ischaemia and feel for pulses. The classical signs of an ischaemic limb, i.e. pain, pallor, pulselessness, paraesthesia, 'perishing cold' and paralysis may be present. Occupation will suggest repetitive strain injury and there will usually be little to find on examination. Horner's syndrome (ptosis, miosis, enophthalmos and anhidrosis) suggests Pancoast's tumour. With bone tumours there will be localised swelling and tenderness. With compartment syndrome there will be a swollen tender compartment in the forearm, paraesthesia and paralysis. Pulses may be normal initially; later they are reduced or absent.

GENERAL INVESTIGATIONS

- **FBC, ESR**
  WCC ↑ infection, e.g. osteomyelitis or cervical spine TB. ESR ↑ infection and malignancy.
- **CRP**
  ↑ Infection/inflammatory cause.
- **Cervical spine X-ray**
  Cervical spondylosis, bony metastases, cervical spine fractures.
- **CXR**
  Malignancy resulting in bone secondary. Pancoast's tumour (apical lung tumour spreading to involve brachial plexus). Cervical rib (13 ribs).
- **ECG**
  Cardiac ischaemia.
- **Cardiac enzymes**
  Cardiac ischaemia

SPECIFIC INVESTIGATIONS

- **CT**
  Cervical disc lesions, tumours.
- **MRI**
  Cervical disc lesions, tumours.
- **Nerve conduction studies**
  Brachial plexus lesions, peripheral neuropathy, carpal tunnel syndrome.
- **Duplex Doppler**
  Arterial or venous lesions.
- **Arteriography**
  Arterial lesions.
- **Venography**
  Venous lesions, e.g. axillary vein thrombosis.

ARM SWELLINGS

Swelling may be localised or generalised. Localised swellings may be related to joints or fractures. Localised swellings around joints are covered in the section on joint disorders (page 250). This section includes only those conditions that may cause generalised swelling of the arm.

CAUSES

Trauma

Infection
- Cellulitis
- Lymphangitis

Lymphoedema
- Congenital
- Acquired
  - Axillary node lesions
    - Carcinoma
    - Infection, e.g. filariasis
    - Excision
    - Radiotherapy

Axilliary vein thrombosis

Other
- Reflex sympathetic dystrophy (Sudek's atrophy)

HISTORY

A history of trauma will be obvious in many cases, although pathological fractures may occur with little trauma. Reflex sympathetic dystrophy may follow trauma e.g. Colles' fracture. Congenital lymphoedema of the arm is rare; however, secondary lymphoedema is not and a history of carcinoma of the breast, operations on the axilla, or radiotherapy to the axilla should be sought. There may be a history of a puncture wound or flea bite, suggesting cellulitis or lymphangitis. Streptococcal cellulitis is common following puncture wounds in patients who already have lymphoedema of a limb. Axillary vein thrombosis may come on after excessive or unusual exercise and has been nicknamed 'effort thrombosis'. An example is a patient who has been painting a ceiling who is not used to doing that sort of thing.

It may occur in patients with cervical ribs or thoracic inlet obstruction. Thrombosis may also occur following insertion of a central line.

EXAMINATION

There may be localised swelling and tenderness together with crepitus associated with a fracture. There may be generalised non-pitting oedema suggestive of lymphoedema. Examination of the axilla may reveal a mass of lymph nodes, a scar suggestive of previous surgery or the skin changes of previous radiotherapy. Examination of the breast may reveal the site of a primary tumour that has resulted in secondary axillary lymphadenopathy. With axillary vein thrombosis there will be swelling, cyanosis and prominent dilated veins on the arm. With cellulitis there may be redness and heat in the arm, and in lymphangitis there may be red, inflamed streaks along the line of lymphatic vessels. With reflex sympathetic dystrophy the limb becomes painful, swollen and stiff with a reddened, smooth, shiny appearance to the skin.

GENERAL INVESTIGATIONS

- **FBC, ESR**
  Hb ↓ tumour. WCC ↑ infection. ESR ↑ tumour or infection.
- **Swab**
  C&S of any lesion that may have resulted in cellulitis or lymphangitis.
- **CXR**
  Cervical rib (associated with axillary vein thrombosis).
- **Arm X-ray**
  Patchy porosis of bone with reflex sympathetic dystrophy. Possible foreign body associated with cellulitis.

SPECIFIC INVESTIGATIONS

- **US or CT**
  Axillary mass.
- **Mammography**
  Breast carcinoma – axillary lymphadenopathy.
- **Duplex Doppler**
  Axillary vein thrombosis.
- **Venography**
  Axillary vein thrombosis.

ASCITES

Ascites is the accumulation of excess free fluid in the peritoneal cavity.

CAUSES

Hepatic
- Cirrhosis
- Hepatic tumours

Malignant disease
- Carcinomatosis
- Abdominal/pelvic tumour (primary or secondary)
- Pseudomyxoma peritonei
- Primary mesothelioma

Cardiac
- Cardiac failure
- Constrictive pericarditis
- Tricuspid incompetence

Renal
- Nephrotic syndrome

Peritonitis
- Tuberculosis
- Spontaneous bacterial

Venous obstruction
- Budd–Chiari syndrome
- Veno-occlusive disease
- Hepatic portal vein obstruction
- Inferior vena cava obstruction

Gastrointestinal
- Malabsorption
- Pancreatitis
- Bile ascites

HISTORY

Symptoms
Patients with ascites can present with abdominal discomfort, increasing abdominal girth, weight gain and ankle or sacral swelling.

Onset

The development of ascites is usually gradual, but sudden onset can result from acute decompensation of liver cirrhosis, malignancy, portal or splenic vein thrombosis and Budd–Chiari syndrome.

Past medical history

Any history of malignancy in the abdomen or pelvis is relevant; however, abdominal metastasis can also result in ascites, especially from breast, ovarian, prostatic, testicular and haematological malignancies. Cirrhosis of the liver may result from alcoholism, previous hepatitis, Wilson's disease primary and secondary biliary cirrhosis and haemochromatosis. A previous history of tuberculosis should raise suspicion of secondary disease.

Associated symptoms

Shortness of breath can result from splinting of the diaphragm due to tense ascites itself, or secondarily as part of the syndrome of cardiac failure when it is the underlying cause.

EXAMINATION

Classical findings are shifting dullness and a fluid thrill. As liver disease and carcinomatosis account for 90% of the cases presenting with ascites, a detailed examination of all systems is required. The next commonest causes are cardiac failure and nephrotic syndrome.

Inspection

Evidence of liver disease would be suggested by the presence of jaundice, spider naevi, loss of body hair, gynaecomastia, palmar erythema, caput medusae. The JVP is elevated in the presence of cardiac failure, and a prominent v wave is seen with tricuspid regurgitation. Further elevation of the JVP on inspiration (Kussmaul's sign) may be observed with a pericardial effusion.

Palpation

Careful abdominal examination should be performed to look for possible abdominal or pelvic tumours. 'Dipping' may be required to feel masses in the presence of gross ascites. Hepatomegaly and splenomegaly can occur with portal hypertension and hepatic and haematological malignancies. Displacement of the apex beat with cardiomegaly may result from cardiac failure. Pedal oedema occurs with cirrhosis, cardiac failure, malabsorption, obstruction of

lymphatic flow due to intra-abdominal or pelvic tumours, and
nephrotic syndrome.

Auscultation

A third heart sound, systolic murmurs (functional tricuspid and
mitral regurgitation) and crepitations (pulmonary oedema) may
be audible with cardiac failure. Heart sounds are muffled with
pericardial effusions. A pericardial friction rub or knock is
occasionally audible in pericarditis.

Percussion

Dullness of the lung bases occurs with pulmonary oedema and
pleural effusions (which may occur secondary to ascites).

Internal examination

A rectal examination may reveal ulceration or a fixed mass
suggestive of a carcinoma. In women, an adnexal mass PV may be
the first indication of a pelvic tumour.

GENERAL INVESTIGATIONS

History and examination findings may reveal the underlying cause.
General investigations can be used to confirm or indicate the
possible aetiology.

- **Urine dipstick**
  Will be strongly positive for protein in nephrotic syndrome. If so,
  a 24-hour urine collection for protein should be undertaken:
  more than 3.5 g/24 hours is indicative of nephrotic syndrome.
- **FBC**
  A raised white count may indicate an infective aetiology but a
  differential white count is more specific.
- **U&Es**
  Elevated urea and creatinine implies severe renal impairment,
  and may occur as a component of hepatorenal syndrome, which
  is renal impairment secondary to liver failure.
- **LFTs**
  May be deranged in the presence of liver disease. The serum
  albumin will be able to indicate hypoalbuminaemia but the
  underlying cause must still be sought.
- **CXR**
  Findings suggestive of cardiac failure are cardiomegaly, upper
  venous diversion of blood, the presence of Kerley B lines,
  pulmonary oedema and pleural effusions. Occasionally the

presence of carcinoma may be suggested by a lesion in the lung fields.

- **US abdomen/pelvis**
  In addition to confirming the presence of ascites, US will detect any intra-abdominal masses that are not palpable on clinical examination, and visualise fatty deposits in the liver in the presence of cirrhosis. Dilated collateral veins may be seen in conditions that result in obstruction of the venous outflow of the liver, including cirrhosis and Budd–Chiari syndrome.
- **Abdominal paracentesis**
  Aspiration of the ascitic fluid is very useful to help determine the underlying cause. A sample should be sent to microbiology, clinical chemistry and pathology.

Ascitic fluid

Appearance

Chylous   The milky white appearance of chylous ascites is due to obstruction of the lymphatic ducts.

Bile-stained   Is suggestive of bile peritonitis.

Haemorrhagic   Can occur in malignancy, trauma and tuberculosis.

Straw-coloured   The usual appearance with most other causes.

Biochemistry

Protein   The ascitic protein levels are often used to classify the ascites as a transudate or an exudate; however this may not always be reliable. A transudate would be ascitic fluid with the protein concentration of less than 25 g/l in the sample or 11 g/l lower than the serum protein level, while an exudate is the opposite.

Amylase   Is usually elevated in pancreatic ascites.

Glucose   Low in bacterial infections.

Triglyceride   Elevated in chylous ascites, may indicate obstruction of drainage of the thoracic duct.

Bilirubin   Elevated in bile ascites.

Microbiology
Gram and Ziehl–Neelsen staining with cultures may be positive with a bacterial aetiology.

Cytology
WCC Neutrophilia is suggestive of a bacterial peritonitis, while tuberculous peritonitis usually results in a lymphocytosis. Malignant cells may be identified and a primary source may possibly be located.

SPECIFIC INVESTIGATIONS

- **Echocardiography**
  Cardiac failure will manifest as a dilated and poorly contracting ventricle with a reduced ejection fraction. A pericardial effusion is visible as an echo-free space between the left ventricle and the pericardium. Tricuspid regurgitation can be visualised with colour-flow Doppler imaging.
- **Liver biopsy**
  Will be able to confirm and may be able to ascertain the underlying cause of liver cirrhosis.
- **Renal biopsy**
  Reveals the underlying cause of nephrotic syndrome.
- **Portal venography**
  Is indicated if obstruction to the venous outflow of the liver is suspected and can confirm Budd–Chiari syndrome and veno-occlusive disease.

▶ AXILLARY SWELLINGS

The great majority of axillary swellings are enlarged lymph nodes. Axillary nodes are often enlarged due to secondary deposits from carcinoma of the breast. Most axillary swellings are easily diagnosed on clinical examination alone.

CAUSES

Superficial
- Acute abscess
- Sebaceous cyst
- Lipoma
- Hidradenitis suppurativa

Deep
- Chronic abscess, e.g. tuberculosis (rare)
- Lymphadenopathy
- Lipoma
- Axillary artery aneurysm
- Breast lump (in the axillary tail)

HISTORY

Superficial

Acute abscess
This presents as a tender swelling in the skin. There may be a purulent discharge. Common in diabetics.

Sebaceous cyst
A sebaceous cyst will present as a firm swelling in the skin, often with a punctum. It may be tender if it becomes inflamed and there may be discharge from it.

Lipoma
This presents as a soft lobulated swelling in the subcutaneous tissue.

Hidradenitis suppurativa
The patient presents with multiple tender swellings in the superficial tissue of the axilla, the infection occurring in the apocrine sweat glands. A purulent discharge usually occurs. There may be a history of diabetes.

Deep

Chronic abscess
Check for a history of tuberculosis. There may be night sweats.

Lymphadenopathy (page 305)

The patient may have noticed a lump in the axilla, which may be tender or non-tender. Check for a site of infection or malignancy in the region of drainage of the nodes, i.e. the arm, the chest wall and the abdominal wall as far down as, and including, the umbilicus, the skin of the back as far down as the iliac crest, and the breast. Has the patient noticed any lumps elsewhere? Check for malaise, pyrexia, night sweats, cough. There may be a history of bruising or epistaxis to suggest a blood dyscrasia. Is there any evidence of scratches on the arm to suggest cat scratch disease?

Lipoma

Occasionally the patient may notice a firm swelling which appears intermittently, slipping out from under cover of the muscles.

Axillary artery aneurysm

This is rare. The patient may notice a pulsatile swelling under the arm. When the swelling becomes large, the patient may notice the arm moving away from the side of the body with each heart beat. Occasionally there may be symptoms in the hand due to distal embolisation.

Breast lumps

Occasionally a lump in the medial wall of the axilla may be a swelling in the axillary tail of the breast, e.g. fibroadenoma or carcinoma.

EXAMINATION

Superficial

Acute abscess
There may be a tender, red, fluctuant swelling with purulent discharge.

Lipoma
There will be a soft, lobulated swelling in the subcutaneous tissue.

Sebaceous cyst
A small, well-defined swelling in the skin. A punctum may be visible. If it is infected, the surrounding skin will be red and the lesion tender. Discharge may be present.

Hidradenitis suppurativa

Multiple tender swellings with surrounding erythema and discharge of pus are present.

Deep

Chronic abscess

A fluctuant swelling presents in the axilla. With tuberculosis there may be little or no signs of inflammation.

Lymphadenopathy

Single discrete node, e.g. lymphoma. Numerous hard nodes or matting of nodes (carcinoma). Tender fluctuant nodes (abscess). Check for infection or tumour in the area of drainage of the lymphatics. Examine the breast. Check all other sites of nodes, e.g. cervical, inguinal; check for hepatosplenomegaly.

Lipoma

Deep lipomas are usually intermuscular and may be felt only in certain positions. They may slip in and out between the pectoral muscles. They may be firmer and not have the lobulated feel of a more superficial lipoma.

Axillary artery aneurysm

A pulsatile mass will be palpable within the axilla. Check the distal circulation. If an axillary artery aneurysm is large, when the patient stands with the arms by the sides, the arm moves away from the side of the body as the lump pulsates.

Breast lumps

A lump on the medial wall of the axilla may be a lump in the axillary tail of the breast.

GENERAL INVESTIGATIONS

- **FBC, ESR**

  Hb ↓ malignant disease. WCC ↑ infection or leukaemia. ESR ↑ infection and malignancy. Platelets ↓ leukaemia.
- **Swab**

  C&S, microscopy of any discharge.

SPECIAL INVESTIGATIONS

- **CXR**

  TB.

- **US**
  Lymphadenopathy, lipoma, aneurysm.
- **Mantoux test**
  TB.
- **FNAC**
  Benign versus malignant.
- **Mammography**
  Carcinoma of the breast.
- **Arteriography**
  Assess distal circulation with axillary artery aneurysm.

▶ BACKACHE

Backache is one of the most common complaints seen in general practice and orthopaedic clinics. It accounts for about 20% of referrals to orthopaedic clinics. Most causes are either traumatic or degenerative but other causes are numerous and may occur as a result of pathology in almost any system of the body.

CAUSES

Congenital
- Kyphoscoliosis
- Spina bifida
- Spondylolisthesis

Acquired

Traumatic
- Vertebral fractures
- Ligamentous injury
- Joint strain
- Muscle tears

Infective
- Osteomyelitis – acute and chronic
- TB
- Discitis

Inflammatory
- Ankylosing spondylitis
- Rheumatology disorders

Neoplastic
- Primary tumours (rare)
- Metastases (common)

Degenerative
- Osteoarthritis
- Intervertebral disc lesions

Metabolic
- Osteoporosis
- Osteomalacia

Endocrine
- Cushing's disease (osteoporosis)

Idiopathic
- Paget's disease
- Scheuermann's disease

Psychogenic
- Psychosomatic backache (common)

Visceral
- Penetrating peptic ulcer
- Carcinoma of the pancreas
- Carcinoma of the rectum

Vascular
- Aortic aneurysm
- Acute aortic dissection

Renal
- Carcinoma of the kidney
- Renal calculus
- Inflammatory disease

Gynaecological
- Uterine tumours
- Pelvic inflammatory disease
- Endometriosis

HISTORY

Congenital

The diagnosis is usually apparent from the history, although with spondylolisthesis the symptoms, i.e. low lumbar backache, worse on standing, may not present until late childhood or early adult life.

Acquired

General

Is the onset sudden (trauma-related, disc lesions) or gradual (degenerative disease)? Are there neurological symptoms and is the bladder affected? Are the patient's symptoms worse on movement and relieved by rest, suggesting a mechanical cause? Is the pain severe and unrelenting, supporting a malignant cause? Are the symptoms related to systems other than the musculoskeletal system, e.g. abdominal pain, dysuria or menorrhagia?

Traumatic

There will usually be a clear history of trauma. Care must be taken in moving the patient. Neurological sequelae may be obvious.

Infective

There may be a history of tuberculosis; the patient may have had night sweats or cough. Osteomyelitis of the spine may also occur in diabetes and the immunocompromised, in which case the organism is more commonly *Staphylococcus aureus*. With spinal tuberculosis the patient is usually young and complains of malaise, fever, pain, tenderness and limitation of movement of the spine. Discitis usually presents with mild back ache accompanied by leg pain.

Inflammatory

Ankylosing spondylitis usually affects young adult males. The sacroiliac joints are affected initially, then the whole spine. The patient usually presents with lumbar stiffness, especially when rising in the morning. Iritis and plantar fasciitis may also occur. Rheumatology disorders may present with symptoms in other joints.

Neoplastic

The patient is usually unwell with severe unrelenting pain, often localised to a particular area of the spine. There may be a past history of a primary tumour (e.g. bronchus, breast, thyroid, prostate or kidney), or the primary may not be apparent. The pain may have been of sudden onset with a pathological fracture resulting in a collapsed vertebra. Rarely paraplegia may be a presenting symptom. Myeloma may present with backache.

Degenerative

Osteoarthritis usually presents in the older patient, with pain made worse on movement and relieved by rest. With intervertebral disc lesions there is usually sudden onset of pain radiating down the back of the leg (sciatica). The pain is worse on movement, coughing and straining. Neurological symptoms may be present, e.g. weakness of a limb, bladder symptoms.

Metabolic

Osteoporosis is commonest in postmenopausal women. Bone pain and pathological fractures occur. Osteomalacia may occur in adults with a history of gastrectomy, steatorrhoea, renal failure or anticonvulsant therapy.

Endocrine

There may be a history of Cushing's disease or long-term steroid therapy.

Idiopathic

Paget's disease of bone may cause backache. This usually occurs over the age of 40 years. The patient may have noted other changes, e.g. enlargement of the face, or bowing of the leg. Scheuermann's disease is osteochondritis of the spine. It causes backache in adolescence. The patient may present because the parents have noticed round shoulders.

Psychogenic

This is very common. Check for malingering, anxiety, depression and compensation neurosis.

Visceral

With penetrating peptic ulcer the patient complains of epigastric pain radiating straight through to the back. The pain may be relieved by food and antacids. With carcinoma of the pancreas the patient will describe a boring pain in the back, which is unrelenting. There will be a history of anorexia and weight loss. The patient may be jaundiced. With carcinoma of the rectum invasion of the sacrum and the sacral plexus may occur, causing low back pain with sciatica.

Vascular

Aortic aneurysm may cause back pain by eroding into the vertebral bodies. Alternatively it may cause severe back pain due to rupture. The patient may have noticed a pulsation in the abdomen. Acute aortic dissection usually gives a severe tearing back pain associated with chest pain. The patient is usually shocked.

Renal

There is usually a dull, boring ache with carcinoma of the kidney. The patient may also complain of haematuria. With ureteric colic the pain radiates from loin to groin and is severe, the patient being unable to get into a comfortable position. Inflammatory disease of the kidney presents with upper lumbar back pain. The patient may be feverish with rigors, and complain of frequency and dysuria.

Gynaecological

The pain is usually low back pain associated with pelvic discomfort. The patient may also complain of dysmenorrhoea, menorrhagia or postmenopausal bleeding.

EXAMINATION

General

Acute cord compression will cause bilateral leg pain with lower motor neurone signs at the level of the compression, and upper motor neurone signs below. Check for sphincter disturbance. Acute cauda equina compression causes root pain in the legs, saddle anaesthesia, and disturbances of bladder and bowel function.

In any patient with acute backache the above signs should be sought and, if found, the appropriate urgent referral made to a neurosurgeon or spinal surgeon.

Congenital

Kyphoscoliosis and spina bifida are usually obvious on examination. With spondylolisthesis a 'step' may be palpable in the line of the spinous processes, with a skin crease below. It usually involves L5 slipping on S1, or less commonly, L4 slipping on L5. Occasionally there are neurological signs in the limbs.

Acquired

Traumatic

This will usually be obvious. Careful positioning of the patient and full neurological examination should be carried out. Always check for associated injuries.

Infective

With acute osteomyelitis there is pyrexia, malaise, and local tenderness and spasm. With chronic osteomyelitis, e.g. due to tuberculosis, there will be wasting of the paraspinal muscles, spasm and restricted movements. There may be a localised kyphosis or 'gibbus' due to vertebral collapse. A psoas abscess may be present in the groin. Paraplegia may occur. With discitis there will be reduced movement of the spine.

Inflammatory

The patient with ankylosing spondylitis will present with a stiff spine. There will be flexion of the hips and spine. In the advanced case the patient cannot raise the head to see in front. Check for iritis and plantar fasciitis. Rheumatological disease will also present with problems in other joints.

Neoplastic

With myeloma, in addition to backache there may be pain in the ribs, long bones and skull. Bone tenderness will be present with secondary deposits. Palpate along the spine for tenderness. Check the chest, thyroid, breast, kidney and prostate for malignancy. Check for any neurological signs.

Degenerative

There will be limitation of movement of the spine with osteoarthritis. With acute disc lesion there will be limitation of spine movement, lordosis and neurological symptoms of the lower limbs. Carry out a full neurological examination.

Metabolic

With osteoporosis, usually there will be only localised bone tenderness. There may be evidence of recent vertebral collapse. With osteomalacia, apart from bone pain, there may be proximal myopathy resulting in a waddling gait.

Endocrine

There may be signs of Cushing's disease or prolonged steroid therapy, e.g. cushingoid facies, buffalo hump, proximal myopathy, abdominal striae, etc.

Idiopathic

In Paget's disease check for changes in the skull, long bones (bowing of the tibia). Compressive symptoms due to skull enlargement may result in blindness, deafness or cranial nerve entrapment. There may be signs of high-output cardiac failure due to vascularity of bone. In Scheuermann's disease there will be a smooth, thoracic kyphosis and below this a compensatory lumbar lordosis. The chest is flat.

Psychogenic

This is often difficult to assess. Signs may vary from examination to examination. There may be exaggeration of symptoms during the examination. It is best to watch from a distance as the patient leaves the consulting room. The gait, posture and demeanour may suddenly change!

Visceral

Check for epigastric tenderness or mass. Jaundice may be present in pancreatic cancer, and the gall bladder may be palpable (Courvoisier's law). Carry out a digital rectal examination to check for rectal carcinoma.

Vascular

A pulsatile abdominal mass may be palpable. The patient may be shocked. With acute aortic dissection, there may be shock with disparity of pulses in the extremities.

Renal

Check for renal masses or loin tenderness.

Gynaecological

Check for pelvic masses. Carry out bimanual examination.

GENERAL INVESTIGATIONS

- **FBC, ESR**
  Hb ↓ malignancy, peptic ulceration. WCC ↑ infection, e.g. osteomyelitis. ESR ↑ malignancy, e.g. myeloma or secondary deposits. TB. Ankylosing spondylitis.
- **CRP**
  ↑ Infection, inflammation.
- **U&Es**
  May be abnormal in renal disease.
- **LFTs**
  Bilirubin and alkaline phosphatase will be raised in biliary tract obstruction related to carcinoma of the head of the pancreas. Alkaline phosphatase may also be raised in Paget's disease, osteomalacia and secondary deposits in bone. This is bony alkaline phosphatase that is raised and isoenzymes will need checking.
- **CXR**
  Primary tumour, e.g. bronchial carcinoma. Secondary tumours.
- **Spine X-ray**
  Trauma – fractures. Osteoarthritis – narrowed disc spaces and osteophytes. Prolapsed intervertebral disc – mild scoliosis, loss of lumbar lordosis, loss of disc space, Schmorl's node. Spondylolisthesis – decapitated 'Scottie dog' sign. Scheuermann's disease – wedging of vertebra and irregularity of vertebral end plates. Chronic osteomyelitis – erosion of joint surfaces, destruction of bone and intervertebral discs, soft tissue shadows, e.g. psoas abscess. Myeloma – punched-out lesions. Secondary deposits – osteolytic or osteosclerotic (prostate). Osteoporosis – thinned bones, vertebral collapse. Ankylosing spondylitis – 'bamboo' spine; irregularity, sclerosis and fusion of sacroiliac joints. Paget's disease of bone – 'sclerotic' white vertebrae.
- **US**
  Aortic aneurysm. Renal lesions. Uterine lesions.

SPECIFIC INVESTIGATIONS

- **PSA**
  Prostatic carcinoma.
- **Serum calcium**
  Raised in malignancy, myeloma, and bony metastases.

- **Bence Jones protein**
  May be raised in myeloma.
- **Plasma protein electrophoresis**
  Monoclonal gammopathy in myeloma.
- **CT**
  Pancreatic lesions. Aortic lesions. Pelvic lesions.
- **Technetium scan**
  Hot spots with bony secondaries. Occasional hot spots with inflammatory disease.
- **MRI**
  Location of disc lesion. Spinal tumour. Spinal compression.

▶ BREAST LUMPS

A lump in the breast is a common clinical presentation. In every case of a breast lump, carcinoma must be excluded.

CAUSES

Discrete lumps

Malignant
- Carcinoma
- Phylloides tumour (some behave in benign fashion)

Benign
- Fibroadenoma
- Cyst (in cystic mastitis)
- Galactocele
- Fat necrosis
- Lipoma
- Duct ectasia
- Tuberculous abscess
- Sebaceous cyst

Generalised swelling
- Pregnancy
- Lactation
- Puberty
- Mastitis

Swellings behind the breast
- Retromammary abscess from chest disease
- Tietze's disease
- Rib deformities
- Chondroma of the costal cartilages

HISTORY

A diagnosis of carcinoma is suggested by a strong family history, nulliparous state, early menarche, late menopause, history of cystic hyperplasia. The patient may have found a breast lump (carcinoma is painless in 85% of cases) or may have noticed nipple retraction, skin dimpling, axillary swelling. Jaundice may have occurred due to liver secondaries or porta hepatis node involvement. Bone pain may be due to secondary deposits and pathological fractures. Breathlessness may be due to lung secondaries or a pleural effusion. Personality change, fits, headaches suggest cerebral metastases. A patient who presents in pregnancy or lactation may have mastitis, abscess or galactocele. A history of trauma suggests fat necrosis. A patient in the fifth decade with retroareolar pain, nipple retraction and a thick, creamy nipple discharge suggests duct ectasia. The patient presenting between the ages of 15 and 25 years with a non-tender swelling suggests fibroadenoma. A patient with a history of painful breasts may have one of the conditions described under breast pain (page 58). Enquiries should be made of a past history of TB, as rarely a tuberculous abscess may form within the breast or erode through the chest wall from the lung.

EXAMINATION

Carcinoma

Hard irregular swelling. May be fixed to the skin or fixed deeply. Skin dimpling. Nipple retraction. Peau d'orange. Paget's disease of the nipple. Axillary lymphadenopathy. Supraclavicular lymphadenopathy. Hepatomegaly. Pathological fractures – spine, ribs, long bones.

Phylloides tumour

Mobile mass may become very large.

Fibroadenoma

Smooth, rounded, mobile mass. Breast 'mouse' (so called because it darts about under the examining fingers).

Cyst

Smooth, mobile swelling. May be tender. May be associated with generalised lumpiness of the breast.

Galactocele

Smooth, mobile swelling occurring in the lactating breast.

Fat necrosis

Hard, irregular swelling. May be overlying bruising of the skin or teeth marks! Occasionally the lesion is fixed to the skin and is difficult to distinguish from carcinoma.

Lipoma

Soft, lobulated swelling. Rare on the breast. 'Pseudolipoma' is a bunching of fat between retracted suspensory ligaments of the breast and is associated with an underlying carcinoma.

Duct ectasia

Tender retroareolar area. Retroareolar erythema. Nipple retraction. Thick, creamy nipple discharge.

Sebaceous cyst

Mobile swelling fixed to the skin. May be a punctum. May be infected, with discharge and surrounding redness.

Generalised swellings

Generalised swelling of the breast may occur in pregnancy, lactation and puberty. It may also occur with mastitis, when the breast is enlarged, red, tender and hot.

Swellings behind the breast

These are rare. Tietze's disease is the most common. There will be prominence and tenderness over the second, third and fourth costal cartilages. With retromammary abscess, chest signs may be obvious on percussion and also on auscultation of the chest.

GENERAL INVESTIGATIONS

- **FBC, ESR**
  Hb ↓ widespread malignancy. ↑ WCC breast abscess. ESR ↑ malignancy and tuberculosis.
- **LFTs**
  Alkaline phosphatase ↑ with liver secondaries and bone secondaries (isoenzymes).
- **Serum calcium**
  ↑ in bone secondaries.
- **CXR**
  Secondary deposits in lung and rib. Underlying chest disease, e.g. TB or empyema.

SPECIFIC INVESTIGATIONS

- **FNAC**
  Benign versus malignant. Cystic versus solid.
- **Mammography**
  Infiltrating radio-opaque mass or microcalcification indicates malignancy. Dilated retroareolar ducts and skin indentation suggests duct ectasia. Coarse calcification may occur with long-standing fibroadenomas.

- **Open excision biopsy**
  e.g. fibroadenoma, fat necrosis.
- **US**
  US of breast better than mammography in young women. US of liver for metastases. US guided FNA/core biopsy/Mammotome®
- **CT**
  Abdomen, chest, brain. Metastases.
- **Bone scan**
  Metastases.

▶ BREAST PAIN

Pain in the breast is a common symptom in general surgical practice. Most cases are benign and due to cyclical mastalgia, but occasionally pain may be the presenting symptom of carcinoma.

CAUSES

- Carcinoma (15% of lumps are painful)
- Cyclical mastalgia (fibroadenosis, cystic mastitis)
- Non-cyclical mastalgia
- Duct ectasia
- Fat necrosis
- Breast abscess
- Pregnancy
- Lactation
- Mastitis
- Tietze's disease
- Mondor's disease
- Rib secondaries
- Herpes zoster

HISTORY

Cyclical mastalgia causes soreness, frequently in the upper and outer quadrants of the breast in the week preceding a period. The pain usually disappears after the period and there is freedom from soreness or pain for 2 weeks, when it recommences. Symptoms are common in the 20–45 years age group. Non-cyclical mastalgia may occur and is more common in the 4th and 5th decades. Duct ectasia occurs in the fifth decade. The pain is usually behind the nipple and associated with subareolar erythema and a thick, creamy nipple discharge. Fat necrosis will be suggested by a history of trauma, which occasionally the patient will be embarrassed to admit (the partner's teeth!). Breast abscess or mastitis will be obvious. It usually occurs during pregnancy or lactation but it may occur in a retroareolar position in a patient with duct ectasia. Breast fullness and soreness is a symptom of early pregnancy. Patients may indicate breast pain where the condition is not actively in the breast but behind it. Tietze's disease (costochondritis of the costal cartilages) will present with pain related to the breast. Mondor's disease (superficial thrombophlebitis of the subcutaneous veins of the chest wall) also presents with pain in the breast. It may be associated with an underlying carcinoma. Rib secondaries may also present with pain behind the breast. Herpes zoster may present with pain radiating round into the breast and precedes the development of a vesicular eruption by 2–3 days.

EXAMINATION

A hard, irregular lump is suggestive of carcinoma (this is discussed in the section on breast lumps). Tenderness and lumpiness, occasionally with a smooth, mobile swelling (cyst), is suggestive of cyclical mastalgia. The tenderness and lumpiness is most often palpated in the upper and outer quadrants of the breast. In the early stages of fat necrosis there may be bruising over the breast and the lump is tender. In the later stages it becomes hard and irregular and may be tethered to the skin. Breast abscess will present with redness, swelling, heat and pain in the breast during pregnancy or, more commonly, lactation. The swelling will be fluctuant and usually there is associated fever. Duct ectasia presents with subareolar erythema, tenderness and occasionally a subareolar lump. Nipple retraction may be present in long-standing cases and there may be a thick, creamy discharge that can be expressed from the nipple. Pregnancy will present with fullness of the breast and increased circumareolar pigmentation. In Tietze's disease there will be tenderness, and occasionally swelling, over the second, third and fourth costal cartilages. In Mondor's disease the veins of the chest wall are felt as red, tender cords, often extending on to the anterior axillary fold. The breast should be carefully checked for an underlying mass, as the condition may be associated with carcinoma of the breast. Herpes zoster will usually present with a characteristic vesicular eruption a few days after the pain.

GENERAL INVESTIGATIONS

- **FBC, ESR**
  WCC ↑ mastitis and breast abscess. ESR ↑ widespread carcinoma.
- **LFTs**
  Alkaline phosphatase may be raised with liver or bony secondaries.

- **Serum calcium**
  May be raised with bone secondaries.
- **Swab**
  C&S if there is any discharge from an abscess or from the nipple.
- **CXR**
  Secondaries in lung or ribs. Pleural effusion in carcinoma.

SPECIFIC INVESTIGATIONS

- **βHCG**
  Positive in pregnancy.
- **FNAC**
  Benign versus malignant. Cystic versus solid.
- **Mammography**
  Carcinoma. Duct ectasia.
- **Breast biopsy**
  Benign versus malignant.
- **Bone scan**
  Rib secondaries. Myeloma.

CHEST PAIN

Chest pain is a common presenting symptom of disorders that can range from trivial to life-threatening.

CAUSES

Cardiovascular
- Angina
- Myocardial infarction
- Acute aortic dissection
- Pericarditis

Gastrointestinal
- Reflux oesophagitis
- Oesophageal spasm
- Peptic ulcer disease

Pulmonary
- Pneumonia
- Pulmonary embolism
- Pneumothorax

Musculoskeletal
- Chest wall injuries
- Costochondritis
- Secondary tumours of the rib
- Herpes zoster

Emotional
- Depression

HISTORY

Character
The character of angina is tight and crushing, whilst the pain from aortic dissection has a tearing quality. Oesophageal reflux may be described as a burning pain, and peptic acid-related pain tends to be deep and gnawing.

Location
The pain from angina and oesophageal reflux may be located retrosternally, and they both can radiate to the jaw or down into the left arm. The pain from pericarditis may be centrally located and

radiate to the shoulders (trapezius ridge pain). Pain from aortic dissection often radiates into the back and occasionally into the abdomen (depending on the extent of the dissection). Pulmonary pain can be located anywhere in the thorax.

Precipitating factors

Angina may be precipitated by effort, a defining characteristic. Other known precipitants of angina are emotion, food and cold weather. If angina occurs at rest for more than 20 minutes it should be treated as a myocardial infarction until proven otherwise. Oesophageal reflux is often related to meals and precipitated by changes in posture, such as bending or lying. Pain originating from pericarditis and pulmonary origin is often pleuritic, i.e. worse on inspiration, however, musculoskeletal pain can also be worse on breathing due to movement of the thorax.

Relieving factors

Both oesophageal spasm and angina may be relieved by glyceryl trinitrate (GTN), which relaxes smooth muscle. Antacids will relieve the pain of oesophageal reflux but not angina. The pain associated with pericarditis may be relieved by sitting forwards.

Trauma

A history of a blunt or stretching injury immediately suggests the underlying aetiology of chest wall tenderness and it is important to diagnose rib fractures that can result form more severe trauma. Pathological rib fractures that result from minor injuries may be due to bony metastasis or osteoporosis.

Emotion

Occasionally chest pain is a somatic manifestation of patients with depression or anxiety, but it is essential to exclude all organic causes before accepting depression or anxiety as the underlying cause. Moreover a serious aetiology may coexist.

EXAMINATION

Temperature

Pyrexia can occur with pneumonia, myocardial infarction, pericarditis and herpes zoster infection.

Pulse

Heart rate on its own is not discriminating as pain invariably leads to tachycardia. However, palpating both upper and lower limb pulses may be useful. Occasionally peripheral pulses are absent in patients with aortic dissection.

JVP

The JVP is elevated with congestive cardiac failure and acute right ventricular failure, an occasional complication of inferior myocardial infarction and pulmonary embolism (when more than 60% of the pulmonary vascular supply is occluded).

Palpation of the chest

Chest wall tenderness would imply a musculoskeletal cause. The presence of unilateral tenderness confined to a single or adjacent group of dermatomes would suggest either central (vertebral or spinal origin) or peripheral nerve pathology (herpes zoster infection). The trachea deviates away from the side of a tension pneumothorax, and chest expansion is decreased on the same side for pneumonia and pneumothorax. Dullness to percussion will be noted in an area of consolidation with pneumonia and hyperresonance with pneumothorax (a difficult sign to interpret).

Auscultation of the chest

The unilateral absence of breath sounds is consistent with a pneumothorax; more localised loss occurs over an effusion. Bronchial breath sounds are audible over a segment of consolidation and sometimes above the level of an effusion. Localised areas of crepitations are audible with lobar pneumonia, whereas widespread crepitations suggest multilobar involvement or pulmonary oedema secondary to left ventricular failure (from myocardial infarction).

A friction rub may be auscultated with both pericardial and pleuritic disease, but only a pericardial rub will be present when the patient holds the breath.

Lower limbs

Hemiparesis can occur with aortic dissection, and a hot, swollen, tender calf or thigh may give a clue to an underlying deep vein thrombosis. Measurements of the mid-thigh or mid-calf circumference may demonstrate a larger circumference on the side of a DVT. Less reliably, pain is found on dorsiflexion of the foot (Homans' sign).

GENERAL INVESTIGATIONS

- **FBC**
  An elevated white cell count will be expected with a pneumonia, and to a lesser extent in a myocardial infarction.

- **Serum cardiac markers**
  Following a myocardial infarction, cardiac troponin rises within 6 hours and remains elevated for up to 2 weeks.
- **ECG**
  Angina or a myocardial infarct will result in ECG changes following the anatomical pattern of coronary vascular insufficiency. Involvement of the left main coronary artery would result in ECG changes of ischaemia or infarction in the anterior (V3–4) and left lateral (V4–6) leads. Involvement of the left anterior descending artery will be reflected in the anterior leads, and insufficiency of the posterior descending artery will produce changes in the inferior leads (II, III, aVF). Changes suggestive of ischaemia or non ST elevation myocardial infarction (NSTEMI) are ST segment depression and T wave inversion. Elevated serum cardiac markers distinguish NSTEMI from angina. ST segment elevation infarcts (STEMI) by definition produce ST segment elevation and Q wave formation in the corresponding leads. Pulmonary emboli usually result in non-specific ECG changes such as tachycardia, right axis deviation, right ventricular strain and atrial fibrillation. Occasionally one may find the S1Q3T3 pattern (S wave in lead I, Q wave and an inverted T wave in lead III), indicative of right heart strain.
- **CXR**
  The line of the pleura with absence of lung markings distal to it is the usual finding for a pneumothorax. Areas of consolidation on a chest film may be confined to a lobe or widespread in bronchopneumonia. The classic wedge-shaped shadow (base is distal) of a pulmonary embolus is rare, and occurs only if pulmonary infarction resulted. Dissection of the aorta may widen its width, causing a bulge to appear at the right mediastinal border. Rib fractures or secondary deposits in ribs may be visible.

SPECIFIC INVESTIGATIONS

- **V/Q scan**
  Will show a mismatch in the majority of pulmonary emboli.
- **Pulmonary angiography**
  Pulmonary emboli will be delineated. It is possible to visualise the site and extent of the embolism and it may also be possible to extract the emboli using a catheter.

- **CT aortography**
  Confirm and assess the extent and site of the dissection of the aorta.
- **Upper GI endoscopy**
  Oesophagitis.
- **Oesophageal manometry**
  Abnormal oesophageal pressures.

▶ CLOTTING DISORDERS

Congenital disorders of clotting usually present with complications related to prolonged blood loss, whereas acquired disorders are usually discovered during coagulation testing.

CAUSES

Congenital
- Haemophilia
- von Willebrand's disease

Acquired
- Vitamin K deficiency
  - Haemorrhagic disease of the newborn
  - Obstructive jaundice
  - Fat malabsorption
- Liver disease
- Disseminated intravascular coagulation
- Autoimmune diseases, e.g. SLE
- Massive transfusion
- Drugs – heparin, warfarin, thrombolytic therapy

HISTORY

Onset and duration

The duration of symptoms and age of presentation is very useful in determining the underlying aetiology. Bleeding in the first few days of life occurs as a result of deficient vitamin K synthesis by the neonatal liver, due to immaturity. Patients with haemophilia usually present at a young age with excessive blood loss following injuries or surgical procedures, such as circumcision. Muscle haematomas and painful haemarthroses may be accompanying features.

Past medical history

Concomitant disease constitutes the majority of causes of acquired coagulation disturbances. As coagulation factors are synthesised in the liver, disease of the liver naturally predisposes to clotting abnormalities. Vitamin K is a fat-soluble vitamin essential for the production of clotting factors II, VII, IX and X. Conditions, such as obstructive jaundice, pancreatic or small bowel disease, that impair the absorption of fat will result in decreased production of the aforementioned factors.

Patients with SLE may produce antibodies such as the lupus anticoagulant, which, although prolonging clotting in *in vitro* testing, predisposes to thrombosis *in vivo*.

Severe infections, malignancy, obstetric complications and burns may give rise to DIC. This is characterised by widespread consumption of clotting factors and platelets, resulting in severe coagulation disturbances.

Drug history

Coagulation abnormalities may be iatrogenic. Therapeutic anticoagulation is achieved with heparin and warfarin. Thrombolytic agents produce severe derangement of clotting as a side-effect of therapy. Coagulation disturbances can result from dilution from massive blood transfusions (when the patient's entire circulating volume has been replaced by transfusion within 24 hours).

EXAMINATION

A general examination is performed to identify any stigmata from haemophilia. Early-onset osteoarthritis and pseudotumours may result from episodes of repeated haemorrhage. Skin necrosis and haematomas may be seen with warfarin overdosage. In acquired coagulation disorders signs of liver disease may bring attention to the underlying disorder.

GENERAL INVESTIGATIONS

● **FBC**
  Low platelet count or abnormal platelet function results in prolonged bleeding time but not clotting results.

Disorder	PT	APTT	TT
Haemophilia	N	↑	N
von Willebrand's disease	N	↑	N
Liver disease	↑	↑	N
Warfarin/vitamin K deficiency	↑	↑	N
Heparin	N or ↑	↑	↑
DIC	↑	↑	↑

- **Clotting screen**
  PT, APTT and TT are measured. Abnormalities are listed in the table on page 67.
- **Bleeding time**
  Allows the differentiation of a primary clotting disorder (normal bleeding time) and platelet disorders causing prolonged bleeding.

SPECIFIC INVESTIGATIONS

- **Clotting factor assays**
  Clotting factor assays are required to differentiate between haemophilia A, haemophilia B and von Willebrand's disease. Low levels of factor VIII are found in both haemophilia A and von Willebrand's disease. Low levels of factor IX indicate haemophilia B. As the name implies, von Willebrand's factor is low in von Willebrand's disease and the bleeding time is also prolonged.
- **Fibrinogen and fibrin degradation products**
  With DIC, the platelet count and serum fibrinogen levels are low, whereas the fibrin degradation products such as D-dimers are increased.

CLUBBING

Clubbing is the selective bulbous enlargement of the distal segments of fingers or toes due to proliferation of connective tissues.

CAUSES

Respiratory
- Bronchial carcinoma
- Chronic suppurative lung disease
  - Bronchiectasis
  - Lung abscess
  - Empyema
  - Cystic fibrosis
- Fibrosing alveolitis

Cardiovascular
- Infective endocarditis
- Congenital cyanotic heart disease

Gastrointestinal
- Cirrhosis
- Ulcerative colitis
- Crohn's disease
- Coeliac disease

Other
- Familial
- Graves' disease (hyperthyroidism)

Clubbing is present, with loss of the normal angle between the base of the nail and the nailfold. In the presence of clubbing, when the fingernails from each hand are placed together, the gap is lost and this is known as Shamroth's sign. Other features are increased curvature of the nailbed (in all directions), sponginess or fluctuation, and expansion of the end of the digit to resemble a drumstick.

HISTORY

A systematic approach to the history is required to determine the cause of clubbing. Respiratory, cardiovascular and gastrointestinal system enquires should be made in an attempt to determine the underlying cause. A detailed discussion on the diagnosis of congenital cyanotic heart disease (tetralogy of Fallot, transposition of great arteries, total anomalous pulmonary venous drainage) is beyond the scope of this text.

Duration

The duration of clubbing may give an indication of the underlying aetiology. Clubbing present since infancy would suggest a familial trait or congenital cyanotic heart disease. Alternatively, it may be a secondary manifestation of hereditary disorders such as coeliac disease and cystic fibrosis.

Respiratory symptoms

A history of cough, haemoptysis, dyspnoea and weight loss in a chronic smoker should alert the clinician to the diagnosis of bronchial carcinoma. Symptoms of metastasis (bone pain, jaundice) and paraneoplastic involvement (neuropathy, thirst and polyuria from hypercalcaemia) should also be ascertained. With bronchial carcinoma, clubbing may be part of a generalised arthritic manifestation of hypertrophic pulmonary osteoarthropathy.

Cough productive of copious amounts of purulent sputum is usually the main complaint with bronchiectasis. With a chronic lung abscess or empyema, the symptoms are often less specific and may be preceded by a history of pneumonia or aspiration secondary to neurological disorders, dysphagia or alcoholism. Patients may present with a persistent low-grade pyrexia, malaise, weight loss and productive cough.

Gastrointestinal symptoms

Malaise, diarrhoea, abdominal pain and weight loss are experienced by most patients with inflammatory bowel disease and coeliac disease. The presence of aphthous ulceration, fistulae and perianal sepsis are suggestive of Crohn's disease. Predominantly rectal involvement with tenesmus, mucus and blood PR is more characteristic of ulcerative colitis; however, differentiation based on the history alone can be very difficult. Symptoms of coeliac disease tend to be very variable and non-specific, with non-bloody diarrhoea with steatorrhoea.

Heavy alcohol consumption or previous infection with hepatitis B will predispose to cirrhosis of the liver. Patients may complain of jaundice, abdominal distension due to ascites (page 37), upper gastrointestinal haemorrhage due to varices or bruising from impaired clotting (page 66). Severely affected individuals may present with encephalopathy or even coma (page 74).

Family history

A family history of clubbing or cystic fibrosis will suggest a hereditary cause. Approximately 15% of patients with coeliac disease will have an affected first-degree relative.

EXAMINATION

Inspection

The presence of wasting may be accounted for by cachexia of malignancy, chronic lung or gastrointestinal disease. The mucous membranes should be inspected for central cyanosis, which may be a feature of, or sequel to, congenital cyanotic heart disease. Cyanosis may also be noticeable with any of the above causes of severe lung disease. Aphthous ulceration occurs with Crohn's and coeliac disease. A goitre, exophthalmos, ophthalmoplegia and a resting tremor are features of Graves' disease.

With infective endocarditis, splinter haemorrhages, Osler's nodes (raised tender lesions on the pulps of the fingers) and Janeway lesions (flat non-tender macules on the palms and soles) may also be present in addition to clubbing.

Temperature

Pyrexia is notable in several important causes of clubbing, namely suppurative lung disease, infective endocarditis and active inflammatory bowel disease.

Examination of the chest

Auscultation of the precordium may reveal a new or changing murmurs with infective endocarditis. Widespread coarse crepitations of the lungs occur with retained secretions of bronchiectasis. Fine quality end-inspiratory crepitations are suggestive of fibrosing alveolitis. More localised coarse crepitations and dullness to percussion may be found with a lung abscess. Findings suggestive of pleural effusion (unilateral decreased expansion, dullness to percussion and absent breath sounds) may be due to malignancy. However, when this is associated with pyrexia in an ill patient, it should lead to the consideration of a thoracic empyema.

Abdominal examination

On abdominal examination, signs of chronic liver disease (page 38) may be present; however, there may be few specific features to suggest inflammatory bowel disease. When this diagnosis is suspected, a sigmoidoscopy should always be performed. Occasionally, right iliac fossa tenderness or a mass may be found in Crohn's disease. The presence of splenomegaly may indicate portal hypertension with liver disease, or enlargement accompanying infective endocarditis.

GENERAL INVESTIGATIONS

- **FBC**
  Hb ↓ carcinomatosis, inflammatory bowel disease, infective endocarditis. WCC ↑ lung abscess, empyema, inflammatory bowel disease.
- **ESR**
  ↑ carcinoma, inflammatory bowel disease, infective endocarditis.
- **LFTs**
  Liver disease, e.g. cirrhosis.
- **CXR**
  Should be performed if respiratory symptoms are present. Bronchial carcinoma may manifest as a hilar or peripheral opacity, cavitating mass, collapse of a segment of lung due to luminal obstruction, pleural effusion, elevated hemidiaphragm due to phrenic nerve palsy or destruction of an adjacent rib due to invasion. Lung abscesses present as a spherical shadow with a central lucency or air–fluid level. Bronchiectatic lungs have visibly dilated bronchi and multiple areas of consolidation. With fibrosing alveolitis, hazy shadowing of the lung bases produces a honeycomb appearance.

SPECIFIC INVESTIGATIONS

In view of the diverse nature of causes of clubbing, further investigations should be guided by the history and findings on clinical examination.

- **Urinalysis**
  Traces of blood from microemboli in infective endocarditis.
- **Blood cultures (three sets)**
  Infective endocarditis.
- **Echocardiography**
  Useful in the diagnosis of infective endocarditis, especially in the presence of large vegetations.
- **Sigmoidoscopy**
  Inflammatory bowel disease – characteristic findings include erythematous mucosa, areas of haemorrhage, contact bleeding and ulceration.

- **Rectal and colonic biopsy**
  Ulcerative colitis and Crohn's disease.
- **Colonoscopy**
  Inflammatory bowel disease.
- **Barium enema**
  Inflammatory bowel disease.
- **Small bowel enema**
  Crohn's disease.
- **Antireticulin and endomysial antibodies**
  Coeliac disease.
- **Jejunal biopsy**
  Coeliac disease. May reveal subtotal villous atrophy reversible with a gluten-free diet.
- **CT thorax**
  Should be performed if bronchial carcinoma or thoracic empyema is suspected. Also useful to confirm the diagnosis of bronchiectasis and idiopathic pulmonary fibrosis.

▶ COMA

Coma results from sustained impairment of awareness of self and of the environment. It can simply be defined as a state of unconsciousness or numerically categorised as a GCS score of less than 8.

CAUSES

Trauma
- Head injury (diffuse axonal injury)
- Extradural haemorrhage
- Subdural haemorrhage

Metabolic
- Hypothermia
- Hypoglycaemia
- Hyperglycaemia
- Hyponatraemia
- Hypernatraemia
- Diabetic ketoacidosis

Organ failure
- Cardiac/circulatory failure
- Respiratory failure
- Liver failure (encephalopathy)
- Renal failure (uraemic coma)
- Hypothyroidism

Vascular
- Stroke
- Subarachnoid haemorrhage

Infective
- Meningitis
- Encephalitis
- Cerebral malaria

Toxin/drug-induced
- Alcohol
- Overdose (opiates, tricyclics, benzodiazepines)
- Carbon monoxide poisoning

Cerebral
- Brain tumour
- Brain abscess
- Epilepsy

HISTORY

The history for the comatose patient is usually obtained from ambulance crew, relatives, friends or witnesses. Other sources of information are previous hospital notes, records kept by general practitioners, and tablets or prescriptions that have been found at the patient's premises.

Presentation

The circumstances regarding discovery of the patient is usually the first piece of information to be reported. Trauma patients may have been transported from sites of road traffic accidents, fire or have been found assaulted on the street. When teenagers are brought in unconscious from a night club, it is important to exclude alcohol intoxication, resulting hypoglycaemia and the effects of illicit drugs (malignant hyperthermia with 'ecstasy'). Attempted suicides may have an accompanying note, or empty drug bottles may have been recovered from the scene. Carbon monoxide poisoning occurs with suicide attempts in enclosure areas with running engines. Alternatively, it may also result as a complication in victims involved with fires. Patients who have been brought in from outdoors unconscious may also suffer with hypothermia in addition to the primary event.

Onset

When witnessed, information regarding the speed of onset of coma may help in determining a cause. Sudden onset of unconsciousness is characteristic of a seizure or a vascular event.

Trauma

Head injuries are a common cause of coma, but not all causes are due to blunt trauma to the cranium. Diffuse axonal injury results from severe shearing forces on the brain, a sequel to rapid acceleration and deceleration forces. Blunt head injuries may cause extradural haemorrhages as a result of skull fractures with laceration of meningeal arteries. There is usually a history of an injury with transient loss of consciousness, a lucid interval where the patient feels and appears well, followed by drowsiness, headache, vomiting, progressive hemiplegia and eventually coma. Subdural haemorrhages are a consequence of severe trauma with cortical lacerations or less severe trauma with laceration of bridging veins. Chronic subdural haemorrhages may result even in the absence of trauma; elderly patients with cortical atrophy are predisposed to this type of injury.

In addition to head injuries, coma may also complicate any other injuries severe enough to result in circulatory or respiratory insufficiency.

Headache

The onset of severe headache prior to coma may be caused by trauma, subarachnoid haemorrhage (classically patients complain of a sudden onset of blinding headache, the worst ever experienced in their lives) or meningitis (headache associated with photophobia and neck stiffness). Progressive headache, worse in the mornings and associated with vomiting, may due to raised intracranial pressure from a cerebral tumour.

Predisposing factors

The history of a predisposing factor is useful when assessing the comatose patient. The presence of diabetes should lead to the consideration of ketoacidosis (type I diabetics) and hypoglycaemia (oral hypoglycaemic or insulin dosage errors). Patients with known hepatic or renal failure may deteriorate to coma as a result of encephalopathy or uraemia, respectively. Coma may also complicate severe hypothyroidism. Previous suicide attempts or a history of depression should lead to the consideration of drug overdose. Epileptic patients may be in status epilepticus or in a postictal recovery state. Preexisting cardiac or respiratory disease may result in coma as a terminal event.

EXAMINATION

Temperature

Body temperature should be taken in all patients and a series of normal body temperatures can easily exclude hypothermia and hyperpyrexia, which may be a consequence of heat stroke or illicit drug use.

General examination

A thorough inspection should be performed. This will necessitate removal of clothing, log rolling (to examine the back) and a detailed examination of the scalp for bleeding, haematomas and fractures. The presence of bilateral periorbital haematomas or cerebrospinal fluid rhinorrhoea may indicate an anterior fossa fracture of the skull.

Bruising over the mastoid (Battle's sign) or cerebrospinal fluid otorrhoea may be due to a middle cranial fossa fracture. Patients with carbon monoxide poisoning appear bright red. Patients with myxoedema are characteristically obese, with coarse features, dry skin and brittle hair. Inspection of the face often reveals loss of the outer two-thirds of the eyebrow with 'peaches and cream' complexion. The arms should be carefully scrutinised for lacerations and needle puncture sites suggestive of drug abuse. If these are present then consider the possibility of an opiate overdose. Occasionally a petechial rash will be visible on the skin with meningococcal meningitis.

The organ systems should be examined in turn; suspect encephalopathy or uraemia if signs suggestive of liver disease (page 38) or chronic renal failure are present, respectively. The pulse should be examined for arrhythmias, which may precipitate cardiac failure. The JVP may also be elevated. Other causes of JVP distension include tension pneumothorax and cardiac tamponade, both of which may embarrass the circulation and precipitate unconsciousness.

Auscultation of the chest may reveal bilateral crepitations with pulmonary oedema from left ventricular failure, bronchopneumonia, chronic bronchitis or aspiration.

Neurological examination

The neurological examination should begin with the GCS score. Patients who are not involved in trauma can be assessed for neck stiffness. This may result from meningitis or subarachnoid haemorrhage. Trauma patients should have the cervical spine assessed for injury before any manipulation is undertaken. The pupils should be examined for size and light reflex. Pinpoint pupils occur with opiate overdoses, small pupils with brainstem lesions and dilated pupils with cocaine or amphetamine use, hypoglycaemia, postictal states and brainstem death. A unilateral fixed and dilated pupil occurs with an oculomotor nerve lesion, which may result from pressure exerted from intracranial haemorrhage or tumour. Fundoscopy should be performed to identify loss of retinal vein pulsation or frank papilloedema indicating raised intracranial pressure. A limited neurological examination can be performed on comatose patients; this will include assessment of tone, reflexes and the Babinski response. Unilateral increased tone, hyperreflexia and up-going plantar response is indicative of a contralateral upper motor neurone lesion, such as a stroke, intracranial haemorrhage or tumour.

GENERAL INVESTIGATIONS

- **FBC**
  The white cell count will be elevated with meningitis. Viral meningitis is associated with lymphocytosis, and neutrophilia is associated with bacterial meningitis.
- **Blood glucose**
  A bedside blood sugar estimation is very useful to exclude hypoglycaemia, which is an easily correctable cause.
- **Urinalysis**
  The urine should be dipped for ketones which will be present in diabetic ketoacidosis. The urine should also be sent for toxicology analysis if poisoning is suspected.
- **U&Es**
  The urea and creatinine is elevated with renal failure. Disorders of sodium levels will be readily identified.
- **LFTs**
  The bilirubin and transaminases are markedly elevated in liver failure.
- **TFTs**
  $\uparrow$ TSH, $\downarrow$ T_4 with hypothyroidism.
- **Toxicology screen**
  For cases of suspected poisoning and overdose, serum levels of salicylates and paracetamol will be helpful in both diagnosis and treatment. Ethanol levels should also be checked, and carboxyhaemoglobin levels if carbon monoxide poisoning is suspected.
- **ECG**
  An ECG is useful to diagnose arrhythmia and myocardial infarction (page 64); either disorder may compromise the circulation.
- **CXR**
  May reveal pulmonary oedema or lobar consolidation due to infection or aspiration.
- **X-ray cervical spine**
  Exclude fracture in traumatic causes of coma.
- **CT**
  With a history of trauma or clinical signs which suggests head injury a CT scan should be requested (this is in preference to a skull X-ray). Additionally, CT will reveal the presence and location of intracranial bleeding and tumours.

SPECIFIC INVESTIGATIONS

- **Lumbar puncture**

  A lumbar puncture is performed in cases of suspected meningitis and the CSF (which may be turbid) is then sent for microscopy and culture.

- **EEG**

  The EEG is indicated when the diagnosis of epilepsy is suspected. Status epilepticus, however, should be diagnosed and treated clinically. The EEG is also useful in the diagnosis of encephalitis.

▶ CONFUSION

Confusion is a behavioural state of reduced mental clarity, coherence, comprehension and reasoning. The causes may be organic or psychiatric (the reader is referred to a textbook of psychiatry for these conditions). The organic causes are listed below.

CAUSES

Toxins/drugs
- Alcohol intoxication/withdrawal
- Drug intoxication

Hypoxia
- Cardiac failure
- Respiratory disorders

Metabolic disorder
- Hyperglycaemia/hypoglycaemia
- Electrolyte imbalance, e.g. sodium, calcium
- Thiamine deficiency
- Vitamin B_{12} deficiency

Systemic disease
- Renal failure
- Liver failure
- Thyroid disorders

Neurological
- Head injuries
- Epilepsy (postictal)
- Stroke/TIA
- Cerebral metastasis

Infection
- Septicaemia
- Meningitis/encephalitis
- Urinary tract infection
- Respiratory tract infections

HISTORY

Onset
Sudden onset of confusion may be precipitated by head injuries, epilepsy, stroke and metabolic disorders. Systemic infection,

systemic disease and cerebral metastasis tend to pursue a more gradual onset.

Past medical history

Diabetes is associated with abnormalities of glucose levels: high levels may result from poor diabetic control; low levels may be due to drug administration error, missing meals or unaccustomed exercise. A history of thyroid disorder is very relevant and confusion can result from both hyper- and hypothyroidism (myxoedema madness). The presence of coexisting carcinoma may precipitate confusion as a result of cerebral metastasis or the development of hypercalcaemia of malignancy. Encephalopathy is a feature of both liver failure and thiamine deficiency. Renal disease can lead to confusion from uraemic encephalopathy or as a result of a variety of electrolyte disorders. Hypoxia may result from cardiac failure and respiratory disease.

Drug history

Both the use and abrupt withdrawal of benzodiazepines, barbiturates, steroids and illicit drugs can result in confusion. A drug history is especially important in the elderly, as many drugs may precipitate confusion.

Associated symptoms

Confusion with associated motor weakness may be due to a stroke or cerebral metastasis. Sensory deficits may result from thiamine and vitamin B_{12} deficiencies. The elderly are particularly susceptible to confusion precipitated by respiratory or urinary tract infections and may complain of pyrexia, cough with purulent sputum, or dysuria, frequency, offensive smelling urine, pyuria and haematuria, respectively. Occasionally, myocardial infarction may present as confusion in the elderly.

EXAMINATION

Temperature

The presence of pyrexia is suggestive of an infective aetiology, and a careful search for a focus is undertaken when performing the systemic examination.

General

The mental state should be assessed and level of consciousness documented by a GCS score. Careful inspection may reveal scalp lacerations, bleeding or haematoma to suggest the presence of head injury. The antecubital forearm veins may have evidence of needle punctures with intravenous drug abuse.

Systemic examination

Examination of the systems is required to identify general features suggestive of cardiac, respiratory, liver, renal and thyroid diseases.

Neurological examination

The cranial nerves are examined and the presence of nystagmus may be due to acute alcohol intoxication, phenytoin toxicity, barbiturate overdose or cerebellar disease from chronic alcohol abuse. When nystagmus is associated with ocular palsies and ataxia it is suggestive of Wernicke–Korsakoff's syndrome, caused by thiamine deficiency. Isolated cranial nerve abnormalities may also result from meningitis. The motor system is examined and unilateral upper motor neurone weakness may be due to stroke or cerebral metastasis. Sensory neuropathy can result from diabetes, renal failure, alcoholism, carcinoma, thiamine and vitamin B_{12} deficiency. With subacute combined degeneration of the cord from vitamin B_{12} deficiency there is predominant involvement of the posterior columns, with loss of vibration, proprioception and light touch. Classically, loss of ankle jerks and an extensor plantar response accompany this.

GENERAL INVESTIGATIONS

- **BM stix**
  ↑ or ↓ glucose.
- **Blood glucose**
  Hypoglycaemia/hyperglycaemia.
- **Oxygen saturation**
  ↓ with cardiac or respiratory disorder.
- **ABGs**
  - Hypercapnia with respiratory disease. Hypoxaemia.
- **Infection screen**
  Sputum, urine and blood cultures.
- **Toxicology screen**
  Plasma and urine for alcohol or specific drug/toxin.
- **FBC**
  Macrocytic anaemia with vitamin B_{12} deficiency. WCC ↑ infection and infarction. Thick blood film if malaria is suspected.
- **U&Es**
  ↓ or ↑ sodium, ↑ urea and creatinine with renal failure.
- **LFTs**
  ↑ bilirubin and transaminases with liver failure.
- **Serum calcium**
  ↓ or ↑.

- **TFTs**
  Hypothyroidism (myxoedema). Hyperthyroidism.
- **B$_{12}$ assay**
  ↓ with subacute combined degeneration of the cord.
- **ECG**
  To screen for silent myocardial infarction.
- **CXR**
  Bronchial or lobar consolidation – pneumonia.

SPECIFIC INVESTIGATIONS

- **CT head**
  Cerebral metastasis. Stroke. Head injuries.
- **EEG**
  Epilepsy.
- **Lumbar puncture**
  Meningitis.

▶ CONSTIPATION

Constipation is a decreased frequency of abnormally firm motions for a particular patient. It must be related to the patient's normal bowel habit. Acute constipation may be due to acute intestinal obstruction, generalised abdominal disease, or sudden alteration in routine, e.g. admission to hospital. Chronic constipation has a variety of causes. Constipation is a common complaint.

CAUSES

Congenital
- Hirschsprung's disease

Acquired

Obstruction
- Colonic carcinoma
- Diverticular disease
- Extrinsic compression, e.g. pregnancy, ovarian tumours

Painful anus
- Fissure-in-ano
- Perianal abscess
- Strangulated haemorrhoids
- Posthaemorrhoidectomy

Adynamic bowel
- Paralytic ileus
- Senility
- Spinal cord injury

Endocrine
- Diabetes (autonomic neuropathy)
- Myxoedema
- Hyperparathyroidism

Drugs
- Codeine phosphate
- Morphine
- Atropine
- Tricyclic antidepressants
- Laxative abuse

Other
- Anxiety/depression
- Irritable bowel syndrome
- Dietary changes
- Starvation
- Generalised disease

HISTORY

Congenital

Hirschsprung's disease usually presents with constipation from birth. Gross abdominal distension may eventually occur. The condition may not be picked up until well into the teens or even early adult life.

Acquired

Obstruction

There may be rapid onset of constipation, although the onset is usually gradual with the patient complaining of colicky abdominal pain, bloating, weight loss, lethargy and occasionally spurious diarrhoea. Constipation may occur from pressure from adjacent organs, e.g. with pregnancy, ovarian cyst or large fibroids. Diverticular disease with or without stricture may cause constipation.

Painful anus

Pain on defecation may cause a patient to become constipated from fear of defecating because of the pain. The most common cause is fissure-in-ano. Other causes of perianal pain include strangulated haemorrhoids (the patient often giving a past history of haemorrhoids) and perianal abscess, or it may occur posthaemorrhoidectomy.

Adynamic bowel

Paralytic ileus may follow abdominal surgery or abdominal inflammatory conditions. It may also arise following spinal fractures or prolonged bedrest, especially in the elderly. The patient's main complaint will be of a distended abdomen.

Endocrine

Check for a history of diabetes. Diabetic autonomic neuropathy may result in constipation. Myxoedema may cause constipation. Check for other symptoms, e.g. intolerance of cold, and hair and skin changes. Any cause of hypercalcaemia, e.g. hyperparathyroidism, may cause constipation. The patient may also complain of nocturia, nausea, vomiting, abdominal pain and mental disturbance associated with this condition.

Drugs

Take a careful drug history. Chronic laxative abuse may make the bowel 'lazy' and result in constipation.

Other

Patients with anxiety or depression may complain of constipation. With depression, the patient may also complain of a change in sleep pattern, waking early and having difficulty getting back to sleep. With irritable bowel syndrome the patient may complain of constipation or diarrhoea, or both alternating. A change in diet may cause constipation. This is either because the patient is deliberately slimming or else they have some other condition that has reduced their food intake. Generalised disease, which affects the appetite, particularly results in constipation.

EXAMINATION

Obstruction

There will be a distended abdomen with obstructive high-pitched tinkling bowel sounds. The rectum will usually be empty on digital rectal examination. With a diverticular stricture there may be tenderness in the left iliac fossa. With malignancy, a mass may be palpable in the abdomen.

Painful anus

Inspection of the anus may reveal a chronic fissure-in-ano, strangulated haemorrhoids or a perianal abscess. With fissure-in-ano digital rectal examination will be extremely painful, if not impossible. Patients who are posthaemorrhoidectomy may become constipated if appropriate medication has not been given.

Adynamic bowel

The abdomen will be distended and this is often painless distension. Bowel sounds will be absent. There may be signs of recent surgery. A full neurological examination should be carried out if the cause of the ileus is not apparent.

Endocrine

With diabetes there will usually be other complications of diabetes. In myxoedema, check carefully for other signs, e.g. coarse and dry hair, large tongue, hoarse voice, slow relaxing reflexes.

For any patient with constipation a digital rectal examination must be carried out. The rectum may be completely empty with obstruction, or contain rock-hard faecal masses with functional constipation.

GENERAL INVESTIGATIONS

- **FBC, ESR**
  Hb ↓ anaemia associated with bowel carcinoma. WCC ↑ diverticulitis. ESR ↑ carcinoma.
- **U&Es**
  Urea ↑ with dehydration with obstructive causes.
- **LFTs**
  Albumin ↓ in starvation.
- **Sigmoidoscopy**
  Tumour – biopsy. Hirschsprung's disease, biopsy – absence of ganglion cells.
- **AXR**
  Obstruction – dilated bowel.

SPECIFIC INVESTIGATIONS

- **Serum calcium**
  Hyperparathyroidism.
- **TFTs**
  T_4 ↓, TSH ↑ in myxoedema.
- **Blood glucose**
  Diabetes – diabetic autonomic neuropathy.
- **Barium enema**
  Tumours. Diverticular disease.
- **Colonoscopy**
  Tumours. Biopsy.
- **US**
  Tumours, ovarian cysts, fibroids, pregnancy.
- **MRI**
  Spinal trauma. Spinal disease.

▶ CONVULSIONS

A convulsion is a series of involuntary violent contractions of voluntary muscles.

CAUSES

Neurological
- Epilepsy
- Febrile convulsions

Traumatic
- Head injuries
- Neurosurgery

Metabolic
- Glucose
- Calcium
- Sodium
- Hypoxia
- Uraemia

Vascular
- Infarction
- Subarachnoid haemorrhage
- Intracranial haemorrhage

Infective
- Meningitis
- Encephalitis
- Cerebral abscess

Neoplastic
- Brain tumours

Toxin/drug-induced
- Alcoholism/withdrawal
- Amphetamines, cocaine, antipsychotics, 'ecstasy'

HISTORY

Event

When evaluating patients with convulsions it is also important to exclude the causes of syncope (page 414). An accurate description from an observer is invaluable for documentation and may help in differentiating the forms of epileptic seizures. A prodrome or aura may be associated with the onset of a seizure.

Precipitating factors

The history should start with precipitating factors, e.g. causes such as trauma, surgery and drug overdose. Preexisting epilepsy may be obvious.

Headache

Convulsions associated with headaches may be due to trauma, subarachnoid haemorrhage, meningitis or raised intracranial pressure from a tumour. Patients with subarachnoid haemorrhage may also complain of sudden onset of blinding headache. The headache associated with meningitis is often accompanied with neck stiffness and photophobia. In the presence of raised intracranial pressure, the headache tends to be worse in the mornings and on coughing or sneezing. It may be associated with nausea or vomiting. For a fuller description, see page 208.

Associated neurology

Preexisting neurological impairment before the onset of convulsions has important implications. A stroke, subarachnoid haemorrhage or intracranial bleed may precipitate neurological impairment preceding a convulsion. Chronic progressive impairment preceding a seizure may be a result of tumour growth. In the postictal period, transient motor weakness may accompany epilepsy (Todd's palsy). Permanent neurological deficit can be induced by cerebral anoxia from prolonged seizures.

Past medical and drug history

Coexisting disease such as diabetes will predispose to abnormalities of serum glucose concentrations. A drug history should be obtained and specific enquiries are undertaken regarding illicit drug use. The amount of alcohol consumption should be documented. In epileptics, failure to achieve seizure control may arise as a result of poor drug compliance.

EXAMINATION

Temperature

The presence of pyrexia usually suggests an infective aetiology, such as meningitis or cerebral abscess. Examination should also be undertaken to look for the primary focus, such as otitis media or mastoiditis. Convulsions may result as a complication of a pyrexia alone.

General examination

A general examination is performed to look for the presence of head injury and also any injuries that may have resulted as a consequence of the convulsion.

Neurological examination

The primary aim of a neurological examination following a convulsion is to determine the presence of residual neurological deficit. The neurological assessment should include mental state and higher cortical function. If an abnormality is detected the location may be determined by clinical examination to allow focused investigation. However, neurological abnormalities present immediately after a seizure may resolve completely.

GENERAL INVESTIGATIONS

- **BM stix**
  Rapid assessment for hypoglycaemia and hyperglycaemia.
- **FBC**
  WCC ↑ meningitis, encephalitis, cerebral abscess.
- **U&Es**
  ↑ or ↓ sodium, ↑ urea and creatinine – renal failure.
- **Serum calcium**
  ↑ or ↓ calcium.
- **Blood glucose**
  ↑ or ↓ glucose.
- **ABGs**
  Hypoxia.
- **CT head**
  Especially in the presence of neurological deficit. Cerebral tumours – alterations in brain density. Skull fractures. Intracranial bleeding – high-density signal during the first 2 weeks. Subarachnoid haemorrhage – high signal (blood) in the subarachnoid space. Strokes – infarction appears normal in the first 24 hours.

SPECIFIC INVESTIGATIONS

- **Toxicology screen**
  Drug use.
- **EEG**
  Epilepsy.
- **Lumbar puncture**
  Meningitis.

COUGH

Cough is a reflex explosive expiration that prevents aspiration and promotes the removal of secretions and foreign particles from the lung.

CAUSES

Acute
- Inhaled foreign body
- Respiratory tract infection

Chronic

Productive
- Chronic obstructive pulmonary disease (mucoid/purulent)
- Bronchiectasis (purulent)
- Pulmonary oedema (pink, frothy)
- Lung cancer (bloodstained)
- Pulmonary embolism (bloodstained)
- TB (bloodstained)

Non-productive
- Asthma
- Postnasal drip
- Gastro-oesophageal reflux
- Drugs (ACE inhibitors)
- Sarcoidosis

HISTORY

Onset and duration
The onset of a cough may be acute, or chronic (usually defined as a cough that has persisted for more than 3 weeks). Sudden onset of an unrelenting bout of violent coughing may be due to an inhaled foreign body. If this is large enough to occlude the airway, coughing abruptly ceases and is supervened by cyanosis and eventually unconsciousness.

Sputum
The frequency, quantity and appearance of expectorated sputum can be very helpful in the differential diagnosis. Cough continuously productive of purulent sputum is suggestive of chronic bronchitis and bronchiectasis. Expectorated bloodstained sputum tends to be

a complaint of patients with bronchogenic carcinoma, pulmonary embolism and TB.

Smoking history

Smoking alone may cause a chronic cough; however, a long smoking history predisposes to bronchogenic carcinoma and chronic bronchitis.

Associated symptoms

Episodic (or even seasonal) wheezing with shortness of breath is common with asthma. This should be differentiated from the monophonic wheeze, which is suggestive of intraluminal obstruction from foreign bodies or tumour.

Most of the respiratory causes of coughing tend to be accompanied by shortness of breath, but sudden onset of dyspnoea may result from aspiration or pulmonary embolism. Shortness of breath that is worse on recumbency is suggestive of pulmonary oedema; however, asthma may also be worse at night. Weight loss can be a prominent feature with lung tumours and TB.

Pleuritic chest pain may be experienced with pulmonary emboli and pneumonia; unrelenting chest pain is more suggestive of bony metastasis from lung cancer. Retrosternal burning chest pain precipitated by posture suggests gastro-oesophageal reflux disease, and the associated cough is due to aspiration of refluxed material. Frequent clearing of the throat due to nasal discharge or a history of allergy with rhinitis may result in postnasal drip and precipitate coughing.

EXAMINATION

Temperature

The presence of pyrexia usually indicates an infective aetiology; the temperature may also be raised with pulmonary embolism.

Inspection and palpation

With COPD the chest may be barrel-shaped. Patients suffering with lung cancer or TB may appear cachectic. Cyanosis is a feature of pulmonary embolism and COPD. The fingers should be inspected for clubbing (page 69), which is associated with bronchial carcinoma and bronchiectasis. The JVP is raised in congestive cardiac failure. The supraclavicular nodes may be palpable with respiratory tract infections, TB and lung cancer.

Auscultation

On auscultation, coarse crepitations are a feature of broncheictasis and pulmonary oedema. Auscultatory features of bronchial carcinoma are non-specific and may manifest as a pleural effusion (dull to percussion, absent breath sounds, decreased vocal resonance) or segmental collapse of the lung. Widespread wheezing is suggestive of asthma, and a fixed inspiratory wheeze may be heard with bronchial luminal obstruction.

GENERAL INVESTIGATIONS

- **Sputum cultures**
  If a productive cough is present, sputum should be sent for cultures. This will include TB-specific cultures and Ziehl–Neelsen staining.
- **Peak flow**
  Bedside determination of peak expiratory flow rate is useful in the diagnosis of asthma (low peak flow).
- **WCC**
  A raised WCC is a non-specific indicator of infection, as it may also be raised with pulmonary embolism.
- **CXR**
  Very useful and may reveal areas of consolidation with infection. Dilated bronchi with persistent areas of infection is suggestive of bronchiectasis. Apical pulmonary consolidation with calcification and hilar lymphadenopathy is characteristic of TB. The presence of pulmonary oedema is appreciated by bilateral patchy shadowing; this may be accompanied by other radiological features of cardiac failure including cardiomegaly, upper lobe diversion of the pulmonary veins, bilateral pleural effusions and Kerley B lines (1–2 cm horizontal lines in the periphery of the lung fields). Bronchial carcinoma may present as a hilar mass, peripheral mass or with collapse and consolidation of the lung due to airway obstruction. Bilateral hilar lymphadenopathy is suggestive of sarcoidosis.
- **Respiratory function tests**
  Formal respiratory function tests can be used to diagnose airway obstruction (asthma, chronic bronchitis and bronchiectasis) and flow volume loops may reveal fixed airway obstruction.

SPECIFIC INVESTIGATIONS

- **V/Q scan**
  Indicated when the diagnosis of pulmonary embolism is suspected.
- **Pulmonary angiography**
  May be indicated in severely ill patients with suspected pulmonary embolism when surgery or thrombolysis is being considered.
- **CT thorax**
  Useful for the diagnosis and staging of lung cancer; it is also specific for the diagnosis of bronchiectasis.
- **pH studies**
  24-hour pH monitoring may be required when a diagnosis of gastro-oesophgeal reflux disease cannot be made on the history alone.

CYANOSIS

Cyanosis is the abnormal blue discoloration of the skin and mucous membranes resulting from the presence of 5 g/dl or more of reduced haemoglobin in the blood. It is not synonymous with hypoxaemia, which may be present (e.g. anaemia) without cyanosis.

CAUSES

Central cyanosis

Decreased oxygen saturation
- Severe respiratory disease
- Pulmonary oedema
- Pulmonary embolism
- Congenital cyanotic heart disease

Abnormal haemoglobin
- Methaemoglobinaemia
- Sulphaemoglobinaemia

Peripheral cyanosis
- All causes of central cyanosis
- Cold exposure
- Acrocyanosis
- Raynaud's phenomenon
- Arterial occlusion
- Venous occlusion

HISTORY

Central cyanosis

Onset
Cyanosis due to congenital heart disease causing anatomical right to left shunts may have been present from birth or the first few years of life. Immediate onset of cyanosis may be due to pulmonary emboli or cardiac failure. Acute onset of cyanosis may be precipitated by pneumonia and asthma. Patients with COPD develop cyanosis over many years. Accompanying polycythaemia may exacerbate cyanosis in these patients.

Chest pain

Cyanosis associated with pleuritic chest pains may be due to pulmonary emboli or pneumonia. Dull, aching chest tightness is experienced by patients who develop cyanosis from pulmonary oedema as a complication of myocardial infarction.

Dyspnoea

Sudden onset of dyspnoea can occur with pulmonary emboli and pulmonary oedema, while conditions such as asthma produce a more gradual onset.

Past medical history and drug history

Any coexisting respiratory disease is significant, as cyanosis can result from any lung disease of sufficient severity. Consumption of drugs such as phenacetin and sulphonamides may precipitate methaemoglobinaemia and sulphaemoglobinaemia, respectively.

Peripheral cyanosis

General history

Acrocyanosis is a condition in which the hands are persistently blue and cold; it is not associated with pain. Raynaud's phenomenon is the episodic three-colour change that occurs, with arterial vasospasm (white), cyanosis (blue) and reactive hyperaemia (red). It may be idiopathic or be associated with connective tissue diseases, trauma and drugs such as beta blockers.

Peripheral cyanosis may also result from acute arterial occlusion and is accompanied by pain and mottling of the skin. Iliofemoral deep venous thrombosis can produce a painful blue leg, termed phlegmasia cerulea dolens.

EXAMINATION

Temperature

Pneumonia and pulmonary emboli may be associated with pyrexia.

Inspection

It is difficult to detect minor degrees of cyanosis. Central cyanosis produces a blue discoloration of the mucous membranes and digits; peripheral cyanosis produces blue discoloration only of the digits. Episodic peripheral cyanosis may be due to Raynaud's disease and this may be associated with small areas of infarction on the fingertips. The presence of clubbing may be due to congenital cyanotic heart disease. Classically, patients with chronic bronchitis appear cyanosed and obese with poorly expanding barrelled chest. The JVP is elevated with congestive cardiac failure.

Respiratory examination

Poor chest expansion occurs with chronic bronchitis and asthma. Unilateral impairment of expansion may occur with lobar pneumonia; in addition, dullness to percussion is experienced over the area of consolidation. Localised crepitation may be auscultated with lobar pneumonia, but is more widespread with bronchopneumonia, pulmonary oedema and chronic bronchitis. Air entry is poor with chronic bronchitis and asthma. Bronchial breathing may be auscultated over an area of consolidation, and additional sounds such as wheezing may be heard with asthma.

GENERAL INVESTIGATIONS

- **Oxygen saturation**
  Saturation is usually below 85% with cyanosis.
- **ABGs**
  $\downarrow Po_2$ all severe lung disease.
- **FBC**
  Hb $\uparrow$ chronic cyanosis. WCC $\uparrow$ pneumonia and pulmonary embolism.
- **ECG**
  Features of myocardial infarction (pages 63–64). Non-specific ST abnormalities with pulmonary emboli.
- **CXR**
  Pneumonia, pulmonary infarct, cardiac failure (pages 63–64).

SPECIFIC INVESTIGATIONS

- **Sputum and blood cultures**
  Pneumonia.
- **V/Q scan or pulmonary angiography**
  Pulmonary embolus.
- **Echocardiography**
  Pulmonary oedema.
- **Hb spectroscopy**
  Methaemoglobinaemia, sulphaemoglobinaemia.
- **Digital subtraction angiography**
  Acute arterial occlusion.
- **Duplex Doppler or venography**
  Acute venous occlusion.

▶ DEAFNESS

Deafness is loss of hearing and may be divided into 'conductive' and 'sensorineural' to facilitate interpretation of clinical examination.

CAUSES

Conductive deafness

Congenital
- Atresia of the meatus

Acquired
- Obstruction
  - Ear wax
- Infection
  - Otitis externa
  - Otitis media
- Trauma
  - Perforation of the tympanic membrane
  - Barotrauma
- Otosclerosis

Sensorineural deafness

Congenital
- Maternal rubella, toxoplasmosis, cytomegalovirus infection

Acquired
- Age-related
- Ménière's disease
- Infection
  - Mumps
  - Herpes zoster
  - Meningitis
- Trauma
  - Noise-induced
  - Head injuries
- Drugs
  - Aminoglycosides, aspirin, frusemide
- Tumour
  - Acoustic neuroma (vestibular schwannoma)
  - Brain tumours

HISTORY

Duration
Childhood deafness may be hereditary, result from maternal rubella infection or arise as a complication of childhood infection (meningitis, toxoplasma or CMV infection). The duration of symptoms may coincide with the introduction of ototoxic drugs.

Onset
Sudden onset of deafness can result from foreign bodies in the external auditory canal. Deafness usually occurs only if the foreign body perforates the tympanic membrane or disrupts the chain of ossicles. Sudden onset of deafness may also result from trauma, vascular catastrophes or Ménière's disease. Gradual development of deafness occurs with otosclerosis and age.

Pain
Deafness associated with ear pain may be a result of otitis externa, otitis media or infection with herpes zoster. Severe pain is experienced with both direct trauma perforating the tympanic membrane and barotrauma, which can result from a slap on the ear or scuba diving.

Precipitating factors
A history of trauma is usually obvious. Sensorineural deafness can result as a complication of mumps or from prolonged exposure to high noise levels.

Associated symptoms
Tinnitus in combination with episodic deafness and vertigo occur with Ménière's disease. When tinnitus occurs with deafness alone, consider otosclerosis, noise exposure, ototoxic drugs and acoustic neuroma.

Drug history
Offending drugs can easily be determined from a drug history.

EXAMINATION

Examination of the ear
On inspection, the vesicles of herpes zoster or presence of otitis externa may be obvious. With otitis externa, the skin appears erythematous with scaling and exudation. Tenderness will be elicited by movement of the pinna or compression of the tragus.

Otoscopic examination will identify ear wax or foreign bodies occluding the external auditory canal. With a patent ear canal, the tympanic membrane may be visualised, traumatic perforations may be seen as a tear of tympanum accompanied with blood. Injection, erythema or frank perforation of the tympanic membrane can result from otitis media.

Assessment of hearing

Crude tests of hearing can be performed with conversational voice, whispered voice or measuring how far away from the ear the ticking of a watch can be heard.

Rinne's test is performed with a 512 Hz tuning fork; mastoid or bone conduction (BC) is compared against air conduction (AC). Air conduction is normally better than bone conduction. Weber's test is performed holding the base of the struck tuning fork against the centre of the forehead. Normally the sound is heard equally in both ears (see table).

Deafness	Rinne's test	Weber's test
Sensorineural	AC > BC	Heard in good ear
Conductive	BC > AC	Heard in deaf ear

General examination

A complete neurological examination is performed. Nystagmus may be present with Ménière's disease; rarely acoustic neuromas may affect the facial nerve, producing unilateral facial paralysis; and motor or sensory deficits can result from brain tumours. Examination should also include the nose and throat, as nasopharyngeal sepsis may be a factor predisposing to middle ear infection.

GENERAL INVESTIGATIONS

- **Pure tone audiometry**
  Allows accurate measurements of hearing levels with bone and air conduction.

SPECIFIC INVESTIGATIONS

- **Speech audiometry**
  Impaired speech discrimination in the 50–80% range occurs with conductive deafness, and 0–50% range with sensorineural causes.
- **Electric response audiometry**
  Assessment of hearing in babies.
- **Impedance tympanometry**
  Increased impedance (reduced compliance) with otitis media with effusion.
- **MRI**
  Acoustic neuroma, brain tumour.

DIARRHOEA

Diarrhoea is an increased frequency of abnormally loose motions for a particular patient. The diagnosis of diarrhoea must be related to the patient's normal bowel habit. Acute diarrhoea in adults is most likely to be due to infection.

CAUSES

Intestinal

Infective enteritis
Non-specific, Bacterial
- *Campylobacter* spp
- *Salmonella* spp
- *Escherichia coli*
- Staphylococci
- *Shigella* spp
- *Vibrio cholerae*
- *Clostridium difficile*
- *Yersinia enterocolitica*

Viral, Fungal, Protozoal
- *Cryptosporidium* spp
- *Giardia lamblia*
- *Entamoeba histolytica*

Inflammatory
- Ulcerative colitis
- Crohn's disease

Malabsorption
- Coeliac disease
- Blind loop syndrome
- Short bowel syndrome
- Radiation

Neoplastic
- Carcinoma
- Villous adenoma

Other intestinal
- Diverticular disease
- Irritable bowel syndrome
- Faecal impaction – spurious diarrhoea

- Ileocolic fistula
- Ischaemic colitis

Gastric
- Postvagotomy

Pancreatic
- Chronic pancreatitis
- Cystic fibrosis
- Carcinoma
- Pancreatic resection

Endocrine
- Thyrotoxicosis
- Carcinoid syndrome
- Zollinger–Ellison syndrome
- Vipoma (rare)
- Medullary thyroid cancer

Drug-induced
- Antibiotics
- Laxatives
- Magnesium-containing antacids
- Cytotoxic agents

Other
- Anxiety
- Diet

HISTORY

Infective enteritis
There is usually colicky abdominal pain and diarrhoea. The diarrhoea may be bloody. Cholera presents with cramping abdominal pain, vomiting and severe diarrhoea, described as 'rice water' stools. There may be fever, rapid dehydration, collapse and death. In infective enteritis check for ingestion of any unusual food or whether anyone else has been affected in the family. Check for a history of foreign travel.

Inflammatory bowel disease
Both Crohn's disease and ulcerative colitis present with frequent diarrhoea with blood, and occasionally mucus and pus, associated with colicky abdominal pain. The patient may be toxic and febrile, with abdominal pain and distension if toxic dilatation of the colon has occurred.

Malabsorption

In addition to diarrhoea there may be offensive stools, which are fatty and float, i.e. steatorrhoea. Has the patient had any previous surgery for resection of the bowel to suggest short bowel syndrome, or any bypass surgery to suggest blind loop syndrome? Is there any history of abdominal radiotherapy?

Neoplastic

Carcinoma may cause diarrhoea associated with colicky abdominal pain and the passage of blood and mucus PR. The diarrhoea may be spurious, liquefied stools only passing through an area of obstruction, with faecal masses behind the obstruction. Loose watery mucus passed frequently may be associated with a villous adenoma, the patient complaining of weakness associated with hypokalaemia due to the passage of excessive mucus rich in potassium.

Other intestinal

Diverticular disease may cause diarrhoea. The condition usually occurs in the older patient. The patient will also complain of associated colicky abdominal pain and pain usually in the left iliac fossa. Irritable bowel syndrome may cause similar symptoms to diverticular disease but occurs in the younger patient. Faecal impaction may result in spurious diarrhoea, while an ileocolic fistula associated with diverticular disease or rectosigmoid carcinoma is also associated with diarrhoea. Ischaemic colitis usually presents in an elderly patient with colicky abdominal pain, diarrhoea and passage of dark-red blood PR.

Gastric

Check for a history of gastric surgery. Destruction of the pylorus or section of the vagus nerve may result in diarrhoea, often associated with dumping.

Pancreatic lesions

These may result in diarrhoea or steatorrhoea. Check for a history of cystic fibrosis. The patient may have chronic pancreatitis, in which case there may be chronic back pain associated with epigastric pain and weight loss. Check for a history of pancreatic surgery. Patients with carcinoma of the pancreas may also present with diarrhoea.

Endocrine disorders

Check for a history of thyroid disease. The patient may prefer cold weather and complain of sweating, anxiety, tremor, and have obvious eye signs. They may also have noticed a goitre. Carcinoid syndrome may present as flushing (especially after alcohol, coffee and certain foods), asthma and loud bowel sounds, i.e. borborygmi. Patients with Zollinger–Ellison syndrome may have a past history of recurrent peptic ulceration, with haematemesis or melaena in addition to diarrhoea. Vipoma is rare but presents with severe watery diarrhoea associated with potassium loss, with weakness due to hypokalaemia. Check if the patient has a goitre, as diarrhoea may be associated with medullary carcinoma of the thyroid. Symptoms and signs of hyperparathyroidism and phaeochromocytoma may also be present (MEN syndrome).

Drugs
Take a careful drug history, especially for recent antibiotics, laxative abuse, the ingestion of magnesium-containing antacids or recent cytotoxic agents.

Other
Anxiety and dietary changes may lead to diarrhoea. A careful history should be taken, particularly looking at any recent changes in diet.

EXAMINATION

Infective enteritis
The patient may be dehydrated or collapsed. Check for tachycardia and hypotension. There may be abdominal tenderness and distension. Digital rectal examination may reveal blood and pus on the examining glove.

Inflammatory bowel disease
There may be little to find except for mild, localised tenderness. In toxic dilatation there will be fever, malaise, abdominal distension, vomiting and localised tenderness. Perforation may occur with peritonitis. An abdominal mass may be palpable with Crohn's disease.

Neoplastic
There may be abdominal distension if obstruction has occurred. There may be a palpable abdominal mass. Digital rectal examination may reveal a carcinoma or a villous adenoma.

Other intestinal
With diverticular disease there may be little to find other than tenderness in the left iliac fossa. The findings are similar in irritable bowel syndrome. With faecal impaction, rock-hard faecal masses

may be palpated in the abdomen and may be felt on digital rectal examination. There may be little to find with an ileocolic fistula. With ischaemic colitis there will be tenderness and guarding in the left side of the abdomen. Rectal examination will reveal dark-red blood.

Gastric

Other than a scar and history of gastric surgery there may be nothing else to find on examination.

Pancreatic

There may be epigastric tenderness or a palpable mass in the epigastrium with pancreatic carcinoma.

Endocrine

With thyrotoxicosis there will be tachycardia, sweating, brisk reflexes, eye signs and a goitre. With carcinoid syndrome there may be hepatomegaly and signs of tricuspid incompetence and pulmonary stenosis. In Zollinger–Ellison syndrome there may be little to find on examination. With vipoma, other than weakness due to hypokalaemia, there may also be little to find on examination. With medullary carcinoma of the thyroid there will be a palpable goitre.

GENERAL INVESTIGATIONS

- **FBC, ESR**
  Hb ↓ bleeding. PCV ↑ dehydration. WCC ↑ infection. ESR ↑ inflammation, tumour.
- **U&Es**
  Urea ↑ dehydration. Potassium ↓ severe diarrhoea, villous adenoma.
- **LFTs**
  Alkaline phosphatase ↑ with liver metastases.
- **Stool culture and microscopy**
  Infective causes. Microscopy for parasites.
- **Sigmoidoscopy**
  Carcinoma, inflammatory bowel disease, villous adenoma, pseudomembranous colitis.
- **Barium enema**
  Tumours, colitis, diverticular disease.
- **Colonoscopy**
  Tumours, colitis (extent and severity), diverticular disease.

SPECIFIC INVESTIGATIONS

- **TFTs**
  T_4 ↑, TSH ↓ in thyrotoxicosis.
- **24-hour urine**
  5HIAA ↑ in carcinoid.
- **US**
  Carcinoid. Liver metastases.
- **Serum gastrin**
  Zollinger–Ellison syndrome.
- **Serum calcitonin**
  Medullary carcinoma of the thyroid.
- **Serum vasoactive intestinal peptide**
  Raised in vipoma.
- **Faecal fats**
  Malabsorption.
- **Duodenal/jejunal biopsy**
  Malabsorption – coeliac disease.
- **Small bowel enema**
  Crohn's disease.

DIZZINESS

Spatial disorientation may be expressed by the patient as dizziness, vertigo or feeling 'light-headed'. True vertigo is not experienced as a sensation of movement but as tilting or sloping of the environment.

CAUSES

Episodic
- Ménière's disease*
- Benign paroxysmal positional vertigo
- Recurrent posterior circulation TIAs
- Arrhythmia
- Postural hypotension
- Migraine
- Anxiety
- Hyperventilation

Constant
- Acute onset
- Labyrinthitis*
- Head injuries*
- Vestibular neuronitis
- Posterior circulation CVA

Gradual onset
- Cerebellopontine angle tumour*
- Ototoxicity – aminoglycosides*
- Multiple sclerosis

HISTORY

General
The causes above are listed according to speed of onset and duration of symptoms. Conditions that are accompanied by additional audiological symptoms, such as tinnitus, are marked with an asterisk.

Precipitating factors
Causes of dizziness that are precipitated by movements of the head include BPPV, labyrinthitis and head injuries. Patients with BPPV complain of short episodes of dizziness accompanying

*Indicates causes accompanied by audiological symptoms.

changes in the position of the head. Labyrinthitis may result either as a complication of systemic viral infection or from extension of a cholesteatoma due to chronic suppurative otitis media. A history of trauma is usually obvious. Postural dizziness precipitated by rising from a lying position may be caused by orthostatic hypotension.

Associated symptoms

Dizziness may be precipitated by arrhythmia and patients may complain of associated palpitations. It may also be experienced with migraine attacks and patients may complain of associated unilateral throbbing headache, nausea, vomiting and photophobia. Ménière's disease is diagnosed with a history of episodic severe vertigo with continuous tinnitus and hearing loss. Patients with vertebrobasilar insufficiency from cervical spondylosis may complain of dizziness with extension of the neck. With posterior circulation TIAs, sudden onset of dizziness is caused by ischaemia of the lateral brainstem or cerebellum. This may be accompanied by syncope, nausea, vomiting, visual field defects and diplopia. Severe progressive vomiting and ataxia may also result from intracerebellar haemorrhage, a neurosurgical emergency. Patients with anxiety disorders may experience attacks of dizziness, tinnitus and tremor, with or without accompanying hyperventilation. Certainly hyperventilation alone is sufficient to precipitate dizziness. Vertigo is a prominent feature of multiple sclerosis when demyelination occurs in the brainstem; this may be accompanied by dysarthria and cranial nerve palsies. Young age would favour the diagnosis of demyelination over ischaemia. Tumours of the cerebellopontine angle tend to present gradually, dizziness may be mild and this may be accompanied by numbness and paralysis to the face due to trigeminal and facial nerve involvement. There are no precipitating factors for vestibular neuronitis, the dizziness is not associated with nausea or tinnitus.

Drug history

Numerous drugs have ototoxic effects; perhaps the most commonly known are aminoglycosides and frusemide.

EXAMINATION

Assessment of nystagmus, hearing and positional testing provide the most amount of information when determining the cause of dizziness.

Multidirectional nystagmus results from diffuse cerebellar

disease, while unidirectional nystagmus occurs either with ipsilateral cerebellar disease (multiple sclerosis, posterior circulation TIA/CVA) or contralateral vestibular disease (Ménière's, labyrinthitis, acoustic neuroma). On lateral gaze, nystagmus of the abducting eye with failure of adduction of the opposite eye is due to internuclear ophthalmoplegia, classically caused by brainstem demyelination.

Hearing is assessed with Rinne's and Weber's tests (page 100). Sensorineural hearing loss may be caused by Ménière's, acoustic neuroma and drug-induced ototoxicity. Hearing loss accompanied by trigeminal and facial nerve palsy may be due to tumour effects at the cerebellopontine angle.

Specific positional tests, such as the Hallpike test, are performed to assess the integrity of the vestibulo-ocular and labyrinthine pathways. Patients with BPPV usually complain of vertigo and exhibit delayed nystagmus that fatigues on repeated testing.

A complete neurological examination is then undertaken. Homonymous hemianopia can result from posterior circulation infarcts and brainstem lesions such as demyelination, and stroke may give rise to combinations of ipsilateral cranial nerve palsies and motor or sensory deficits of the face. In addition, pale optic discs due to optic atrophy may be seen in multiple sclerosis. Patients with cerebellar disease will exhibit an intention tremor when performing the finger–nose test. In addition to a broad-based ataxic gait, they may also exhibit nystagmus, dysdiadochokinesia and dysarthria.

When a cardiovascular cause is suspected, the pulse is assessed for irregularities of rhythm, which may suggest atrial fibrillation. The blood pressure is measured both lying and standing to screen for postural hypotension, and potential sites for emboli, such as the cardiac valves and the carotid vessels, are auscultated for murmurs and bruits, respectively.

GENERAL INVESTIGATIONS

Most causes of dizziness can be diagnosed on history and clinical examination.

- **FBC**
  Hb ↑ predisposes to CVA. WCC ↑ infection.
- **ESR**
  ↑ CVA, malignancy, infection.

SPECIFIC INVESTIGATIONS

- **24-hour ECG**
  To screen for arrhythmia.
- **Audiometry**
  Allows assessment and classification of any accompanying hearing loss.
- **Carotid Dopplers**
  To evaluate patency of the vessel and to screen for the presence of plaque (TIAs).
- **CT head**
  Stroke, cerebellar haemorrhage, evaluation of severe head injuries.
- **MRI**
  Acoustic neuroma and other cerebellopontine angle tumours, demyelination with multiple sclerosis.

DYSPHAGIA

Dysphagia means difficulty in swallowing. It may or may not be associated with pain on swallowing. Dysphagia may be associated with ingestion of solids or liquids, or both. Dysphagia should be distinguished from pain alone on swallowing (odynophagia), which does not interfere with the act of swallowing.

CAUSES

Congenital
- Oesophageal atresia

Acquired

In the lumen
- Food bolus
- Foreign body

In the wall
- Inflammatory stricture
  - Gastro-oesophageal reflux
  - Caustic stricture
  - Candidiasis
- Achalasia
- Carcinoma
- Plummer–Vinson syndrome
- Irradiation
- Scleroderma
- Chagas' disease (rare)

Outside the wall
- Goitre
- Pharyngeal pouch
- Mediastinal tumours
  - Bronchial carcinoma
  - Lymphadenopathy
- Enlarged left atrium (mitral stenosis)
- Thoracic aortic aneurysm
- Paraoesophageal (rolling) hiatus hernia
- Dysphagia lusoria (rare)

Neuromuscular disorders
- Bulbar palsy
- Guillain–Barré syndrome

- CVA
- Motor neurone disease
- Myasthenia gravis

HISTORY

Congenital

Oesophageal atresia

This may be associated with maternal polyhydramnios. The newborn baby will show dribbling of saliva, inability to swallow feeds, production of frothy mucus, choking attacks, cyanotic attacks and chest infections.

Acquired

In the lumen

There may be a history of ingestion of a foreign body. In children this is often a coin. In elderly patients it may be false teeth. Occasionally the history may not be forthcoming. In the case of a food bolus it is unusual for this to cause dysphagia without there being some form of underlying stricture.

In the wall

With a caustic stricture there is usually a history of caustic ingestion, except in the psychiatrically disturbed, where the history may not be apparent. There will be sudden onset of pain and dysphagia, which may improve with appropriate treatment only to recur after several months due to a stricture. Patients with inflammatory stricture due to gastro-oesophageal reflux associated with a hiatus hernia will have a history of retrosternal burning pain and acid reflux which is worse on recumbency or bending down. The dysphagia is usually of gradual onset and the patient may localise the site of dysphagia to the level of the lower end of the sternum. Oesophageal candidiasis may cause dysphagia and this usually occurs in the immunocompromised patient. Achalasia is a disorder where there is degeneration of the oesophageal myenteric plexus resulting in loss of peristaltic contraction in the oesophagus and failure of the lower oesophageal sphincter to relax in response to swallowing. It usually presents between 30 and 50 years of age. The dysphagia may be intermittent and then gets progressively worse. It may be worse for liquids than for solids. Fluid regurgitation at night may result in aspiration pneumonitis. With carcinoma the dysphagia is usually of rapid onset. Initially it is for solids, then for fluids. There may be associated weight loss, anorexia and symptoms of anaemia. There may be a history of achalasia or Barrett's oesophagus. Dysphagia with food sticking at the upper end of the oesophagus in a middle-aged female may suggest Plummer–Vinson syndrome. This is due to a web in the upper oesophagus (postcricoid web). The condition is premalignant. A history of radiotherapy to chest or mediastinum may suggest an irradiation stricture. With scleroderma, the patient may have noticed changes in the skin, around the lips, in the fingers (sclerodactyly) or may have a past history of Raynaud's phenomenon. Chagas' disease is extremely rare and is associated with degeneration of the myenteric plexus associated with trypanosomal infection. The symptoms are identical with those of achalasia.

Outside the wall
The presence of a large goitre will be obvious. With the pharyngeal pouch, patients are usually of middle age or elderly. They may have noticed a swelling, usually in the left posterior triangle of the neck. They may also have dysphagia localised behind the manubrium associated with the pouch pressing on the oesophagus. On lying down there is regurgitation of food with coughing. The patient may also have halitosis. With bronchial carcinoma there may be direct pressure on the oesophagus from the tumour or via mediastinal lymph node secondaries. There may be a history of bronchial carcinoma or the patient may present with haemoptysis. With dysphagia from mediastinal lymphadenopathy, the patient may have noticed enlarged swellings at other sites, e.g. axilla or groin. Dysphagia from pressure of an enlarged left atrium may be associated with mitral stenosis and there may be a past history of this. With a paraoesophageal (rolling) hernia the dysphagia may be intermittent, due to a full stomach pressing on the adjacent oesophagus. Hiccups may occur due to irritation of the diaphragm.

Neuromuscular
There will usually be a history of Guillain–Barré syndrome, poliomyelitis, motor neurone disease, myasthenia gravis or a CVA.

EXAMINATION

With oesophageal atresia an orogastric tube is passed and it will arrest at the site of the obstruction.

In many cases of dysphagia there will be nothing to find on examination. With a goitre there will be an obvious swelling which

moves on swallowing. With pharyngeal pouch there may be
a palpable swelling low down in the posterior triangle of the
neck (usually left), which gurgles on palpation. With carcinoma
there may be signs of weight loss, a palpable liver due to metastases,
or cervical lymphadenopathy due to metastases. With
Plummer–Vinson syndrome check for koilonychia, angular cheilitis
and glossitis. With irradiation stricture there may be changes in the
skin consistent with previous radiotherapy. With scleroderma there
may be calcinosis of the subcutaneous tissue, Raynaud's
phenomenon, sclerodactyly and telangiectasia. With dysphagia due
to an enlarged left atrium in mitral stenosis there may be signs of
mitral stenosis, e.g. peripheral cyanosis, malar flush, left
parasternal heave, tapping apex beat, opening snap and mid-
diastolic murmur best heard at the apex. A variety of neurological
abnormalities will be associated with dysphagia of neuromuscular
origin.

GENERAL INVESTIGATIONS

- **FBC, ESR**
  Hb ↓ associated with carcinoma but may also occur with
  oesophagitis associated with peptic strictures. Anaemia may
  also be associated with Plummer–Vinson syndrome. ESR ↑ in
  malignancy and scleroderma.
- **U&Es**
  Dehydration.
- **LFTs**
  Alkaline phosphatase ↑ in liver secondaries.
- **CXR**
  Foreign body if radio-opaque. Air–fluid level in achalasia.
  Gastric air bubble in chest in paraoesophageal hernia. Hilar
  lymphadenopathy. Bronchial carcinoma. Widened mediastinum
  with aortic aneurysm. Large left atrium (double shadow behind
  the heart) – mitral stenosis.
- **ECG**
  Left atrial hypertrophy.

SPECIFIC INVESTIGATIONS

- **Barium swallow**
  Pharyngeal pouch (never OGD as it may perforate the pouch),
  stricture, achalasia, external compression.

- **OGD**
  Foreign body. Food bolus. Candidiasis. Benign versus malignant stricture. Plummer–Vinson syndrome – postcricoid web. Biopsy – benign lesion versus malignant lesion, absence of myenteric plexus in achalasia.
- **CT**
  Goitre. Mediastinal nodes. Spread of malignancy. Tumour staging. Aortic aneurysm. Dysphagia lusoria (abnormally placed arteries causing external compression).

▶ DYSPNOEA

Dyspnoea is the uncomfortable awareness of breathing.

CAUSES

Sudden (seconds to minutes)
- Pneumothorax
- Pulmonary oedema
- Pulmonary embolism
- Aspiration
- Anaphylaxis
- Anxiety
- Chest trauma

Acute (hours to days)
- Asthma
- Respiratory tract infection
- Lung tumours
- Pleural effusion
- Metabolic acidosis

Chronic (months to years)
- Chronic airflow limitation (COPD)
- Cardiac failure
- Fibrosing alveolitis
- Anaemia
- Arrhythmia
- Valvular heart disease
- Chest wall deformities
- Neuromuscular disorders
- Cystic fibrosis
- Pulmonary hypertension

HISTORY

Many cardiac or respiratory diseases of sufficient severity produce
dyspnoea. When considering chronic respiratory causes you may
relate them anatomically to diseases of the pulmonary vasculature,
airways, interstitium and chest wall. When approaching a patient
with dyspnoea it is important to ensure that the Airway, Breathing
and Circulation (ABC) are attended to before continuing with the
diagnostic process.

Onset

The speed of onset is a useful indicator of the disease process. Classification by speed of onset narrows the differential diagnosis in urgent clinical situations.

Precipitating factors

An obvious precipitating factor may be present, such as trauma causing either fractured ribs or a pneumothorax. Aspiration of a foreign body may be determined from the history; however, aspiration of vomit is more difficult as it usually occurs in patients with decreased consciousness levels or who have lost the gag reflex. Dyspnoea on recumbency is caused by cardiac failure; occasionally patients may complain of waking up at night gasping for breath when they slide down the pillows (paroxysmal nocturnal dyspnoea). Dyspnoea associated with asthma may be seasonal (grass pollen) or perennial (house dust mite faecal proteins), depending on the precipitating allergen. A history of severe allergy should lead to the consideration of anaphylaxis. Stressful events can precipitate asthma attacks but may also cause anxious patients to hyperventilate.

Relieving factors

Dyspnoea resulting from cardiac failure may be relieved by sitting upright, and, when due to asthma, by beta agonists.

Associated factors

Cough productive of (green, yellow, rusty) sputum indicates the presence of a chest infection. This may be the primary cause or it may exacerbate dyspnoea in patients with an existing condition such as asthma, COPD or cardiac failure. Bloodstained sputum may result from a chest infection (especially TB), pulmonary embolism or a tumour. Wheezing may result from asthma or aspiration of a foreign body.

EXAMINATION

Inspection

Cyanosis, which is observed from the fingertips (peripheral) or in the mucous membranes (central), is an indicator of severe underlying disease. Decreased consciousness level may indicate a life-threatening situation. However, it may also be the presenting feature of patients with a metabolic acidosis (diabetic ketoacidosis). Kyphosis severe enough to cause dyspnoea should be evident on general inspection. Patients with COPD may appear barrel-chested and cyanosed or thin and tachypnoeic (with pursed-lip breathing) accompanied by the prominent use of the accessory musculature.

The respiratory rate *per se* may not be very specific, but extremes may be indicators of severity of the underlying disease. The respiratory rate should be carefully counted and not just estimated.

The hands should be inspected for clubbing, as it is associated with bronchial carcinoma and fibrosing alveolitis (page 69).

Pulse

A change in rate or regularity of rhythm may indicate an arrhythmia as a precipitating factor (usually in preexisting heart or lung disease). The rate itself is not, however, very specific to the underlying aetiology.

JVP

Acute elevation of the JVP suggests tension pneumothorax, pulmonary embolism or tricuspid regurgitation (prominent v waves). Chronic elevation results from congestive heart failure or any chronic lung disease with right heart failure (cor pulmonale).

Temperature

An elevated temperature may occur with a chest infection and pulmonary embolism.

Trachea

The trachea deviates away from the side of a tension pneumothorax, pleural effusion and any large mass. It deviates to the side of a collapsed segment which can result with obstruction of the bronchial lumen from tumour or foreign bodies.

Expansion

May be reduced on the side of an area of consolidation (infection), pneumothorax and effusion. It may be reduced bilaterally in patients with COPD.

Percussion

The area overlying consolidation, effusion or collapse is dull to percussion. Hyperresonance is often described on the affected side of a pneumothorax; however, a 'relative dullness' of the unaffected side is the usual initial finding.

Auscultation of the precordium

Auscultation may reveal murmurs associated with valvular heart disease. The presence of a third heart sound is consistent with cardiac failure, and quiet heart sounds may be due to an overexpanded chest from COPD.

Breath sounds

Localised reduction in the intensity of breath sounds occurs over areas with consolidation or collapse of the lung; however, it may be reduced generally with asthma and COPD.

Added sounds

Wheezing may be appreciated in a localised area following intraluminal airway obstruction from inhaled foreign body or tumour. Generalised wheezing usually occurs with asthma. When a history of preexisting asthma is not evident, then consider anaphylaxis. Localised crepitations may be auscultated over areas of pulmonary consolidation. Extensive bilateral crepitations occur with fibrosing alveolitis (fine inspiratory), pulmonary oedema and bronchopneumonia.

GENERAL INVESTIGATIONS

- **FBC**
  Hb ↓ points to anaemia as the primary cause or as an exacerbating factor of underlying disease. Hb ↑ (polycythaemia) may be seen in chronic lung disease. WCC ↑ usually indicates infection, but it can also occur with other conditions, such as pulmonary embolism.
- **Peak expiratory flow rate**
  This simple bedside test allows you to evaluate airflow limitation. A reduced flow rate may indicate asthma or chronic airflow limitation.
- **ECG**
  Arrhythmias are readily appreciated on the ECG; atrial fibrillation or supraventricular tachycardia may precipitate dyspnoea in patients with preexisting heart or lung disease. However, an arrhythmia may be a manifestation of the underlying cause, such as myocardial infarction, pulmonary embolism and hypoxia. ST segment elevations occur with myocardial infarction and are also a non-specific finding in pulmonary embolism. Right bundle-branch block may occur in the presence of long-standing lung disease.
- **Pulse oximetry**
  Although low saturation *per se* is not very discriminatory, acute severe impairment of oxygen saturation is associated with pulmonary embolus and pneumothorax. Postexercise desaturation is helpful if opportunistic pneumonia is suspected.

- **ABGs**
  Useful to quantify severity of the disease and subtype of respiratory failure. Normal levels of oxygenation, however, are not useful to exclude respiratory or cardiac disease. Low levels of bicarbonate indicate metabolic acidosis and should lead to the investigation of the underlying cause, such as diabetic ketoacidosis. An alkalosis (high pH) with low $P\text{CO}_2$ and high $P\text{O}_2$ points to hyperventilation. CO_2 retention may result from chronic lung disease (type II respiratory failure) or may indicate the need for ventilation with coexisting hypoxia in asthmatics.

- **Serum cardiac markers**
  Cardiac troponin or CK-MB is elevated with myocardial infarction in the setting of acute left ventricular failure.

- **CXR**
  Hyperinflation of the lungs (if the hemidiaphragm is below the seventh rib anteriorly or the twelfth rib posteriorly) is a feature of emphysema, and may also result from asthma. Areas of consolidation are seen on a plain film; however, radiographic changes of a chest infection may lag behind in time with the clinical findings. The presence of cardiac failure is appreciated by cardiomegaly, upper lobe diversion of the pulmonary veins, bilateral pleural effusions, Kerley B lines (1–2 cm horizontal lines in the periphery of the lung fields) and patchy pulmonary oedema. A pneumothorax may be diagnosed by identifying the line of the pleura and the absence of lung markings beyond it. Bronchial carcinoma may present as a hilar mass, peripheral opacity or collapse and consolidation of the lung due to airways obstruction.

SPECIFIC INVESTIGATIONS

- **Sputum and blood cultures**
  Should be taken if an infective aetiology (pneumonia, lung abscess) is suspected, preferably before antibiotics are administered.

- **Respiratory function tests**
  Apart from physiological measurements of the lung, spirometry allows classification of restrictive or obstructive lung defects. It can also provide information regarding severity of the disease and the response to inhaled bronchodilators. Flow volume loops can indicate fixed airways obstruction (plateau in the expiration phase), which can result from foreign body or intraluminal tumour. Restrictive pattern of ventilatory impairment is

characterised by a normal FEV1 to FVC ratio and a reduced vital capacity. It is characteristic of pulmonary fibrosis, infiltrative lung disease and restriction of chest wall motion. Obstructive pattern of ventilatory impairment is characterised by a reduced FEV1 to FVC ratio and a normal vital capacity. It is characteristic of asthma, COPD, bronchiectasis and cystic fibrosis.

- **Bronchoscopy**

  Bronchoscopy should be performed if aspiration of a foreign body is suspected, the procedure can be both diagnostic and therapeutic. Intraluminal bronchial carcinomas may be visualised and biopsied. Bronchoscopy also allows collection of specimens for culture in the diagnosis of pneumonia.

- **CT thorax**

  Complete visualisation of the thorax by CT is useful to evaluate masses of unknown aetiology, and for staging of bronchial carcinoma. High-resolution CT is useful for evaluating pulmonary fibrosis.

- **Echocardiography**

  An echocardiogram is indicated if cardiac failure or valvular heart disease is suspected. A large pulmonary embolus can be diagnosed by a finding of right heart failure and elevated pulmonary artery pressures. Elevated pulmonary artery pressures can also be caused by pulmonary hypertension causing dyspnoea. Although a proportion are idiopathic, known causes are congenital heart disease, any severe lung disease and recurrent pulmonary emboli.

- **V/Q scan**

  Majority of pulmonary emboli may be diagnosed by V/Q scanning.

- **Pulmonary angiography**

  Is indicated if the V/Q scan is inconclusive due to preexisting disease, or when urgent interventions such as thrombolysis or thrombectomy are planned.

▶ EAR DISORDERS

Ear disorders are common in general practice. Earache is a frequent complaint. It may represent intrinsic ear disease or it may be due to referred pain from the oral cavity or pharynx. Causes of deafness are dealt with on page 98.

CAUSES

Local

External ear
- Trauma
- Boils
- Inclusion dermoid
- Malignant disease

External auditory meatus
- Otitis externa
- Furuncle
- Malignant disease (rare)

Middle ear
- Acute otitis media
- Chronic otitis media
- Mastoiditis

Referred pain
- Dental problems
- Carcinoma of the posterior third of the tongue
- Pharynx
  - Tonsillitis
  - Pharyngitis
  - Quinsy
  - Foreign body

Neurological
- Herpes zoster
- Glossopharyngeal neuralgia

HISTORY

Local

External ear

Trauma may cause subperichondral haematoma. This is usually caused by a shearing blow. The patient will present with bruising and a swelling. If the swelling is not drained, repeated trauma occurs, and this will lead to the condition of 'cauliflower ear', often seen in rugby players. Avulsion of the ear is rare but may occur in major trauma. Occasionally, cellulitis and swelling of the ear occur due to bites, either animal or human. The patient may complain of a swelling on the lobe of the ear. Enquire whether there has been any recent ear-piercing, as inclusion dermoids may result. Ulcers may arise on the pinna as a result of malignant disease, the most common being squamous cell carcinomas and rodent ulcers.

External auditory meatus

The patient may complain of irritation, discharge, pain and occasionally deafness. Inflammation may spread out on to the pinna. There may be a history of poking the ear with a matchstick or hairgrip to remove wax. It may occur in those who swim frequently at public baths. With a furuncle (boil) in the external auditory meatus, the patient will present with extreme pain and throbbing. The pain is made worse by inserting an auriscope into the meatus. There may be a history of a foreign body inserted into the external auditory meatus. The patient is most commonly a child. Seeds or pips may have been inserted into the ear. In adults it is often matchsticks, cotton-wool buds or paperclips that have been inserted to remove wax from the ear. Occasionally an insect gets into the ear. There is usually pain and discharge. Malignant disease of the external auditory meatus is rare. When advanced, it may cause intractable pain, bloodstained discharge, and may invade the middle ear, facial nerve or the temporomandibular joint. The patient may present with a facial palsy.

Middle ear

Acute otitis media usually occurs in children. There may be a preceding history of common cold, tonsillitis, adenoiditis or infectious disease of childhood. In adults there may be a history of sinusitis, trauma, air flight or temporal bone fracture. The patient presents with severe earache, often with deafness, and appears flushed and ill. Chronic otitis media presents with a history of deafness, discomfort in the ear, tinnitus and occasionally problems with the balance. Acute mastoiditis is a complication of otitis media. It is rare nowadays because of antibiotics. Occasionally children still present with pain, discharge (creamy and profuse) and deafness, with swelling behind the ear.

Referred pain

Check for a history of dental problems. In the elderly there may be carcinoma of the posterior third of the tongue. A classical picture of this used to be the elderly man spitting blood with a piece of cotton wool in his ear. Check for a history of tonsillitis or pharyngitis or difficulty in swallowing due to quinsy. Occasionally a foreign body lodged in the pharynx may be responsible. Other malignant disease of the pharynx may cause referred pain. Check for a history of dysphagia.

Neurological

Herpes zoster of the geniculate ganglion may give rise to lesions of the external auditory meatus, pinna and sometimes the palate. Glossopharyngeal neuralgia presents with very severe pain radiating from throat to tongue and into the ear.

EXAMINATION

Local

External ear

With trauma there may be obvious subperichondral haematomas. Bites will result in cellulitis and swelling of the ear. Inclusion dermoids usually follow ear-piercing and present as lumps in the lobe of the ear adjacent to the area of piercing. Malignant disease will usually present as an ulcer, either with a typical appearance of a rodent ulcer or the everted edges of a squamous cell carcinoma.

External auditory meatus

There is often inflammation at the entry to the meatus. The meatus is tender and there is moist debris, oedema and redness of the meatal wall on examination with an auriscope. A furuncle (boil) is extremely painful. Examination with the auriscope will reveal the tense, tender boil or even pus in the external auditory meatus. A foreign body is usually obvious on examination with the auriscope, as is malignant disease.

Middle ear

With acute otitis media the patient is usually flushed and ill, often with a temperature of 39–40°. Examination of the tympanic membrane shows loss of lustre and disruption of the light reflex.

There is redness, fullness and bulging of the drum. There may be signs of perforation with otorrhoea, with a mucoid, purulent or bloodstained discharge. Chronic otitis media shows fluid in the middle ear (glue ear), with discoloration and often retraction of the tympanic membrane. Tuning-fork test will reveal conductive deafness. In acute mastoiditis the child is usually ill with a high pyrexia. There is tenderness over the mastoid process and postauricular swelling. The tympanic membrane may be red and bulging or perforated with discharge.

Referred pain

Examine for dental problems. Examine the posterior third of the tongue for carcinoma. Inspect the throat with a mirror looking for tonsillitis, pharyngitis, quinsy, foreign body or malignancy.

Neurological

With herpes zoster there will be vesicles in the meatus, on the pinna and sometimes on the palate and fauces. This will have been preceded by severe otalgia. With glossopharyngeal neuralgia there may be a trigger area in the throat in the same way as there is a trigger area that may initiate trigeminal neuralgia.

GENERAL INVESTIGATIONS

The majority of ear disorders can be diagnosed on clinical examination alone.

- **Hb, FBC, ESR**
  Hb ↓ malignant disease. WCC ↑ acute otitis media. Acute mastoiditis. ESR ↑ malignancy and infection.
- **Swab**
  C&S. Otitis externa. Otitis media with discharge. Furuncle. Tonsillitis.
- **Biopsy**
  Malignant disease of the pinna and external auditory meatus. Carcinoma of the posterior third of the tongue.
- **Skull X-ray**
  Opacity and coalescence of the air cells in mastoiditis.
- **CT**
  Malignancy. Mastoiditis.

► EYE DISORDERS

Most eye disorders tend to present as the 'red eye'. It is the single most common ophthalmic complaint encountered by general practitioners.

CAUSES

Eyelids
- Blepharitis
- Stye (hordeolum)
- Meibomian cyst
- Xanthelasma
- Entropion
- Ectropion

Eye

Surface
- Trauma
- Foreign body

Conjunctiva
- Conjunctivitis
  - Bacterial
  - Viral
  - Chlamydial
  - Allergic
  - Subconjunctival haemorrhage

Sclera
- Episcleritis
- Scleritis

Cornea
- Corneal abrasion
- Corneal ulceration (keratitis)
  - Bacterial
  - Viral
  - Fungal

Iris and ciliary body
- Iridocyclitis (uveitis)

Intraocular
- Acute angle-closure glaucoma

HISTORY

Pain

Most disorders of the eye present with pain. Sudden onset of unilateral eye pain and lacrimation may be due to a foreign body. Patients with infective conjunctivitis tend to complain of a soreness rather than true pain. Patients with blepharitis complain of a foreign body sensation or grittiness, whereas patients with allergic conjunctivitis (hayfever, acute allergy or atopy) tend to complain of itching rather than pain. Severe pain is experienced with corneal abrasions, ulcers, angle-closure glaucoma, herpes zoster ophthalmicus, uveitis and scleritis. Patients with the latter two conditions experience exacerbation of pain on palpating the globe. A stye is a suppurative inflammation of an eyelash follicle. It is common and extremely painful. A meibomian cyst is an infection of a meibomian gland which is in the posterior half of the eyelid margin. Following inflammation of a meibomian gland, it may either resolve spontaneously or leave a pea-size swelling known as a chalazion. Entropion is the rolling inwards of the lid margin. The eyelashes irritate the conjunctiva and cornea, causing a painful red eye. The opposite condition is known as ectropion and usually results in a watery eye. Subconjunctival haemorrhages are usually spontaneous and, although they may present with impressive chemosis (soft-tissue swelling), they are not usually painful.

Visual disturbance

Impairment of vision can occur with corneal ulceration, uveitis and acute angle-closure glaucoma. This is usually associated with photophobia. In addition, patients with glaucoma may perceive halos around lights due to corneal oedema.

Discharge

Documenting the presence, amount and colour of any discharge originating from the eye is important. A purulent discharge is associated with bacterial and chlamydial conjunctivitis, and a clear discharge with allergic and viral conjunctivitis.

Past medical history

A history of atopy or hayfever may be present in patients with allergic conjunctivitis. Previous herpes infection on the face may be the only clue with dendritic corneal ulceration. Conjunctivitis, urethritis and arthritis form the triad of Reiter's syndrome caused by *Chlamydia trachomatis* infection. A history of contact lens use is important, as patients may develop sight-threatening infections acutely.

Scleritis is a deeper and more severe inflammatory process compared with episcleritis. It tends to be associated with connective tissue diseases, such as rheumatoid disease and SLE.

Uveitis is associated with inflammatory bowel disease, psoriasis, ankylosing spondylitis and sarcoidosis. Orbital congestion may be seen in patients with thyroid disorders. Xanthelasma are fatty plaques in the skin of the eyelids. Extensive or multiple xanthelasma may indicate abnormalities of cholesterol metabolism, diabetes or arterial disease.

EXAMINATION

Visual acuity should be assessed with correcting spectacles or pinhole, and documented with reference to a Snellen chart. Conditions that present with visual impairment are corneal ulceration, uveitis and glaucoma. Patients with these conditions should be referred to an ophthalmologist. The eyelids should be carefully inspected. Swelling of the upper eyelid with redness may indicate a stye. There may be a bead of pus apparent at the infected hair follicle. The upper eyelid is everted to inspect for a meibomian cyst and foreign bodies. Papillae (conjunctival elevations with a vessel in the centre) are seen with allergic conjunctivitis, and follicles (collections of lymphocytes) may be visible with viral or chlamydial infection. Ectropion and entropion are usually obvious: in the former the lower eyelid is everted and in the latter it is inverted, the eyelashes scratch the conjunctiva and cornea giving rise to a red, watery eye. A similar effect is produced by trichiasis, which is caused by irregular pointing lashes. Xanthelasma are fatty plaques in the skin of the eyelids. They look like masses of yellow opaque fat. They are not painful or tender.

Inspection is then undertaken to identify the presence of any foreign bodies on the surface of the eye. Areas of erythema should be carefully assessed. Diffuse erythema, maximal in the fornices, is a feature of conjunctivitis. Localised areas of segmental erythema may be due to episcleritis, but if it is maximal near the limbus it may be a focal keratitis. Scleritis produces a brawny red discoloration, while a deep crimson–red area is observed with subconjunctival haemorrhage. Marked erythema adjacent to the iris is known as a ciliary flush and occurs with anterior uveitis and glaucoma.

Attention is then focused on to the cornea. Ulceration of the cornea may not be visible without fluorescein staining. Infection may extend to the anterior chamber, and a collection of pus (hypopyon) can present as a white fluid level. Loss of brightness of the cornea occurs with glaucoma due to corneal oedema.

The pupil is examined and the resting position noted. A constricted pupil may result from ciliary spasm with uveitis and it rests in a fixed, semidilated position with glaucoma.

Fluorescein staining should be performed and the eye is then viewed with a blue filtered light: corneal abrasions or ulcerations glow green.

GENERAL INVESTIGATIONS

● **Swab**
  Microscopy and C&S for infective organisms, e.g. stye, bacterial, viral and chlamydial conjunctivitis.
● **Rose bengal staining**
  To assess dead or damaged cells. It is useful in outlining a dendritic ulcer with herpes simplex infection.
● **Blood glucose**
  Infections are often associated with diabetes, as are xanthelasma.

SPECIFIC INVESTIGATIONS

● **Intraocular pressure measurements**
  ↑ glaucoma, uveitis.
● **Corneal scrape**
  For infective lesions.

▶ FACIAL PAIN

Most patients are able to distinguish between pain arising from the cranium, which is termed headache, and that of the face, which is covered here under the heading of facial pain.

CAUSES

Local

Sinus
- Sinusitis
- Carcinoma

Ear
- Otitis media
- Otitis externa

Mastoid
- Mastoiditis

Teeth
- Dental abscess

Skin
- Herpes zoster

Parotid gland
- Mumps
- Parotitis
- Tumour

General
- Trigeminal neuralgia
- Temporal arteritis
- Tumour
  - Nasopharyngeal carcinoma

HISTORY

In the majority, facial pain originates from local structures. Therefore when formulating a differential diagnosis, consider the conditions affecting the anatomical structures of the face.

Site

The site of pain is perhaps the most useful feature when discriminating between the causes. Although local tenderness may direct the clinician to the affected site, do not forget to consider referred pain from adjacent structures. Pain in the region of the ear may be referred from the skin, teeth, tonsils, pharynx, larynx or neck. Tenderness over the maxilla may be due to sinusitis, dental abscess or carcinoma.

Character

Patients with trigeminal neuralgia often describe paroxysms of sharp, severe pains in the distribution of the trigeminal nerve or major divisions. Pains associated with infections of structures such as the teeth, mastoid and ear often have a dull, aching quality.

Precipitating factors

Pain precipitated by food or chewing action may be due to a dental abscess, salivary gland disorder, salivary duct disorder, temporomandibular joint disorder or jaw claudication due to temporal arteritis. Pain arising from most structures is aggravated by touch; however, with trigeminal neuralgia, even the slightest stroking of the skin is sufficient to produce intense pain.

Associated symptoms

Tears may result when the lacrimal duct is obstructed by nasopharyngeal carcinoma. Complaints of otorrhoea and hearing loss should direct the clinician to infections affecting the ear or mastoid. Nasal obstruction and rhinorrhoea occurs with maxillary sinusitis and carcinoma of the maxillary antrum. This may be accompanied by unilateral epistaxis. Swelling of the cheek may be experienced with dental abscesses and maxillary carcinoma. Proximal muscle weakness and pain usually accompany temporal arteritis due to associated polymyalgia rheumatica. Paraesthesia in the distribution of the trigeminal nerve often precedes the rash of herpes zoster.

EXAMINATION

Inspection

A thorough inspection of the face, salivary glands, ear, nose and throat may produce a wealth of information. This involves the use of specific equipment such as the otoscope and nasal speculum. Unilateral erythema and vesicles in the distribution of the trigeminal nerve may be striking with herpes zoster infection but may not be present in the early stages of the disease. Localised areas of erythema or swelling may also correspond to the site of infection, such as the sinus, ear, mastoid and parotid gland. Postauricular swelling and downward displacement of the pinna may be observed with mastoiditis. Maxillary swelling and erythema can be caused by dental abscess or maxillary carcinoma. With otitis media, injection or perforation of the tympanic membrane may be visualised with an otoscope. Nasopharyngeal carcinoma may be seen on direct inspection of the nose and throat. Features of facial paralysis may be seen with infiltration of the facial nerve by tumours of the parotid gland.

Palpation

Gentle stroking of the skin of the face will precipitate severe pains with trigeminal neuralgia. Tenderness may be elicited over the frontal bone with frontal sinusitis, and over the maxilla with maxillary sinusitis. With dental abscesses, pain is elicited over the maxilla or mandible. Mastoid tenderness occurs with mastoiditis or otitis media, and parotid tenderness can result from either mumps or parotitis. Tenderness along the course of the superficial temporal artery is suggestive of temporal arteritis. Movement of the pinna produces pain with otitis externa.

Palpation of the superficial lymph nodes of the neck may reveal lymphadenopathy in the distribution of the lymph drainage of structures affected by infection or carcinoma.

GENERAL INVESTIGATIONS

- **FBC**
  Hb ↓ malignancy. WCC ↑ infection.
- **ESR**
  ↑ malignancy and temporal arteritis.
- **X-rays**
  X-rays of the sinuses show mucosal thickening with air–fluid levels in sinusitis. Occasionally total opacification is seen with sinusitis and mastoiditis on mastoid films. In carcinoma of the sinuses there may be complete opacification of the sinus and destruction of the adjacent bone. CT will reveal the extent of invasion.

SPECIFIC INVESTIGATIONS

- **CT**
  Carcinoma of the sinuses, nasopharyngeal carcinoma, parotid conditions. Extent of tumour and degree of invasion will be apparent.
- **MRI**
  Tumours – extent and invasion.
- Sialography
  Parotid conditions, e.g. duct stones, sialectasis.
- **FNAC**
  Parotid tumours.

▶ FACIAL SWELLINGS

Facial swelling is a common presenting complaint. It may be generalised or localised. Many cases are due to trauma or infection but it may be a sign of systemic disease.

CAUSES

Traumatic
- Facial fractures
- Insect bites

Infective
- Erysipelas
- Dental infection
- Sinusitis
- Parotitis

Neoplastic
- Parotid
- Sinuses
- Jaw
- Mediastinal tumours

Vascular
- Superior vena caval thrombosis
- Cavernous sinus thrombosis

Endocrine
- Cushing's syndrome
- Cretinism
- Acromegaly

Metabolic
- Endocrine
- Renal failure

Drug-induced
- Steroids

Other
- Allergic reactions
- Angioneurotic oedema
- Paget's disease

HISTORY

Traumatic

Usually obvious history of trauma. Swelling may be severe, with bruising and closure of the palpebral fissures. Insect bites may cause swelling due to allergy or infection. The patient may not be aware of an insect bite.

Infective

Erysipelas is an uncommon skin infection caused by streptococci. Pain and redness are apparent usually over the cheek. Pyrexia and malaise may occur. Dental infections are common (see jaw pain and swelling, page 245) and are often initially localised but the side of the face may swell. There is severe associated throbbing pain. Sinusitis presents with constant unilateral pain over the frontal or maxillary sinuses. There is usually puffiness of the skin overlying the sinus. Parotitis presents with pain and swelling over the gland. If this is due to obstruction in the duct, the swelling occurs during eating, when the patient salivates, and regresses afterwards. Bilateral parotitis occurs with mumps.

Neoplastic

Neoplasia may affect the parotids, sinuses and jaw. There is usually localised swelling with carcinoma of the sinuses. The patient complains of a blocked nose and a bloodstained discharge, which may be foul-smelling. With neoplastic lesions of the jaws there is usually deep-seated boring pain in relation to the swelling. Mediastinal tumours compress the superior vena cava and may cause suffusion of the face and facial oedema.

Vascular

Superior vena caval thrombosis may occur. This is rare and there may have been long-term central venous cannulation. There is cyanotic suffusion of the face with facial oedema. Cavernous sinus thrombosis usually presents following a history of infection of the face or in the sinuses. There may be a history of immunosuppression or diabetes. The patient complains of pain in the eye and forehead, with swelling around the eye and a protruding eye. The swelling may eventually involve the whole of the side of the face. Double vision occurs as a result of cranial nerve involvement.

Endocrine

Cushing's syndrome presents with swelling of the face (moon face) with a typical red appearance. Facial swelling is also seen in acromegaly. The patient will usually complain of an increase in shoe size and large hands. There may also be a hoarse voice, protrusion of the jaw and cardiac failure. Cretinism is associated with a puffy swollen face and enlargement and protrusion of the tongue.

Metabolic

Puffiness around the eyelids usually indicates renal failure.

Drugs

History of steroid therapy.

Other

Allergic reactions to drugs, especially antibiotics, or blood transfusions may result in periorbital or facial oedema. Take a careful drug history. Angioneurotic oedema chiefly affects the eyelids and lips. Recurrent attacks of sudden onset of burning and irritation. A family history suggest the diagnosis. Paget's disease often presents with painful enlargement of the skull, femur and clavicles and bowing of the tibia. The patient notices an increase in hat size. The forehead appears enlarged and prominent.

EXAMINATION

Traumatic

Fractures are usually obvious. Check pupillary reaction and test the cranial nerves. Insect-bite puncture wounds may be obvious but often they are not. There is often surrounding cellulitis and oedema.

Infective

Erysipelas presents as a red, tender area with well-demarcated margins raised above the surrounding normal skin. The patient is usually pyrexial. Dental abscesses are usually obvious, with local tenderness and oedema. Sinusitis is largely diagnosed from the history, with localised tenderness and swelling. With parotitis the gland is swollen and tender if infection has occurred, with occasionally redness over the skin. It may be unilateral or bilateral. Examine the orifice of the parotid duct for stone or stenosis.

Neoplastic

Neoplasia of the parotid usually presents as an enlarged, irregular, firm or hard swelling. There may have been a preexisting pleomorphic adenoma. Test the integrity of the facial nerve, which may be affected by carcinoma. Carcinoma of the maxillary sinus may present with swelling over the sinus. Jaw swellings are considered on page 245. Superior vena caval obstruction presents with facial oedema and cyanotic suffusion of the face. Examine the chest.

Vascular

Superior vena caval thrombosis presents in a similar way to obstruction. With cavernous sinus thrombosis there will be oedema, redness and swelling around the orbit, spreading on to the face. Exophthalmos will be present. Test for paresis of cranial nerves III, IV and VI. The patient will usually be pyrexial and ill.

Endocrine

In Cushing's syndrome there will be moon face, and usually other features such as striae, buffalo hump, proximal myopathy. In cretinism there is a broad, flat face, the eyes are wide apart and the tongue protrudes from the mouth. In acromegaly there is a large face with overgrowth of the soft tissues of the face, nose, lips and tongue. The patient will have large hands and a large protuberant jaw (prognathism).

Metabolic

In renal failure the swelling usually occurs around the eyes. There may also be peripheral oedema and hypertension. There is usually a bronze–lemon tinge to the skin in chronic renal failure.

Drugs

Steroid therapy gives an appearance similar to Cushing's syndrome (see above).

Other

In allergic reactions there is often swelling of the eyes, lips and face, with urticaria of other areas on the body. Laryngeal oedema and bronchospasm may occur. Angioneurotic oedema is usually diagnosed from the history. Examination will reveal swellings of the eyelids and lips, with burning and irritation. In Paget's disease there is an enlargement of the skull, with the vault of the skull bulging outwards above the eyes. Deafness may occur. Occasionally there is compression of the cranial nerves. Test the cranial nerves. High output cardiac failure may be present.

GENERAL INVESTIGATIONS

- **FBC, ESR**
  Hb ↓ malignancy. WCC ↑ infection, e.g. sinusitis, cavernous sinus thrombosis. ESR ↑ infection, malignancy.

- **U&Es**
  Urea and creatinine ↑ in renal failure.
- **Skull X-rays**
  Fractures. Sinusitis – opaque sinus. Malignancy – opaque sinus and erosion of bone. Bone tumours. Paget's disease. Pituitary fossa – acromegaly, Cushing's disease.
- **CXR**
  Mediastinal tumour. Primary bronchial carcinoma with inappropriate secretion of ACTH leading to Cushing's syndrome.
- **Swab**
  C&S – infection e.g. erysipelas, insect bites.

SPECIFIC INVESTIGATIONS

- **Hand X-ray**
  Acromegaly.
- **CT**
  Acromegaly. Cushing's disease. Fractures. Mediastinal tumours. Carcinoma of the air sinuses. Parotid tumours. Cavernous sinus thrombosis.
- **Sialography**
  Parotid conditions, e.g. stone in parotid duct.
- **TFTs**
  Cretinism.
- **Plasma cortisol**
  Cushing's syndrome.
- **Glucose tolerance test with growth hormone assay**
  Acromegaly.

FACIAL ULCERS

Most facial ulcers are serious. Malignant facial ulcers are common in patients who work outdoors and are exposed to ultraviolet light. Lesions of the lips have been dealt with elsewhere (page 300) and will not be included.

CAUSES

Traumatic
- Physical
- Chemical
- Irradiation
- Dermatitis artefacta
- Neuropathy – anaesthetic areas after surgery for trigeminal neuralgia
- Bites

Neoplastic
- Basal cell carcinoma (rodent ulcer)
- Squamous cell carcinoma
- Malignant melanoma

Infective
- Herpes simplex
- Herpes zoster
- Keratoacanthoma
- Syphilis (rare)
  - Chancre
  - Gumma
- Leishmaniasis (rare)

Other
- Pyoderma gangrenosum

HISTORY

A history of trauma should be sought. This may be as minor as scratching a spot. Self-inflicted injury resulting in dermatitis artefacta may be suspected when other causes have been excluded. Has the patient had radiotherapy in the past to suggest irradiation causes? Anaesthetic skin is easily traumatised. In the case of the face, anaesthesia may have arisen following surgery to the trigeminal ganglion for trigeminal neuralgia. Syringobulbia is a rare cause of facial anaesthesia. Check for a history of bites, either insect, animal or human, which may become infected and ulcerate.

Malignant ulcers are usually on exposed areas of the face. Check the patient's occupation. Malignancy is more common in outdoor workers exposed to ultraviolet light. Most rodent ulcers occur above a line drawn from the angle of the mouth to the lobe of the ear. Their incidence increases with increasing age. Malignant ulcers are usually painless unless they become infected. They may be pigmented and there may be a history of a change in a preexisting mole to suggest malignant melanoma. These changes include: change in size; change in colour, with deepening pigmentation; bleeding or ulceration; itching; inflammatory 'halo'; satellite nodules; palpable regional lymph nodes.

Infection may be due to herpes simplex, which may spread from around the lips or nose. The patient will complain of an itchy, burning red area on which vesicles form and then crust over and ulcerate. Herpes zoster may arise in the distribution of the trigeminal nerve. Pain precedes malaise and fever by a few days. Vesicles develop later and may ulcerate. Syphilis is rare and may give rise to either a chancre or gumma (see lip lesions, page 300). Leishmaniasis is spread by sandflies and there would be a history of travel to India, Africa, the Middle East or the Mediterranean. There would be a history of bite leaving an itchy papule, leading to an ulcer. Keratoacanthoma may be due to a virus. It resembles a squamous cell carcinoma, from which it needs to be carefully distinguished. It occurs in adults as a rapidly growing lump with a central core filled with keratin. It usually takes 2–3 weeks to grow and often resolves spontaneously over several months. A history of inflammatory bowel disease will suggest pyoderma gangrenosum.

EXAMINATION

Benign ulcers

These usually have a sloping edge. Check the face for normal sensation to pain and temperature.

Malignant ulcers

Basal cell carcinomas (rodent ulcers) usually have a raised, rolled, pearly margin. They may become very large and erode deeply and locally. They do not metastasise and therefore local lymph nodes should not be enlarged unless the lesion becomes infected. Squamous cell carcinoma presents as an ulcerated lesion with an everted edge. Metastasis occurs to local lymph nodes and these may be palpable. Care should be taken to distinguish a squamous cell carcinoma from a keratoacanthoma, which is a benign, fast-growing, self-limiting papule surmounted by a keratin plug (it resembles a small volcano with a crater). Malignant melanomas vary in colour from pinkish-brown to black. They may develop a purplish hue due to a rich blood supply. There may be a brownish-pink 'halo' around the lesion or there may be 'satellite' nodules. The local lymph nodes may be enlarged. Early metastases may occur to the liver and therefore patients should be examined for hepatomegaly.

Infective

The characteristic lesions of herpes simplex will be seen around the lips and nose. In immunosuppressed patients, these lesions may coalesce and become infected. Ophthalmic herpes zoster will be recognised by its characteristic distribution in the ophthalmic division of the trigeminal nerve. It may affect the cornea.
A syphilitic chancre begins as a macule, becoming a painless, hard ulcer, which is very infectious. It develops rapidly and is associated with enlargement of the local lymph nodes. A gumma occurring on the face is uncommon. It appears as a punched out ulcer with a wash-leather base. Cutaneous leishmaniasis (oriental sore) develops at the site of a sandfly bite, commencing as an itchy papule from which the crusts may separate, leaving an ulcer with deep perpendicular edges. Pyoderma gangrenosum presents with a nodule or pustule, which ulcerates with tender, reddish, blue necrotic edges.

GENERAL INVESTIGATIONS

- **FBC, ESR**
  WCC ↑ infected ulcer. ESR ↑ malignancy, syphilis.
- **LFTs**
  Alkaline phosphatase may be raised with liver secondaries, e.g. malignant melanoma.
- **Swab**
  C&S from infected ulcer. Dark-ground illumination microscopy for *Treponema pallidum*.
- **Biopsy**
  Benign versus malignant. Keratoacanthoma versus squamous cell carcinoma. In the case of malignant melanoma, excision biopsy is required.

SPECIFIC INVESTIGATIONS

- **VDRL**
  Syphilis.
- **Aspiration of lesion**
  Leishmaniasis – protozoal organism may be seen by microscopy in aspirates from fluid at the edge of the ulcer.
- **Viral culture**
  Herpes simplex, herpes zoster (rarely needed – diagnosis usually obvious clinically).
- **Antibody titres**
  Herpes simplex, herpes zoster (rarely needed – diagnosis usually obvious clinically).

FAECAL INCONTINENCE

Faecal incontinence implies loss of voluntary control of passage of faeces from the anus. Faecal soiling of the clothes occurs, which is socially embarrassing for the patient. Any disease process that interferes with rectal sensation or affects function of the anorectal musculature may produce incontinence. However, incontinence may still occur with normal sphincters and pelvic floor, for example in severe diarrhoea.

CAUSES

Normal sphincters and pelvic floor
- Severe diarrhoea, e.g. infection, inflammatory bowel disease
- Faecal impaction

Abnormal sphincters and/or pelvic floor

Congenital
- Anorectal anomalies, meningomyelocele

Acquired
Traumatic
- Iatrogenic
  - Internal sphincter surgery, e.g. anal dilatation or sphincterotomy
  - Fistula-in-ano surgery
  - Obstetric – traumatic childbirth
- Pelvic fractures
- Impalement
Neurological
- Spinal injuries
- Spinal tumours
- Peripheral neuropathy
- Stroke
- Dementia
- Multiple sclerosis
Other
- Fistula-in-ano
- Rectal prolapse
- Extensive anorectal carcinoma
- Radiotherapy
- Lymphogranuloma venereum

HISTORY

Is there a history of trauma, e.g. pelvic fractures, impalement injuries? Probably the commonest cause of faecal incontinence is gastroenteritis. The history will be obvious. A history of inflammatory bowel disease may be elicited. Other important factors to elicit in the history are recent anorectal surgery; recent difficult childbirth – long duration of labour, forceps delivery, forceful delivery, perineal tears, episiotomy; predisposition to peripheral neuropathy, e.g. diabetes mellitus, vitamin B_{12} deficiency, alcoholism or medication. A history of constipation may suggest faecal impaction. A history of a recent stroke, dementia or neurological illness will usually be obvious.

EXAMINATION

Soiling of the underwear may be apparent at examination. Digital rectal examination will demonstrate any reduction in anal tone and the inability to sustain a voluntary contraction. It may be possible to feel the defect in the anorectal ring. Faecal impaction may well also be obvious on digital rectal examination. Is there any evidence of trauma or infection? Rectal prolapse may be apparent or descend during straining. Look for evidence of a fistula-in-ano or extensive anorectal cancer. Full neurological examination will often be necessary.

GENERAL INVESTIGATIONS

- **FBC, ESR**
  Macrocytic anaemia may be associated with vitamin B_{12} deficiency (peripheral neuropathy).
- **LFTs**
  Deranged in alcoholism, which may be a cause of peripheral neuropathy.
- **Blood glucose**
  Neuropathy of diabetes mellitus.
- **Sigmoidoscopy**
  Biopsy.
- **Proctoscopy**
  Biopsy.

SPECIFIC INVESTIGATIONS

- **Endoanal US**
  May show defect in anorectal musculature.
- **Anorectal manometry**
  May demonstrate cause of incontinence.
- **EMG**
- **MRI**
  Defects in anorectal musculature. Pelvic malignancy. Spinal tumours.

▶ FINGER LESIONS

Lesions of the fingers are common. The fingers are important tactile organs and hand function may be impaired. Painful finger lesions are dealt with on page 151.

CAUSES

Congenital
- Absent digit
- Extra digit
- Syndactyly (fusion of digits)
- Camptodactyly

Acquired

Traumatic/degenerative
- Implantation dermoid
- Dupuytren's contracture
- Trigger finger
- Mallet finger
- Swan-neck deformity
- Boutonnière deformity
- Heberden's nodes
- Mucous cyst

Metabolic
- Tophaceous gout
- Ectopic calcification (chronic renal failure)

Connective tissue disease
- Calcinosis in CREST syndrome

Neoplastic
- Subungual melanoma
- Enchondroma

HISTORY

Congenital
These lesions will be recognisable at birth. They may be associated with other congenital abnormalities.

Acquired

Traumatic/degenerative

Implantation dermoid   Cysts occur where skin is forcibly implanted into the subcutaneous tissue as a result of injury. There is a likely to be a history of injury, often minor e.g. pinprick. Implantation dermoid used to be common in ladies who sewed – hence the use of protective thimbles. The patient complains of small painful swellings on the finger tips.

Dupuytren's contracture   In the early phases the patient may merely complain of a nodule in the palm near the base of the ring finger. Eventually the patient complains of being unable to extend fully the MCP joint at the ring, and later, the little finger. It affects the patient's grip. Patient complains of difficulty dressing – either poke themselves in the eye while brushing hair or catch finger on trouser pocket. There may be a family history. Check also for a history of epilepsy, cirrhosis or diabetes.

Trigger finger   The patient complains that the finger 'jumps' or 'clicks' as it moves. It may get stuck in the flexed position. There is not usually a history of injury.

Mallet finger   This results from injury to the extensor tendon of the terminal phalanx. There is usually a history of injury. It occurs if the tip of the finger is forcibly flexed during active extension (stubbed) , e.g. catching a cricket ball. The finger adopts a position in which the distal phalanx is flexed.

Swan-neck deformity   The patient complains of deformity of the distal finger.

Boutonnière deformity   This is the opposite of swan-neck deformity. Again, the patient merely complains of a deformity of the distal finger.

Heberden's nodes   The patient complains of swelling close to the distal finger joints, i.e. swelling and deformity of the knuckles. There may be a history of osteoarthritis elsewhere.

Mucous cyst   The patient complains of a swelling over the dorsum of the DIP joint. It may discharge.

Metabolic

Tophaceous gout   There may be a history of gout. Deposits of uric acid occur in joints or soft tissues and the patient complains of swellings on the fingers.

Ectopic calcification The patient complains of hard, whitish, subcutaneous swellings. There may be a history of hyperparathyroidism, hypercalcaemia, or chronic renal failure.

Connective tissue disease

CREST syndrome The patient complains of white deposits in the pulps of the fingers.

Neoplastic

Subungual melanoma This occurs as a pigmented lesion beneath the nail. There is no history of trauma as with a subungual haematoma, which may also appear pigmented when the bruise organises. Unlike subungual haematoma, a melanoma does not grow out with the nail. Eventually the melanoma may lift the nail and ulcerate.

Enchondroma The patient notices a bony, hard, swelling along the finger. It may occur beneath the nail and result in deformity of the nail (subungual exostosis).

EXAMINATION

Congenital

Congenital anomalies of the fingers will be obvious at birth. With camptodactyly there is painless flexion deformity at the PIP joint of the little finger. Check for other associated congenital anomalies.

Acquired

Traumatic/degenerative

Implantation dermoid. Examination reveals small firm spherical swellings in the subcutaneous tissues of the finger tips.

Dupuytren's contracture Examination may reveal only a firm painless nodule in the palmar fascia near the base of the ring finger. Puckering of skin of the palm may be obvious. Eventually the MCP joint and PIP joint become flexed. The DIP joint remains extended. Garrod's knuckle pads on dorsum of PIP joints. Check for signs of diabetes or liver disease. Occasionally the condition is associated with Peyronie's disease of the penis.

Trigger finger The patient may be able to demonstrate how the finger sticks and then snaps out in extension. Thickening of the tendon and the tendon sheath may be felt over the head of the metacarpal bone.

Mallet finger The distal phalanx of the affected finger remains flexed at about 20° when the patient tries to straighten the finger.

Swan-neck deformity There is hyperextension of the PIP joint and flexion of the distal interphalangeal joint.

Boutonnière deformity This is the opposite of swan-neck deformity. Flexion of the PIP joint occurs, with hyperextension of the DIP joint. It develops when the PIP joint pokes through a rupture of the centre of the extensor expansion.

Heberden's nodes These are bony swellings on the dorsal surface of the fingers just distal to the DIP.

Mucous cyst Swelling on the dorsum of the DIP joint. Discharge may be apparent. May be groove in nail due to pressure on nail bed.

Metabolic

Tophaceous gout Swellings, often multi-lobulated, occur on the fingers. They contain toothpaste-like infiltrates of uric acid crystals.

Ectopic calcification Firm to hard, yellow–white deposits of calcium occur in the subcutaneous tissues.

Connective tissue disease

CREST syndrome Small, hard, subcutaenous nodules in the finger pulps and on the dorsal aspects of the fingers.

Neoplastic

Subungal melanoma A subungal melanoma is seen as a brown lesion with an indistinct edge. Occasionally it may be quite extensive and have lifted the nail.

Enchondroma This is a painless, hard swelling on the bone. The surface of it is usually smooth. It may occur under the nail and lift the nail.

GENERAL INVESTIGATIONS

The diagnosis of most of these lesions is made on clinical examination alone.

- **FBC, ESR**
  Hb ↓, ESR ↑ in disseminated malignancy from subungal melanoma.

- **Blood glucose**
  Diabetes (Dupuytren's).
- **LFTs**
  Cirrhosis (Dupuytren's).
- **Serum calcium**
  Hypercalcaemia – ectopic calcification. Hyperparathyroidism.
- **Serum uric acid**
  Gout.
- **Rheumatoid factor**
  Rheumatoid arthritis – swan-neck deformity. Boutonnière deformity.
- **Finger X-ray**
  Heberden's nodes. Enchondroma. Mucous cyst – degenerative/osteoarthritic changes in the DIP joint. Ectopic calcification. Calcinosis. Erosion of phalangeal bone with tophaceous gout.
- **Biopsy**
  Excision biopsy for malignant melanoma.

FINGER PAIN

A painful finger is a common presenting symptom. This may vary from an obvious local lesion to part of a generalised disease, e.g. rheumatoid arthritis. Impairment of the function of even a single finger may grossly impair the overall function of the hand.

CAUSES

Traumatic
- Fractures
- Subungual haematoma

Inflammatory/infective
- Paronychia
- Pulp space infection
- Tendon sheath infection

Neoplastic
- Glomus tumour
- Bone tumour
- Secondary deposits in bone (rare)

Degenerative
- Rheumatoid arthritis

Vascular
- Chilblains
- Small vessel disease
  - Raynaud's phenomenon
  - Buerger's disease
  - Diabetes
  - Emboli

Metabolic
- Gout

Autoimmune
- Scleroderma

Referred pain
- Cervical lesions

HISTORY

Traumatic

There will be a history of trauma, often a crushing injury. Subungual haematoma results from 'trapping' of the nail. It is extremely painful, as a bruise comes up between the nail and the nail bed.

Inflammatory/infective

Paronychia

This presents as a painful, tender spot close to the nail. It throbs and may keep the patient awake. There may be a history of picking the skin around the nail. Pus may exude from the side of the nail.

Pulp space infection

This occurs in the pulp space of the fingertip. There may be a history of penetrating injury, e.g. a prick with a sharp object. There is pain, redness and swelling and the finger throbs.

Tendon sheath infection

There may be a history of a direct puncture wound or there may be a preceding pulp space infection, which has extended into a tendon sheath. The patient presents with a red, tender and painful finger held in slight flexion at the IP and MCP joint.

Neoplastic

Glomus tumour

This is a rare lesion but is very painful. The patient complains of severe pain every time the nail is touched, the most common site being below the nail.

Primary and secondary bone tumours

These are rare in the phalanges. Pain and swelling occurs and there may be a history of a primary tumour, e.g. breast, bronchus, thyroid, kidney or prostate.

Degenerative

Rheumatoid arthritis

Women are more commonly affected than men. The usual symptoms are pain, swelling and stiffness of the fingers. General malaise may occur. The patient may complain of deformities of the fingers.

Vascular

Chilblains

The simplest vascular problem that effects the fingers is chilblains. Women are more affected than men. The patient complains of a swelling on the side or backs of the fingers, which develops rapidly after exposure to cold. The lesion is painful and itches. The lesions are usually multiple and occur most commonly in winter.

Small vessel disease

Ischaemia results in pain, discoloration, ulceration or frank gangrene. The patient may complain of sudden onset of a cold, painful finger, or frank gangrene may be apparent. There may be a history of Raynaud's phenomenon, Buerger's disease, diabetes or scleroderma. There may be cardiac disease, peripheral vascular disease or a cervical rib to suggest embolism. With Raynaud's phenomenon there are often the characteristic changes of sudden onset of pallor induced by exposure to the cold, followed by cyanosis, followed by sudden vasodilatation with a painful, tingling, red digit.

Metabolic

Gout

Gout usually affects the first MTP joint but may affect any joint. The patient will complain of sudden onset of pain, swelling and redness in relation to a joint. There may be a previous history of gout. There may be a family history. An attack may be precipitated by trauma, starvation, infection, diuretics, cytotoxic or immunosuppressive drugs. Gouty tophi may be present.

Autoimmune

Scleroderma

Females are affected more than males. There may be thickening of the fingers. The patient may also complain of Raynaud's phenomenon and splits and ulcers of the fingertips. There may be a change in facial appearance and the patient may complain of dysphagia.

Referred pain

Cervical lesions

The patient may complain of pain or tingling in the fingers. There may be a history of cervical spondylosis or other previous problems with the cervical spine.

EXAMINATION

Traumatic

Deformity, redness and swelling to suggest a fracture will be obvious. 'Trapping' of the nail or a blow to it will cause a collection of blood under the nail. The diagnosis is usually obvious from the history and the patient will be in considerable pain.

Inflammatory/infective

Paronychia
The skin at the base and side of the nail is red, shiny and bulging. A bead of pus may be seen discharging from under the nail.

Pulp space infection
There is swelling and redness over the pulp of the finger. A pus-filled blister may be seen. If the tension is not rapidly relieved it may either discharge into the tendon sheath or may cause pressure necrosis and osteomyelitis of the distal part of the terminal phalanx.

Tendon sheath infection
The finger is acutely painful and held in slight flexion. It is red and swollen and exquisitely tender along the line of the tendon sheath.

Neoplastic

Glomus tumours
These are rare. They are angioneuromyomas. If the tumour occurs under the nail (most common site), there is a small purple–red spot below the nail.

Primary and secondary tumours
These are rare. There is palpable bony swelling, which may or may not be tender.

Degenerative

Rheumatoid arthritis
The finger joints enlarge and become fusiform. Joint deformities occur, with ulnar deviation at the wrist and hyperextension of the proximal interphalangeal joints. There is wasting of muscles of the hand.

Vascular

Chilblains
These usually occur on the dorsum and side of the fingers. The skin over the swelling is reddish–blue. The swellings are oedematous and may burst and ulcerate. There are usually chilblains on the ankles and feet as well as on the fingers.

Small vessel disease
In ischaemic patients there may be pallor, cyanosis or even frank gangrene of a finger. Ischaemic ulcers may be apparent on the

fingertips. The pulp of the fingers may be wasted. Palpate for a cervical rib. Check the pulse for atrial fibrillation (emboli).

Metabolic

Gout

Acute inflammation of a joint occurs, the skin being tense, shiny, hot and red over the joint. The presence of gouty tophi locally or elsewhere, e.g. on the ears, suggests the diagnosis.

Autoimmune

Scleroderma

The skin of the hands has a thickened, white, waxy appearance. The fingers appear swollen with thickened skin, while the pulps of the fingers may be wasted. Small subcutaneous nodules, which are hard, may be palpable. These are due to calcinosis. Look for other signs of scleroderma, e.g. the skin of the face looks tight and shiny and is puckered around the mouth. There may be multiple telangiectasia over the face. Evidence of weight loss due to dysphagia may be present.

Referred pain

Cervical spondylosis

Check sensation in the fingers. Check also the range of neck movements and the reflexes in the upper limbs.

GENERAL INVESTIGATIONS

- **FBC, ESR**
  Hb ↓ anaemia of chronic disease, e.g. rheumatoid arthritis. WCC ↑, e.g. tendon sheath infection. ESR ↑, e.g. rheumatoid arthritis.
- **U&Es**
  Urea and creatinine raised in chronic renal failure, which may be associated with gout or scleroderma.
- **Rheumatoid factor**
  Rheumatoid arthritis.
- **Blood glucose**
  Diabetes.
- **ECG**
  Atrial fibrillation – emboli.
- **Hand X-ray**
  Rheumatoid arthritis. Bone lesions. Pulp space infection – pressure necrosis with osteomyelitis of the distal part of the terminal phalanx.

- **CXR with thoracic inlet**
  Cervical rib – Raynaud's phenomenon, emboli.
- **Cervical spine X-ray**
  Cervical spondylosis with referred pain.

SPECIFIC INVESTIGATIONS

- **Serum uric acid**
  Gout.
- **Autoantibody screen**
  Autoimmune disease.
- **Cold agglutinins**
  Raynaud's disease.
- **Echocardiography**
  Cardiac disease – embolism.
- **Arteriography**
  Arterial lesions. Mural thrombus from aneurysms leading to emboli. Peripheral vascular disease.

FOOT DEFORMITIES

These are not common. The deformity will often be apparent at birth but occasionally does not present until the child starts walking. A deformity of the foot and ankle is normally referred to as 'talipes'. Other terms may qualify the word talipes, e.g. varus (inverted heel), valgus (everted heel) and equinus (foot plantar-flexed). Deformities of the toes are dealt with under toe lesions (page 424).

CAUSES

Talipes equinovarus (congenital clubfoot)

Metatarsus adductus (intoeing)

Pes planus (flatfoot)

Pes cavus (high-arch foot)
- Idiopathic
- Neuropathic
- Spastic dysplegia
- Spina bifida
- Spina bifida occulta
- Poliomyelitis
- Charcot–Marie–Tooth disease (hereditary motor and sensory neuropathy)
- Friedreich's ataxia

Acquired talipes

Upper motor neurone lesion
- Spastic paresis
- Cerebrovascular accident

Lower motor neurone lesion
- Spina bifida
- Poliomyelitis
- Amyotrophic lateral sclerosis
- Cerebellar lesions
- Friedreich's ataxia

Muscular disease
- Muscular dystrophy
- Volkmann's ischaemic contracture

Trauma
- Fractures
- Burns

HISTORY

Talipes equinovarus
Apparent at birth. The child is born with clubfoot. Picked up on routine postnatal examination.

Metatarsus adductus
Common cause of intoeing in children. Only the forefoot is adducted and not the hind foot.

Pes planus
All children are flatfooted and the arches are not fully developed until the age of 10. The parents may notice an abnormality of gait and perhaps rapid and uneven wear and tear of the shoes. Pain is rare.

Pes cavus
There is accentuation of the longitudinal arch of the foot. There may be pain and discomfort. Again, the condition may be noted by the child's parent. There may be no specific cause. Alternatively there may be a history of spina bifida, spina bifida occulta, poliomyelitis, or rarely Friedreich's ataxia, for which there will be a family history, Charcot–Marie–Tooth disease begins at puberty with foot drop and weakness in the legs.

Acquired talipes
There are a variety of causes of upper and lower motor neurone lesions giving rise to acquired talipes. Check for a history of spastic paresis, cerebrovascular accident, spina bifida, poliomyelitis. There may be a family history of Friedreich's ataxia. The patient may be known to have muscular dystrophy. With Volkmann's ischaemic contracture there will be a history of ischaemia of the calf muscles, e.g. from supracondylar fracture of the femur with popliteal artery damage.

Trauma
There will usually be an obvious history of trauma or of burns causing contractures.

EXAMINATION

Talipes equinovarus

This will usually be apparent in the newborn. There is an equinus deformity, i.e. the hindfoot is drawn up with a tight Achilles tendon; varus deformity – the sole faces inwards; and adduction of the forefoot – the inner border of the forefoot is concave and points upwards.

Metatarsus adductus

The hind foot is normal with a normal sized heel. The forefoot is adducted.

Pes planus

The longitudinal arch is flattened and the medial border of the foot rests on the ground.

Pes cavus

The high arch is clearly visible. The toes are clawed due to hyperextension of the MTP joints and flexion of the IP joints. The patient cannot straighten the toes. Callosities usually develop under the metatarsal heads. Check for spina bifida, spina bifida occulta (hairy patch over lumbar spine), poliomyelitis. With Charcot–Marie–Tooth disease there will be foot drop and also atrophy of the peroneal muscles. With Friedreich's ataxia there will be other signs, e.g. ataxia, dysarthria and nystagmus.

Acquired talipes

Check for upper motor neurone and lower motor neurone lesions. Friedreich's ataxia (see above). Volkmann's ischaemic contracture will demonstrate firmness and wasting of the calf muscles together with clawing of the foot.

Trauma

The deformity will depend on the type and severity of trauma. Scarring and contractures of burns will be obvious.

GENERAL INVESTIGATIONS

The diagnosis of nearly all the above conditions is made on history and clinical examination.

- **Foot X-rays**
  May help with assessment.

▶ FOOT PAIN

Pain in the foot is a common presenting complaint. The majority of causes are related to either postural problems or arthritis.

CAUSES

Traumatic
- Fractures
  - March fracture

Infective
- Cellulitis
- Osteomyelitis
- Pyogenic arthritis

Inflammatory
- Rheumatoid arthritis
- Plantar fasciitis
- Reiter's disease
- Osteochondritis of the navicular bone (Köhler's disease)
- Osteochondritis of the metatarsal head (Freiberg's disease)

Vascular
- Ischaemia
- Ulcers

Metabolic
- Gout

Degenerative
- Osteoarthritis
- Flatfoot
- Other foot deformities (page 157)

Other
- Metatarsalgia
- Morton's metatarsalgia
- Plantar warts
- Corns and callosities
- Referred pain, e.g. disc lesions, neuropathies

HISTORY

Traumatic

History of trauma, e.g. heavy object falling on foot, crush injuries. Fatigue or march fractures may occur with prolonged walking, e.g. as in soldiers marching. Severe pain may result. It usually affects the second metatarsal.

Infective

Cellulitis may occur following a puncture wound, e.g. standing on nail, insect bite. The history will usually be apparent. The patient will present with a painful, red, swollen foot. Osteomyelitis is rare but may follow blood-borne infection, e.g. with salmonella, or local infection, especially in diabetics. There will be pain, tenderness, swelling and redness over the affected bone. Pyogenic arthritis is rare but presents with a painful, red, swollen joint.

Inflammatory

The foot is commonly involved in rheumatoid arthritis. Deformities are multiple and severe eventually. There are usually signs of rheumatoid arthritis elsewhere. Plantar fasciitis causes pain under the heel. The patient is often middle-aged. It may also be associated with Reiter's disease. The pain is often worse on standing after a period of rest. Osteochondritis may affect the second metatarsal head (Freiberg's disease) or the navicular bone (Köhler's disease). Pain, tenderness and swelling occur in relation to the particular bone.

Vascular

There may be a history of intermittent claudication progressing to ischaemic rest pain. The patient complains of severe pain in the foot, usually in bed at night, which is relieved by hanging the foot out of bed. The patient may also complain of ulcers and discoloration of the foot. Gangrene may be apparent. Check for a history of smoking, diabetes.

Metabolic

Gout classically affects the first MTP joint but other joints of the foot may be affected. There is acute onset of pain, redness and swelling. There may be a previous history. Attacks may be precipitated by trauma, surgery, infection or drugs, e.g. diuretics. There may also be a history of leukaemia, polycythaemia, and cytotoxic or immunosuppressive therapy.

Degenerative

Osteoarthritis, flatfoot, or other foot deformities (page 157) may cause foot pain. Hallux rigidus, i.e. primary osteoarthritis of the MTP joint of the great toe, causes pain and stiffness.

Other

Metatarsalgia causes pain under the metatarsal heads. It is most common in middle-aged females. Excessive standing triggers the symptoms. Morton's metatarsalgia is caused by a digital neuroma. It most often affects the nerve running between the third and fourth metatarsal heads. It is commonest in women aged 40–50 years. Sharp intermittent pains shoot into the toes, usually occurring only when shoes are worn. Plantar warts are painful. The patient will usually have noticed the wart. They are common in the region of the metatarsal head, great toe and heel. Corns and callosities over pressure points may be painful. They are often associated with deformities of the foot. Referred pain to the foot may occur due to spinal lesions. A history of backache or weakness in the limb may be relevant.

EXAMINATION

Traumatic

Pain, tenderness, swelling, deformity or crepitus will be present with fractures. With march fractures there may be localised tenderness and oedema on the dorsum of the foot.

Infective

Cellulitis, osteomyelitis and pyogenic arthritis will be associated with fever, malaise, and swelling, redness and tenderness of the foot.

Inflammatory

Rheumatoid arthritis may be associated with signs elsewhere, e.g. hands. In the foot there may be pes planus, hallux valgus, clawing of the toes, and subluxation at the MTP joints. With plantar fasciitis there is usually localised tenderness over the undersurface of the os calcis. With Reiter's disease there may be urethritis and conjunctivitis. Freiberg's disease and Köhler's disease present with swelling and tenderness over the relevant bone.

Vascular

Look for signs of ischaemia, e.g. pallor, paraesthesia, loss of pulses, ulcers, gangrene.

Metabolic

With gout there will be swelling, redness, and tenderness of the first MTP joint. Gouty tophi may be present elsewhere.

Degenerative

Osteoarthritis presents with pain and stiffness, e.g. hallux rigidus. Flatfoot and other deformities may be apparent (page 157).

Other

In metatarsalgia there is tenderness under the metatarsal heads. Callosities may be present under the metatarsal heads. In Morton's metatarsalgia, squeezing the forefoot may produce the symptoms. Plantar warts (verruca plantaris) are usually obvious. They present as flat, hyperkeratotic lesions which seem to have been pushed into the skin of the sole of the foot. In contrast to callosities, pressure over them causes pain. If referred pain is suspected, a full neurological examination should be carried out.

GENERAL INVESTIGATIONS

- **FBC, ESR**
  Hb ↓ anaemia of chronic disease, e.g. rheumatoid arthritis. WCC ↑ infection, e.g. cellulitis, osteomyelitis. ESR ↑ rheumatoid arthritis.
- **Blood glucose**
  Diabetes.
- **Foot X-ray**
  Fractures (march fractures may not be apparent until callus forms, therefore the need for repeat X-ray). Osteomyelitis – normal in early stages, osteoporosis, subperiosteal new bone, sequestration. Rheumatoid arthritis. Osteoarthritis. Osteochondritis – dense fragments of bone. Foot deformities.

SPECIFIC INVESTIGATIONS

- **Serum uric acid**
  Gout.
- **Blood culture**
  Osteomyelitis.
- **Bone scan**
  Osteomyelitis.

- **CT**
  Spinal lesions – referred pain.
- **MRI**
  Spinal lesions – referred pain.
- **Duplex Doppler**
  Vascular disease.
- **Arteriography**
  Vascular disease. Site of disease. Small vessel versus large vessel disease.

FOOT ULCERS

Ulcers on the feet are common. The majority of them are of vascular or neuropathic origin.

CAUSES

Vascular

Large vessel disease
- Arteriosclerosis
- Embolism

Small vessel disease
- Diabetes
- Buerger's disease
- Raynaud's disease
- Embolism
- Vasculitis, e.g. SLE, rheumatoid arthritis, scleroderma

Neuropathic

Peripheral nerve lesions
- Diabetes
- Peripheral nerve injuries
- Leprosy
- Alcoholism

Spinal cord lesions
- Spina bifida
- Tabes dorsalis
- Syringomyelia

Neoplastic
- Squamous cell carcinoma
- Malignant melanoma

Traumatic
- Ill-fitting footwear

Infective
- Madura foot (rare)

HISTORY

Vascular

Ischaemic ulcers are common in the elderly. They are painful and do not bleed much. They show no signs of healing. There is often a history of intermittent claudication and rest pain. Check for a history of diabetes. In the younger patient, diabetes, Buerger's disease or Raynaud's disease may be responsible. Check for a history of cardiac disease, which may suggest embolism leading to ischaemic ulceration. Proximal arterial disease, e.g. aneurysm, may also cause emboli.

Neuropathic

These are painless ulcers occurring over pressure points. Patients may give a history of neuropathy. They may describe a feeling as though they are walking on cotton wool. Check for a history of diabetes and peripheral nerve lesions. Spinal cord lesions may also be present. In diabetes, ulceration may be associated with both ischaemia and neuropathy.

Neoplastic

Malignant ulcers may occur on the foot. Squamous cell carcinoma is rare but malignant melanoma is not infrequent, especially on the sole of the foot. The patient may have noticed the pigmented lesion, which has changed, with bleeding, itching and ulceration. The patient may also have noticed a lump in the groin, suggesting lymph node secondaries.

Traumatic

Foot ulcers may be caused by minor trauma, e.g. ill-fitting shoes. However, there is usually a history of an underlying predisposing condition, e.g. poor circulation, steroid therapy, neuropathy.

Infective

Pure infective ulcers on the foot are rare. Infections may occur with *Nocardia* species in tropical countries causing Madura foot. Check for a history of foreign travel.

EXAMINATION

Vascular

Ischaemic ulcers are found on the tips of the toes and over the pressure areas. The edge is usually punched out and healing does not occur. The base may contain slough or dead tissue.

Occasionally tendons are seen in the base of the ulcer. Pulses may be absent. Check for atrial fibrillation, which may be associated with embolism as a cause of ischaemic ulceration.

Neuropathic

Neuropathic ulcers are deep, penetrating ulcers. They occur over pressure areas but the surrounding tissues are healthy and have good circulation. The ulcers themselves are painless. Examine the surrounding tissues for blunting of sensation, e.g. absence of pinprick sensation. Pulses are usually present. Carry out a full neurological examination looking for peripheral nerve injuries or evidence of spinal cord lesions.

Neoplastic

Squamous cell carcinomas have an everted edge, often with necrotic material in the base of the ulcer. The edge of the ulcer is hard. Check for inguinal lymphadenopathy. Ulcers associated with malignant melanoma tend to vary from brown to black, although they may be amelanotic. Bleeding and infection may make the surface of the tumour appear wet, soft and boggy. Check for inguinal lymphadenopathy and hepatomegaly.

Traumatic

Traumatic ulcers tend to occur either at pressure points, due to ill-fitting footwear, or at a site of injury. They usually have sloping edges and granulation tissue developing in the base. Always check the circulation, as most traumatic foot ulcers readily heal unless there is an abnormality of the circulation.

Infective

Infective ulcers by themselves are rare. Secondary infection may occur on any type of ulcer. With Madura foot there may be ulceration and bone destruction with little systemic illness.

GENERAL INVESTIGATIONS

- **FBC, ESR**
  Hb ↓ malignant disease. WCC ↑ infection. ESR ↑ malignancy.
- **Blood glucose**
  Diabetes.
- **Swab**
  Microscopy – fungal infection. C&S.

SPECIFIC INVESTIGATIONS

- **Antibody screen**
  Connective tissue disease.
- **Doppler studies**
  Ischaemic ulceration.
- **Arteriography**
  Ischaemic ulceration. Large versus small vessel disease.
- **Nerve conduction studies**
  Neuropathic ulcers.
- **CT**
  Spinal cord lesions.
- **MRI**
  Spinal cord lesions.
- **Biopsy**
  Benign versus malignant.

GAIT ABNORMALITIES

Disorders of gait may be structural or neurological. When assessing gait, it is important to observe the whole patient and not merely the feet.

CAUSES

Structural

- Pain – antalgic gait
- Length discrepancies – short leg gait
- Weak hip abductors – Trendelenburg or waddling gait
- Femoral anteversion – intoe gait

Neurological

- Stroke – hemiplegic gait
- Parkinsons disease – festinant gait
- Peripheral neuropathy – sensory ataxia
- Cerebellar disease – cerebellar ataxia
- Peroneal nerve palsy – foot drop gait
- Frontal lobe lesions – apraxic gait
- Cerebral palsy – scissoring gait

HISTORY

Duration

An abnormality of gait that has been present since birth is usually due to a structural cause or cerebral palsy. Discrepancies of length may originate from disorders affecting joint articulation, bone length or from soft tissue contractures surrounding the joints. Most of the neurological causes of gait abnormalities result from acquired lesions of the central or peripheral nervous systems.

Associated symptoms

Pain is the underlying cause for the antalgic gait and patients will be able to direct you to the site of origin of the pain. Loss of motor function such as paralysis of dorsiflexion of the foot causes the foot drop gait, more extensive paralysis of the arm and leg with the hemiplegic gait may occur with stroke. Paraesthesia, sensory loss or impairment of joint position sense is suggestive of peripheral neuropathy. Patients with sensory apraxia suffer from proprioceptive impairment and have great difficulties walking in the dark when visual cues are lost. A concomitant resting tremor is associated with Parkinson's disease and an intention tremor results from cerebellar disease.

Past medical and drug history

A previous history of trauma to the lower limb is very significant, fractures of the long bones predispose to length abnormalities on healing. Fractures of the fibular neck may disrupt the common peroneal nerve causing foot drop. Frontal lobe contusions may result from severe head injuries. Diabetes, carcinoma and vitamin B deficiencies are associated with peripheral neuropathies. Alcoholism, multiple sclerosis and drugs such as phenytoin are associated with cerebellar impairment. Direct questioning should be undertaken for previous strokes and Parkinson's disease.

EXAMINATION

The clinical examination is divided into three sections. The initial examination of a gait disorder is to determine a structural or neurological cause. If a structural lesion is suspected then it is followed by an orthopaedic examination. Conversely a neurological examination is performed if a neurological lesion is suspected. Once the disorder of gait is defined, the clinical examination should then be tailored to determine the underlying cause.

The asymmetrical gait

The gait is first assessed for symmetry. Apart from the hemiplegic gait, the remaining unilateral gait disorders are structural. The normal gait consists of several phases; there are the swing, heel strike, stance and toe-off phases. The antalgic gait or painful limp is characterised by a decrease in time spent in the stance phase. The Trendelenburg gait is characterised by a downward tilt of the pelvis when the leg is lifted forwards. It may be caused by a painful hip disorder, weakness of the contralateral hip abductors, shortening of the femoral neck or subluxation of the hip joint. With a hemiplegic gait, the leg swings in an outward arc and then back to the midline. A foot drop gait often results in the knee being lifted higher on the affected side.

The symmetrical gait

When analysing the symmetrical gait observe movement of the whole patient. The stooped posture with small shuffling steps and reduced arm swing is characteristic of Parkinson's disease. Patients with apraxia have disjointed movements akin to 'walking on ice', the aetiology is frontal lobe disorder most commonly due to cortical degeneration. Attention is then brought to the movement of the legs, scissoring of the gait due to crossing of the midline when lifting the leg forwards is associated with cerebral palsy. The movements of the feet are then noted, lifting of the knees with slapping of the foot as it contacts with the ground is descriptive of the foot drop gait. The foot is rotated inwards with femoral anteversion. The base of the gait is then analysed, a broad-based gait is characteristic of cerebellar disease and sensory ataxia. With cerebellar disease, patients are unsteady standing with their eyes open, whilst with sensory ataxia the patient is able to stand with their eyes open but not shut (positive Romberg's test).

Orthopaedic examination

An examination of the hip, knee and ankle is required. Measurements are undertaken to determine real and apparent length of the lower limbs. The real length is the distance between the anterior superior iliac spine and the medial malleolus, and the apparent length is the distance between the xiphisternum and the medial malleolus. Any discrepancies will require individual measurements of the femur and tibia to determine the site of shortening. Thomas' test is performed to identify the presence of fixed flexion deformities of the hip that can give rise to apparent shortening. The resting position of both feet can be inspected and internal rotation due to femoral anteversion may be apparent.

Neurological examination

The mask-like facies and resting pill-rolling tremor of Parkinson's disease may be apparent on inspection and examination of the limbs will reveal cog wheel or lead pipe rigidity. Patients with cerebellar disease will exhibit an intention tremor when performing the finger–nose test; in addition to their broad-based ataxic gait they may also exhibit nystagmus, dysdiadochokinesia and dysarthria. With frontal lobe disorders primitive reflexes such as the grasping (the hand of the examiner is grasped when placed or stroked along the patients palm), sucking (sucking action is produced on stroking on side of the mouth) and palmomental reflexes (gentle stroke of the thenar eminence produces dimpling of the chin) are released. Examination of the sensory system may reveal loss of light touch, vibration and proprioception in a glove and stocking distribution with peripheral neuropathy. Unilateral upper motor neuron weakness, hyperreflexia and clasp knife rigidity are features of cortical strokes.

Specific examination

Once the diagnosis of a gait disorder is made, a specific examination is now undertaken to determine the underlying aetiology. For example, with apraxic gait due to frontal lobe disorder a mental state examination is performed to screen for dementia, and fundoscopy is performed to screen for pallioedema, which may be indicative of raised intracranial pressure from a brain tumour.

GENERAL INVESTIGATIONS

The diagnosis of the majority of gait abnormalities is made on clinical history and examination.

SPECIFIC INVESTIGATIONS

- **Local X-rays**
  Structural causes.
- **Nerve conduction studies.**
  Peripheral neuropathy. Peroneal nerve palsy.
- **CT/MRI scans**
  CNS causes e.g. stroke, space-occupying lesions.

GOITRE

A goitre is an enlargement of the thyroid gland. Causes of goitre range from the physiological, when the gland increases in size as a result of increased demand for thyroid hormone, e.g. at puberty, to frank malignant disease, which needs urgent diagnosis and treatment. It is therefore important to be able to distinguish the causes of goitre that require no treatment from those that require urgent thyroidectomy.

CAUSES

Simple (non-toxic) goitre
- Simple hyperplastic goitre
- Multinodular goitre

Toxic goitre
- Diffuse goitre (Graves' disease)
- Toxic nodule
- Toxic multinodular goitre

Neoplastic goitre

Benign
- Adenoma

Malignant
- Papillary
- Follicular
- Anaplastic
- Medullary
- Lymphoma (rare)

Inflammatory
- de Quervain's thyroiditis
- Riedel's thyroiditis

Autoimmune
- Hashimoto's thyroiditis

HISTORY

Simple hyperplastic goitre
The patient presents with a swelling in the neck. Physiological causes include puberty and pregnancy. Iodine deficiency is the

most common cause but is rare in the UK, where iodide is added to table salt.

Multinodular goitre

This is the commonest cause of goitre in the UK. It is more common in women. The usual presentation is a lump in the neck which moves on swallowing, but with a very large gland the patient may complain of dyspnoea or dysphagia.

Toxic goitre

The patient presents with a lump in the neck. He or she may indicate a preference for cold weather, and may also complain of excessive sweating, tiredness, anxiety, increased appetite, weight loss, diarrhoea, palpitations and tremor.

Neoplastic goitre

The patient may present with diffuse enlargement of the thyroid or may have noticed a well-defined swelling in the area of the thyroid gland. Papillary carcinoma occurs in the younger patient (under 35 years) and, in addition to the goitre, the patient may have noticed lymph node swelling in the neck. Follicular carcinoma occurs in middle age (40–60 years). The patient may also complain of bone pain due to metastases. Anaplastic carcinoma occurs in the elderly. Anaplastic carcinoma may present with stridor, dyspnoea and hoarseness. There may be gross lymph node involvement. Medullary carcinoma can present at any age. Check for a family history of medullary carcinoma and symptoms related to phaeochromocytoma and hyperparathyroidism (associated MEN syndrome). Lymphoma of the thyroid is rare and may develop in preexisting autoimmune (Hashimoto's) thyroiditis.

Inflammatory (rare)

The patient may present with a painful swelling of the thyroid associated with malaise or myalgia (de Quervain's thyroiditis). A hard mass associated with dysphagia or dyspnoea may suggest Riedel's thyroiditis.

Autoimmune

Hashimoto's disease presents with a firm goitre. It needs to be distinguished from lymphoma. Eventually the patient becomes hypothyroid, and will complain of intolerance to cold weather, tiredness, a change in voice (hoarseness), weight gain, constipation, and dry skin and dry hair.

EXAMINATION

Simple hyperplastic goitre
The patient is usually euthyroid. The goitre is usually smooth.

Multinodular goitre
The gland is usually smoothly nodular. Occasionally only one nodule may be felt, and is the dominant nodule in a multinodular goitre. Check for tracheal deviation when the gland is large. Percuss for retrosternal extension.

Toxic goitre
Palpation of the gland may reveal a diffuse goitre, a multinodular goitre or a solitary nodule. Check for exophthalmos, lid lag, lid retraction, warm moist palms and tremor. Check for atrial fibrillation. Examine for pretibial myxoedema. Reflexes are brisk. The goitre may have a palpable thrill or a bruit may be heard on auscultation.

Neoplastic goitre
There may be a solitary thyroid nodule (papillary carcinoma) or a more diffuse mass (follicular carcinoma). Anaplastic carcinoma is hard and irregular and invades locally. Check for tracheal deviation. Cervical lymphadenopathy may be present with a papillary carcinoma, when the glands are usually mobile and discrete, and is invariably associated with anaplastic carcinoma, where the glands may be hard and matted. Check for recurrent laryngeal nerve palsy – has the patient got a hoarse voice or is unable to produce an occlusive cough?

Inflammatory
Subacute thyroiditis (rare). There will be a painful, swollen gland. In Riedel's thyroiditis there is a woody, hard goitre, which infiltrates into adjacent muscle. It must be carefully differentiated from anaplastic carcinoma.

Autoimmune
Hashimoto's disease presents with a diffusely enlarged, firm gland. Eventually there may be signs of hypothyroidism. These signs include a pale, waxy skin, periorbital oedema, dry thickened skin and hair, slow pulse, large tongue, peripheral oedema and slow relaxing reflexes. Carpal tunnel syndrome may be present.

GENERAL INVESTIGATIONS

- **FBC, ESR**
  Hb ↓ in disseminated malignancy. ESR ↑ in thyroiditis.
- **TFTs**
  T_4 ↑, TSH ↓ in toxic goitre. T_4 ↓, TSH ↑ in hypothyroidism.
- **Thyroid antibodies**
  Thyroid antibodies will be demonstrated in Hashimoto's disease.
- **CXR**
  Secondary deposits in thyroid carcinoma (follicular, anaplastic).
- **Thoracic inlet X-ray**
  Tracheal compression.
- **US**
  Cystic versus solid. Position of gland.
- **CT scan**
  Position of gland. Compression/invasion of local structures.
- **Radioisotope scan**
  Hot versus cold nodule. Cold nodules may be malignant.
- **FNAC**
  Benign versus malignant.
- **Laryngoscopy**
  Involvement of recurrent laryngeal nerve.

SPECIFIC INVESTIGATIONS

- **Serum calcitonin**
  Calcitonin ↑ in medullary carcinoma.
- **PTH**
  Raised in MEN syndrome.

GROIN SWELLINGS

These are common clinical problems, especially hernias. They are
therefore common in clinical examinations.

CAUSES

Above the inguinal ligament
- Sebaceous cyst
- Lipoma
- Direct inguinal hernia
- Indirect inguinal hernia
- Imperfectly descended testis
- Lipoma of the cord
- Hydrocele of the cord (rare)
- Hydrocele of the canal of Nuck (rare)

Below the inguinal ligament
- Sebaceous cyst
- Lipoma
- Femoral hernia
- Lymph nodes
- Saphena varix
- Femoral artery aneurysm (true or false)
- Imperfectly descended testis
- Neuroma of the femoral nerves (rare)
- Synovioma of the hip joint (rare)
- Obturator hernia (rare)
- Psoas abscess (rare)

HISTORY

Sebaceous cyst
The patient will complain of a mobile lump on the skin. It may be
red and inflamed and discharging.

Lipoma
The patient will present with a soft, painless swelling.

Hernias
A patient with a groin hernia will present with a lump that
disappears on recumbency or may be pushed back (reducible). The
patient may present with a tense, tender lump that will not reduce

and is accompanied by signs and symptoms of intestinal obstruction. Femoral hernia is more common in females. With hernias there is occasionally a history of sudden straining or trauma, following which a lump may become manifest.

Imperfectly descended testis
An imperfectly descended testis may present as a groin swelling. The patient, or, if a child, the mother, will have noticed absence of a testis from the scrotum. Enlargement and pain may indicate malignant change which is more common in an imperfectly descended testis.

Lipoma of the cord
The patient will have noticed a soft swelling in the groin. This is often mistaken for a hernia.

Hydrocele of the cord
This may present as a lump in the inguinal region which does not reduce.

Hydrocele of the canal of Nuck
This is similar to a hydrocele of the spermatic cord but presents in the female. It represents a cyst forming in the processus vaginalis.

Lymph nodes
Lymph nodes may present as swellings below the inguinal ligament. They may be discrete and firm; tender and red; or matted to form a mass. The patient may have noticed a lesion on the leg. Care must be taken to elicit a full history with inguinal lymphadenopathy, as the nodes drain not only the tissues of the leg but also the penis, the scrotal skin, the lower half of the anal canal, the skin of the buttock, and the skin of the lower abdominal wall up to and including the umbilicus. In the female they drain the labia, the lower third of the vagina, and the fundus of the uterus via lymphatics accompanying the round ligament down the inguinal canal. A careful history should therefore be taken of any anorectal disease, e.g. bleeding PR, or gynaecological disease, e.g. bleeding PV to suggest a carcinoma of the uterus.

Saphena varix
A saphena varix is normally associated with varicose veins lower down the leg. The patient will present having noticed a small, soft, bluish mass in the lower part of the groin.

Femoral artery aneurysm
A pulsatile expansile mass suggests a femoral aneurysm. Check for a history of arterial surgery at the groin or arteriography via the

femoral artery, which may suggest the presence of a false aneurysm.

Imperfectly descended testis

An imperfectly descended testis may descend into the upper thigh but its descent is arrested by the attachment of Scarpa's fascia to the deep fascia of the thigh.

Neuroma of the femoral nerve

This is rare and may be associated with anaesthesia or paraesthesia on the anterior aspect of the thigh and inability to extend the knee.

Synovioma of the hip joint

This is rare. The patient complains of a lump deep in the groin which may interfere with hip movement.

Obturator hernia

This is rare. The sac passes through the obturator canal and may present in the groin deep to pectineus. A lump is rarely palpable due to the overlying pectineus. The diagnosis is not usually made until obstruction or strangulation occurs.

EXAMINATION

Sebaceous cyst

This is attached to the skin and a punctum is usually seen at the point of attachment. Sebaceous cysts are firm, spherical and mobile on the underlying tissue. They may be hot, red and tender when inflamed.

Lipoma

The lump will be soft, lobulated, mobile, being fixed neither to the skin nor the underlying tissue. They may be distinguished from hernias in that they are not reducible and do not have a cough impulse.

Hernias

A hernia may be reduced and has an expansile cough impulse. They may be irreducible. Irreducible hernias may be (1) incarcerated – imprisoned in the sac because of adhesions between contents and the wall of the sac; (2) obstructed – small bowel is caught in the sac and intestinal contents cannot pass on; (3) strangulated – the arterial blood supply is cut off and gangrene of the contents ensues. In the last case the lump would be tender, the overlying skin may be red and the patient will be pyrexial with a tachycardia. There will be signs of intestinal obstruction.

It is important to distinguish between an inguinal and a femoral hernia. An inguinal hernia lies above and medial to the pubic tubercle, a femoral hernia below and lateral. An inguinal hernia may be either direct or indirect. An indirect hernia comes down the inguinal canal from the deep inguinal ring. A direct hernia comes through the posterior wall of the canal through Hesselbach's triangle (base – inguinal ligament; lateral border – inferior epigastric artery; medial border – the lateral border of rectus abdominis muscle). Distinction between direct and indirect hernia is made by reducing the hernia and exerting pressure over the deep inguinal ring, asking the patient to cough. If the hernia sac appears medial to the fingers, it is direct. If the hernia appears only after removing the pressure over the deep inguinal ring then it is indirect.

Imperfectly descended testis

An imperfectly descended testis may be in an ectopic position (root of the penis, upper thigh or perineum) or along the normal line of descent. An imperfectly descended testis cannot be felt in the inguinal canal – it is usually too flabby and atrophic and cannot be palpated through the tough overlying external oblique aponeurosis. However, should it become malignant then the hard and irregular testis can be palpated in the inguinal canal. An imperfectly descended testis may also be palpable in the upper thigh below the inguinal ligament. The scrotum will be empty on that side. The testis cannot descend more than a few centimetres into the upper thigh as its descent is prevented by the attachment of Scarpa's fascia to the deep fascia of the thigh below the inguinal ligament. An imperfectly descended testis may also be palpable at the root of the penis or in the perineum.

Lipoma of the cord

This can only be confidently diagnosed at surgery, although there will not be an expansile cough impulse as with a hernia.

Hydrocele of the cord

This is rare. There will be a smooth, palpable swelling along the line of the cord. It does not have a palpable expansile cough impulse. If gentle traction is exerted on the testis, a hydrocele of the cord will be felt to move down the canal. It may transilluminate.

Hydrocele of the canal of Nuck

A swelling, similar to a hydrocele of the cord in the male, occurring in the female is called a hydrocele of the canal of Nuck. Findings will be similar to those of a hydrocele of the cord in the male, except there is nothing to exert traction on!

Femoral hernia

This is more common in females. It lies below and lateral to the pubic tubercle. There will be an expansile cough impulse. It may be reducible. Strangulation of a femoral hernia is not uncommon, particularly one of the Richter's type. A tense, tender, irreducible swelling will be found below and lateral to the pubic tubercle.

Lymph nodes

Lymph nodes are palpable below the inguinal ligament. Classically they are arranged into groups: (1) superficial, with subdivision into horizontal and vertical groups; and (2) deep. In practice it is difficult to distinguish between the groups. Lymph nodes in the groin may be palpable as discrete nodules or they may be hard, irregular and matted together. This type is usually associated with malignant disease. Tender, fluctuant lymph nodes with erythema of the overlying skin are usually associated with lymphadenopathy due to an infective condition. It is important to examine all sites that are drained by these nodes, namely: (1) the skin of the leg, including examination under the toe nails; (2) the skin of the buttock; (3) the skin of the lower abdominal wall up to and including the umbilicus; (4) the skin of the scrotum, penis and glans penis; (5) the labia and lower third of the vagina; (6) the lower half of the anal canal; (7) the fundus of the uterus. It is therefore necessary not only to examine superficial structures but also to carry out a digital rectal examination and a bimanual vaginal examination.

Saphena varix

This is a soft, compressible dilatation at the termination of the saphenous vein. It has a cough impulse and disappears on recumbency. A fluid thrill is felt if the veins lower down the leg are percussed.

Femoral artery aneurysm

A femoral artery aneurysm presents as an expansile pulsatile mass in the line of the femoral artery. Look for a scar in relationship to it, which may suggest a false aneurysm.

Imperfectly descended testis

An imperfectly descended testis may be palpable in the upper thigh below the inguinal ligament. The scrotum will be empty on that side. The testis cannot descend more than a few centimetres into the upper thigh as its descent is prevented by the attachment of Scarpa's fascia to the deep fascia of the thigh below the inguinal ligament.

Neuroma of the femoral nerve

This is rare. It will be palpable along the course of the nerve (lateral to the femoral artery). Test the integrity of the femoral nerve (sensation on the anterior aspect of the thigh; extension of the knee joint).

Synovioma of the hip joint

This is rare. There may be a palpable thickening deep in the groin in relation to the hip joint. Hip joint movements may be limited.

Obturator hernia

This is rare. In a very thin patient a lump may be felt deep in the medial aspect of the groin. More commonly, obturator hernias present with intestinal obstruction and the diagnosis is made at laparotomy.

Psoas abscess

This is rare. It used to be associated with spinal TB, a cold abscess of a vertebral body discharging down the psoas sheath and presenting as a soft fluctuant swelling below the inguinal ligament. Most psoas abscesses nowadays are related to perforation of a hollow viscus retroperitoneally, e.g. the right colon into the psoas sheath.

GENERAL INVESTIGATIONS

The diagnosis of most groin swellings is made on history and physical examination.

- **FBC, ESR**
  Hb ↓ lymph node tumours. WCC ↑ infection in the lymph nodes, strangulated hernia. ESR ↑ lymph node tumours, infection, e.g. TB spine.
- **US**
  Lipoma, imperfectly descended testis, femoral artery aneurysm, psoas abcess.
- **Hip X-ray**
  Osteoarthritis with synovioma.
- **AXR**
  Intestinal obstruction associated with obstructed/strangulated hernia.

SPECIFIC INVESTIGATIONS

- **Duplex Doppler**
  Aneurysm. False aneurysm. Saphena varix.
- **Thoracolumbar spine X-ray**
  TB spine (psoas abcess).
- **CT scan**
  Psoas abscess. TB spine.
- **MRI scan**
  Psoas abscess. TB spine. Cord compression.
- **Herniography**
  Inguinal or femoral hernia.
- **FNAC**
  Lymph node pathology.
- **Biopsy**
  Lymph node pathology.

▶ GUM DISORDERS

Disorders of the gums are common, especially bleeding from the gums. Most disorders that cause bleeding are due to local infective disease but may be a manifestation of systemic disease.

CAUSES

Bleeding
- Dental disease
- Infection
  - Bacterial
  - Viral
  - Fungal
- Blood dyscrasias
- Iatrogenic
  - Anticoagulants
  - Chemotherapy
  - Radiotherapy

Hypertrophy
- Infection associated with dental disease
- Drugs
  - Phenytoin
  - Nifedipine
  - Cyclosporin

Retraction
- Chronic periodontal disease
- Ageing

Others
- Malignancy (ulcers)
- Lead poisoning
- Arsenic poisoning

HISTORY

Periodontal disease is probably the most common factor causing bleeding from the gums. Poor hygiene is usually obvious from the condition of the teeth. Infection will cause the patient to complain of red, inflamed gums, which bleed spontaneously or on brushing the teeth. The patient may have a history of recent malignancy for which they have undergone either chemotherapy, with associated blood dyscrasia, or local radiotherapy. There may be a history of painful lesions in the mouth to suggest herpes simplex. Rarely infectious mononucleosis may cause gingivostomatitis. The patient may present with a pyrexial illness with malaise, lethargy and lymphadenopathy. Abnormalities of the bone marrow, e.g. malignant infiltration, or aplastic anaemia will result in agranulocytosis and thrombocytopenia. Agranulocytosis causes reduced resistance to infection; thrombocytopenia is associated with a bleeding tendency. There may be a generalised illness with malaise and lethargy associated with lymphadenopathy, bruising and spontaneous bleeding from other orifices. There may be a history of haemophilia or von Willebrand's disease. Rarer conditions include scurvy (subclinical vitamin C deficiency may occur in the elderly) and hereditary haemorrhagic telangiectasia. Check for a family history of bleeding disorders. A full drug history should be taken. Check whether the patient is on phenytoin, nifedipine or cyclosporin. Check for occupational exposure to chemicals, especially arsenic and lead.

EXAMINATION

Local

Inspect the gums for signs of inflammation and bleeding. Is it only the gums that are involved or does the condition affect the whole of the oral cavity? Check the condition of the teeth, looking for dental caries or periodontal disease. Is there any evidence of gingival hyperplasia? In gingival hyperplasia the gum hypertrophy predominantly involves the interdental papillae. Is there any localised ulceration of the gum to suggest neoplasia? Is there any evidence of gum retraction? This occurs commonly in ageing but may be associated with chronic periodontal disease. Arsenic and lead are rare causes of gingival bleeding. The gingiva become inflamed, swollen and bleed easily, and, in the case of lead, there is a characteristic blue line at the gingival margin. Other signs of lead poisoning may be present, particularly pigmentation of the skin, vomiting, diarrhoea and hyperkeratosis of the soles of the feet and the palms of the hands. Peripheral neuropathy may be present with arsenic poisoning.

General

Conduct a general examination of the patient. Is there any evidence of systemic disease? Check for lymphadenopathy, hepatosplenomegaly and generalised bruising. Check for telangiectasia.

GENERAL INVESTIGATIONS

- **FBC, ESR**
  Hb ↓ malignancy, malnutrition. WCC ↑ infection. WCC ↓ blood dyscrasias, chemotherapy. ESR ↑ malignancy, infection. Platelets ↓ thrombocytopenia.
- **Swab**
  C&S. Infected ulcers.

SPECIFIC INVESTIGATIONS

- **Clotting screen**
  Dyscrasias, anticoagulants.
- **Vitamin C level**
  Scurvy.
- **Biopsy**
  Malignant ulcers.

GYNAECOMASTIA

Gynaecomastia is enlargement of the male breast. There is an increase in the ductal and connective tissue elements of the breast. The condition should not be confused with fat in the mammary region, which may occur in obese patients and in old age with weight loss. In most cases, gynaecomastia is a result of an increase in the oestrogen:androgen ratio. In many cases the actual mechanism is unknown or the cause is idiopathic.

CAUSES

Physiological

- Neonates
- Puberty
- Old age

Pathological

- Drugs
  - Oestrogens
  - Cyproterone
  - Spironolactone
  - Cimetidine
  - Digitalis
  - Griseofulvin
  - Amphetamines
  - Tricyclic antidepressants
  - Cannabis
- Carcinoma of the male breast
- Liver failure
- Renal failure
- Hyperthyroidism
- Hypogonadism
  - Klinefelter's syndrome
  - Agenesis
- Testicular tumours
- Other tumours
  - Bronchial carcinoma (inappropriate secretion of hormones)
  - Pituitary tumours (e.g. prolactinoma)
- Malnutrition
- Idiopathic

HISTORY

In newborn babies gynaecomastia is associated with placental oestrogens and may be associated with a milky discharge from the nipple (witch's milk). Is the patient pubertal? A minor degree of gynaecomastia occurs in a majority of boys prior to puberty. This often regresses but occasionally remains and is a source of embarrassment. Senescent gynaecomastia occurs in the sixth or later decades.

Most cases of gynaecomastia present as painless, or tender, enlargement of one or both breasts. The majority of pathological causes of gynaecomastia are related to drugs. A careful drug history should be taken. Is there a history to suggest hypogonadism, e.g. undescended testes, bilateral torsion, Klinefelter's syndrome (XXY – tall, female distribution of fat around breast and pelvis, normal male hair distribution, atrophic testes). Has the patient noticed any testicular swelling? Check for a history of alcoholism or hepatitis which might suggest liver failure. Is the patient in chronic renal failure? This will usually be apparent as he will have been on some form of dialysis. Are there any signs of hyperparathyroidism? Has the patient noticed any visual disturbance to suggest a pituitary tumour involving the optic chiasma?

EXAMINATION

Local

One or both breasts may be involved. Enlargement may be considerable, resembling a female breast, but this is rare; it is usually small and localised behind the areolar. The swelling may be soft or hard. In the younger male the hard enlargement is usually confined to a disc of tissue behind the areolar and this usually occurs around puberty. Hard irregular enlargement in an elderly man should raise the diagnosis of carcinoma. Soft or diffuse enlargement is usually associated with drugs.

General

Examine the axillary and supraclavicular lymph node. Examine the testes – atrophic or enlarged (tumour). Check for signs for hyperthyroidism, liver failure or renal failure. The patient may have a CAPD tube or an arteriovenous fistula for treatment of chronic renal failure.

GENERAL INVESTIGATIONS

- **FBC, ESR**
  Hb ↓ anaemia – liver failure. ESR ↑ liver disease.
- **U&Es**
  Renal failure.
- **LFTs**
  Liver failure.
- **TFTs**
  Hyperthyroidism.
- **CXR**
  Primary tumour (bronchial carcinoma with inappropriate
  secretion of hormones).

SPECIFIC INVESTIGATIONS

- **FNAC**
  Carcinoma.
- **Mammography**
  Carcinoma.
- **Chromosome analysis**
  Klinefelter's syndrome.
- **βHCG**
  Testicular tumour.
- **AFP**
  Testicular tumour.
- **Basal serum prolactin**
  Prolactinoma.
- **CT head**
  Pituitary tumour.

▶ HAEMATEMESIS

Haematemesis is the vomiting of blood. This may be frank blood or blood altered by the action of gastric acid and digestive enzymes, i.e. 'coffee grounds'. Haematemesis is usually caused by lesions proximal to the duodenojejunal junction.

CAUSES

Swallowed blood
- Epistaxis
- Haemoptysis

Oesophagus
- Oesophageal varices
- Reflux oesophagitis
- Oesophageal carcinoma

Stomach
- Peptic ulceration
- Mallory–Weiss syndrome
- Acute gastric erosions
- Carcinoma
- Leiomyoma (rare)
- Hereditary haemorrhagic telangiectasia (rare)
- Vascular malformations (rare)

Duodenum
- Peptic ulceration
- Duodenal diverticulae
- Aortoduodenal fistulae
- Invasive pancreatic tumours (rare)
- Haemobilia (rare)

Bleeding disorders
- Liver disease-associated
- Thrombocytopenia
- Haemophilia

Drugs
- Anticoagulants
- Aspirin
- NSAIDs
- Steroids

Others
- Uraemia
- Connective tissue disorders

HISTORY

Swallowed blood

Check for a recent history of epistaxis or haemoptysis.

Oesophagus

There may be a history of excess alcohol consumption or a history of other liver disease to suggest oesophageal varices. Check for retrosternal burning pain and heartburn, which would suggest oesophagitis. Check for a history of dysphagia. The bleeding associated with varices is often torrential; that associated with oesophagitis is minor.

Stomach

History of epigastric pain to suggest peptic ulceration. There may be a history of steroid or NSAID medication. Mallory–Weiss syndrome usually occurs in the younger patient who has had a large meal with much alcohol followed by a forceful vomit. The first vomit contains food, the second contains blood. Acute gastric erosions may occur with stressful illnesses, e.g. major surgery, acute pancreatitis, burns (Curling's ulcer), head injuries (Cushing's ulcer). It is unusual to get a large bleed with a carcinoma. Anaemia is a common presentation, although there may be 'coffee grounds' vomit. Leiomyoma causes a moderate haematemesis. There is usually no preceding history. There will also be no preceding history with vascular malformations. Hereditary haemorrhagic telangiectasia is rare. The patient may present with a history of the condition, or it may be apparent from the telangiectasia around the lips and oral cavity.

Duodenum

Melaena tends to be a more common symptom than haematemesis with duodenal lesions. There may be a history of chronic duodenal ulceration, although often presentation may be acute with little background history. Bleeding from invasive pancreatic tumours is rare. The patient will present with malaise, lethargy, weight loss and vomiting. Haemobilia is rare. Aortoduodenal fistula is rare and usually follows repair of an aneurysm with subsequent infection of the graft. There is massive haematemesis and melaena.

Bleeding disorders

The patient may present with a history of a bleeding disorder, e.g. haemophilia. There may be a history of spontaneous bruising or bleeding from other orifices.

Drugs

There may be a history of anticoagulant, steroid or NSAID therapy. Always question the patient carefully to see whether he or she has bought any proprietary, 'across the counter' preparations that may contain aspirin or NSAIDs.

Others

Uraemia may cause bleeding. Other symptoms such as dyspnoea, nausea, malaise, peripheral oedema or coma may be present. Rarely gastrointestinal bleeding may be a presenting symptom of a connective tissue disease.

Examination

Depending upon the severity of the bleed, there may be shock. The patient will be cold, clammy, with peripheral vasoconstriction; there will be a tachycardia and hypotension.

Swallowed blood

Check for blood around the nose. Examine the chest for a possible cause of haemoptysis.

Oesophagus

There may be little to find on examination except clinical signs of anaemia and weight loss, unless the cause is oesophageal varices. In the latter case there may be jaundice, abdominal distension due to ascites, spider naevi, liver palms, clubbing, gynaecomastia, testicular atrophy, caput medusae, splenomegaly or hepatomegaly.

Stomach

There may be little to find on examination. There may be an epigastric mass with a carcinoma, or a palpable left supraclavicular node (Virchow's node). There may be epigastric tenderness. With hereditary haemorrhagic telangiectasia there may be telangiectasia on the lips and mucous membrane of the mouth.

Duodenum

Again, there may be little to find on examination other than epigastric tenderness. In the rare case where duodenal bleeding comes from an invasive pancreatic carcinoma there may be a palpable mass in the region of the pancreas.

Bleeding disorders

There may be signs of bruising or bleeding from other orifices.

Drugs

The signs will depend on the severity of the bleed and the site of the lesion produced.

Others

There may be signs of uraemia, e.g. pallor, bronze colour of the skin, pulmonary oedema, peripheral oedema, pericarditis, cardiac tamponade, hypertension, retinopathy. Rarely haematemesis may be associated with connective tissue diseases, e.g. polyarteritis nodosa. Other manifestations of polyarteritis nodosa may be apparent, e.g. neuropathies, cardiac disease, skin lesions.

GENERAL INVESTIGATIONS

- **FBC, ESR**
  Hb ↓ anaemia due to chronic bleeding, e.g. from carcinoma. ESR ↑ connective tissue disease.
- **U&Es**
  Urea and creatinine will be raised in uraemia. Urea may be raised due to absorption of blood from the bowel.
- **LFTs**
  Liver failure, oesophageal varices, haemobilia.
- **Clotting screen**
  Liver disease. Bleeding diatheses. Anticoagulants.
- **OGD**
  Will demonstrate most lesions, e.g. varices, oesophagitis, peptic ulcer, gastric erosions, Mallory–Weiss tear, carcinoma and rarer causes of bleeding. Biopsy may be carried out where necessary.

SPECIFIC INVESTIGATIONS

- **Angiography**
  Vascular malformations. Also may diagnose rarer distal duodenal causes, e.g. vascular malformations.
- **US**
  Aortic aneurysm.
- **CXR**
  Chest lesion.
- **CT**
  Aortic graft infection.

▶ HAEMATURIA

Haematuria is the passage of red blood cells in the urine. Care must be taken to distinguish it from other causes of discoloration of urine. All patients with haematuria must be fully investigated. If haematuria has initially been diagnosed on dipstick testing it must always be confirmed by microscopy.

CAUSES

Kidney
- Glomerular disease
- Polycystic kidney
- Carcinoma
- Stone
- Trauma (including renal biopsy)
- TB
- Embolism
- Renal vein thrombosis
- Vascular malformation

Ureter
- Stone
- Neoplasm

Bladder
- Carcinoma
- Stone
- Trauma
- Inflammatory, e.g. cystitis, TB, schistosomiasis

Prostate
- Benign prostatic hypertrophy
- Carcinoma

Urethra
- Trauma
- Stone
- Urethritis
- Neoplasm

General
- Anticoagulant therapy
- Thrombocytopenia

- Haemophilia
- Sickle cell disease
- Malaria
- Strenuous exercise

Red urine

- Haemoglobinuria
- Myoglobinuria
- Acute intermittent porphyria
- Beetroot
- Senna
- Phenolphthalein
- Rifampicin

HISTORY

Is there pain associated with haematuria to suggest infection or inflammation? Painless haematuria is usually associated with tumour or tuberculosis. Total haematuria (throughout the stream) suggests bleeding from the upper urinary tract or bladder. Initial haematuria (at the start of the stream) suggests bleeding from the urethra or the prostate. Terminal haematuria (at the end of the stream) suggests bleeding from the bladder or prostate. Check for a family history of polycystic kidney disease. There may be a history of TB elsewhere. Has there been any recent foreign travel (schistosomiasis)? Is there any pain in the loin to suggest kidney disease, or a history of uteric colic to suggest passage of a stone or clot down the ureter? Bladder disease may be accompanied by suprapubic pain, frequency and dysuria. Check for symptoms of prostatism, i.e. difficulty in starting, poor stream and nocturia. Urethral injury will normally be apparent. It may occur following pelvic fractures or falling astride an object. Is the patient on anticoagulants? Is there any history of blood dyscrasia? Is there evidence of sickle cell disease or exposure to malaria? Strenuous exercise may cause haematuria. Has there been a recent renal biopsy? Discoloration of urine may be due to a variety of causes. Haemoglobinuria may occur with haemolysis and myoglobinuria following crush injuries or ischaemia of muscle. Check for ingestion of any substance that may change the colour of the urine. Acute intermittent porphyria is extremely rare and is accompanied by abdominal pain. If the urine from a patient is allowed to stand in the light it will become purplish–red.

EXAMINATION

Anaemia, weight loss, signs of chronic renal failure. Abdominal examination may reveal a palpable mass, e.g. hypernephroma, distended bladder. Rectal examination may reveal smooth enlargement of the prostate (benign prostatic hypertrophy) or a hard, craggy prostate (carcinoma). Feel along the course of the urethra, e.g. stone or neoplasm. Examine the chest, e.g. TB, secondary deposits from carcinoma of the kidney. Check for any localised bone tenderness, e.g. secondary deposits from carcinoma of the prostate or hypernephroma.

GENERAL INVESTIGATIONS

- **FBC, ESR**
  Hb ↓ gross haematuria, malignancy. Hb ↑ polycythaemia associated with hypernephroma. WCC ↑ infection. Platelets ↓ blood dyscrasias. ESR ↑ malignancy, TB.
- **Urine microscopy**
  Red cells (excludes haemoglobinuria and ingestion of substances that cause discoloration of urine). White cells in infection. Organisms in infection. Cytology.
- **U&Es**
  Renal failure.
- **Clotting screen**
  Anticoagulant therapy. Blood dyscrasias.
- **CXR**
  Metastases (cannonball metastases with hypernephroma). TB.
- **KUB**
  Renal calculus.

SPECIFIC INVESTIGATIONS

- **PSA**
  Prostatic carcinoma.
- **Sickling test**
  Sickle cell disease.
- **IVU**
  Stone. Tumour. TB.
- **US**
  Cystic versus solid. Stone. Urinary tract obstruction.

- **CT**
  Tumour (confirmation and degree of invasion). Cyst. Obstructive uropathy.
- **Cystoscopy**
  Infection. Tumour. Stone.
- **Ureteroscopy**
  Tumour. Obstruction.
- **Selective renal angiography**
  Vascular malformation. Tumour.
- **Renal biopsy**
  Glomerular disease. Tumour.
- **Prostatic biopsy**
  Carcinoma of the prostate.

▶ HAEMOPTYSIS

Haemoptysis is the expectoration of blood or bloodstained sputum. With massive haemoptysis, the main priorities are to secure the airway and initiate emergency resuscitative measures before establishing a diagnosis.

CAUSES

Respiratory
- Bronchial carcinoma
- Pneumonia
- TB
- Chronic bronchitis
- Bronchiectasis
- Pulmonary oedema
- Goodpasture's syndrome
- Wegener's granulomatosis

Vascular
- Pulmonary embolism
- Pulmonary hypertension – mitral stenosis
- Hereditary haemorrhagic telangiectasia

Systemic
- Coagulation disorders

HISTORY

Onset
Sudden onset of haemoptysis can occur with pulmonary embolism and acute respiratory tract infections; the remaining conditions tend to pursue chronic recurrent courses. Although the amount of blood expectorated is not very useful as a discriminating feature, small amounts of blood sufficient to stain the sputum pink are characteristic of pulmonary oedema.

Acute onset of cough with haemoptysis may occur with respiratory tract infections and pulmonary embolism. Associated sputum production may be purulent and long-standing with chronic bronchitis and bronchiectasis. This is accompanied by flecks of blood when lung carcinoma, tuberculosis or mitral stenosis is present.

Dyspnoea

A long history of dyspnoea may be associated with chronic lung disease or mitral stenosis. Acute onset of dyspnoea that occurs with pulmonary embolism may be accompanied by pleuritic chest pain. Dyspnoea that is associated with pulmonary oedema may have a variable speed of onset and is often worse on recumbency.

Weight loss

Progressive weight loss is suggestive of TB or bronchial carcinoma, especially with a background of heavy smoking. Night sweats may be an additional accompanying feature of TB.

Other sites of bleeding

Other bleeding sites should be excluded as haematuria may be due to Goodpasture's syndrome. Epistaxis and haemoptysis occur together with Wegener's granulomatosis and hereditary haemorrhagic telangiectasia. Epistaxis per se may occasionally be confused with haemoptysis when expectorated sputum is mixed with blood originating from the nasal passages.

Past medical and drug history

A careful history is taken to identify a generalised coagulation disorder. This may be congenital, such as haemophilia, or acquired, such as with the use of anticoagulant drugs or in DIC. Previous rheumatic fever predisposes an individual to mitral stenosis. Consider Goodpasture's syndrome and Wegener's granulomatosis in the presence of coexisting renal disease.

EXAMINATION

Inspection

Cachexia is a prominent feature of carcinoma, TB and chronic lung disease. Loss of the nasal bridge and saddling of the nose may be apparent in patients with Wegener's granulomatosis. The presence of clubbing (page 69) is associated with bronchial carcinoma, chronic bronchitis and bronchiectasis. The malar flush characteristic of mitral facies may be present with mitral stenosis. Small dilated blood vessels present on the mucous membranes are features of hereditary haemorrhagic telangiectasia. The JVP may be elevated with a large pulmonary embolus or accompanying congestive cardiac failure secondary to mitral stenosis. The chest may be hyperexpanded with decreased inspiratory movement in chronic bronchitis.

Palpation
During an acute episode, tachycardia is very common. This may be due to the effort of coughing, anxiety or blood loss. The presence of an irregularly irregular heartbeat of atrial fibrillation is associated with mitral stenosis. Moreover, patients with atrial fibrillation are usually on anticoagulant therapy. Supraclavicular lymphadenopathy may be present with pulmonary infections or carcinoma. The calves should be palpated and measured for tenderness and increased girth from deep venous thrombosis, which may give rise to pulmonary emboli.

Percussion and auscultation
Localised crepitations and bronchial breathing may be audible with lobar pneumonia. Generalised coarse crepitations are suggestive of bronchiectasis, pulmonary oedema and chronic bronchitis. Breath sounds tend to be decreased in intensity with chronic bronchitis. Patients with bronchial carcinoma may present with a number of clinical features from the primary tumour, such as wheezing due to large airway obstruction, pulmonary collapse, pleural effusion and superior vena cava obstruction. On auscultation of the mitral area, the loud first heart sound and mid-diastolic rumbling murmur of mitral stenosis is accentuated on expiration with the patient in a left lateral position.

GENERAL INVESTIGATIONS

- **Sputum analysis**
  Sputum should be collected for microscopy, culture and cytology. Infective organisms may be isolated or cytological features of malignancy may be present. When TB is suspected, serial cultures should be taken from sputum, urine, bronchial washings or lung biopsy specimens during bronchoscopy. Polymerase chain reaction amplification techniques may also be performed on cultured specimens to provide a more rapid diagnosis.
- **ECG**
  Sinus tachycardia may be noted with violent coughing, anxiety and blood loss. $S_1Q_3T_3$ is indicative of right heart strain with pulmonary embolism, although non-specific ST abnormalities are more common.
- **FBC**
  Hb $\downarrow$ with chronic haemoptysis resulting in iron deficiency

anaemia. Acute bleeding may not be associated with changes in the blood count until 24 hours later. WCC ↑ may be due to acute bleeding or respiratory tract infection. Monocytosis may be a feature of TB. Platelets ↓ with blood dyscrasias.

- **U&Es**

  The presence of impaired renal function with deranged urea and creatinine estimations may be due to glomerulonephritis from Goodpasture's syndrome or Wegener's granulomatosis. However, prerenal failure may also be precipitated by acute blood loss and volume depletion.

- **Clotting screen**

  A clotting screen is performed to identify any impairment that may prolong the PT or APTT.

- **CXR**

  Bilateral patchy areas of consolidation may be seen on a chest film with bronchopneumonia and pulmonary oedema. Opacification of an entire lobe suggests lobar pneumonia, although pulmonary emboli may have a similar appearance due to the wedge-shaped shadowing of a pulmonary infarct. Recurrent fluffy shadowing may be seen with Goodpasture's syndrome and Wegener's granulomatosis, due to repeated intra-alveolar haemorrhage. The primary focus of tuberculous infection is usually in the middle to upper zones of the lung. This may resolve, with variable amounts of calcification, whereas postprimary TB tends to present with the classical apical shadow. The chest film may be normal with uncomplicated chronic bronchitis; however, with bronchiectasis, visibly dilated bronchi with persistent consolidation may be prominent. With bronchial carcinoma, numerous features may be seen on a chest radiograph, such as a peripheral mass, a hilar mass, collapse of a lobe or pleural effusion. The double right heart border and tenting of the left heart border are all features of enlargement of the left atrium with mitral stenosis. When pulmonary hypertension is present, there may be dilatation of the central pulmonary arteries with right ventricular enlargement.

- **Bronchoscopy**

  Fibreoptic bronchoscopy is useful for locating the site of bleeding. In addition, biopsies of the bleeding site may be sampled for pathological analysis. Multiple arteriovenous malformations will be visible with hereditary haemorrhagic telangiectasia.

SPECIFIC INVESTIGATIONS

- **Mantoux test**

  When TB is suspected an initial dilute Mantoux test (1 in 10 000) may be performed in individuals who have not received BCG immunisation.

- **Urinalysis**

  May reveal the presence of protein and red cell casts with glomerulonephritis due to Goodpasture's syndrome and Wegener's granulomatosis.

- **Antiglomerular basement antibodies**

  Characterises Goodpasture's syndrome.

- **c-ANCA**

  Wegener's granulomatosis is associated with elevated levels.

- **Renal biopsy**

  Will aid in confirming the diagnosis in both Goodpasture's syndrome and Wegener's granulomatosis.

- **Tissue biopsies**

  Majority of lung cancers are diagnosed on CXR; a smaller proportion are diagnosed by cytology. Definitive tissue diagnosis can be made by biopsies from bronchoscopy, mediastinoscopy, CT-guided biopsy or surgical resection.

- **CT thorax**

  Very useful adjunct to the diagnosis of bronchiectasis in cases where the diagnosis cannot confidently be made on the clinical grounds and a chest film. It may also be useful in the staging of lung carcinomas.

- **V/Q scan**

  Useful to diagnose pulmonary embolism, although the pulmonary angiogram is the current 'gold standard'.

- **Echocardiography**

  Allows assessment of left ventricular function with pulmonary oedema. It may also aid in the diagnosis of pulmonary embolism, as right heart failure can occur with large emboli. The integrity of the cardiac valves can be assessed, and valve stenosis with restriction of movement of the mitral valve leaflets can be visualised in mitral stenosis.

HAND DEFORMITIES

Impairment of hand function can lead to severe disability.

CAUSES

Congenital

Failure of formation
- Absent digit
- Radial club hand

Failure of separation
- Syndactyly (fusion of digits)
- Camptodactyly

Duplication
- Extra digit

Primary muscle contractures
- Arthrogryposis multiplex congenita (rare)

Acquired
- Trauma (mal-united fracture)
- Burns
- Dupuytren's contracture
- Rheumatoid arthritis
- Volkmann's ischaemic contracture
- Spinal cord lesions
  - Poliomyelitis
  - Syringomyelia
- Brachial plexus lesions
- Peripheral nerve lesions
- Multiple chondromas (Ollier's disease – rare)

HISTORY

Congenital
These lesions will be recognisable at birth. Arthrogryposis multiplex congenita is due to non-differentiation of mesenchymal tissues, often together with a neurogenic element, the combination producing gross contractures.

Acquired

Trauma and burns
There will be a clear history of previous trauma and burns.

Dupuytren's contracture
In the early phases there will be little deformity, the patient merely complaining of thickening in the palm near the base of the ring finger. Eventually the patient will complain of being unable to straighten the ring and little fingers. The grip is also affected. Check for a history of epilepsy, cirrhosis or diabetes.

Rheumatoid arthritis
By the time the hand is deformed the patient is usually well aware of the diagnosis. There is pain and swelling of the joints with weakness of the hand, together with gross deformity.

Volkmann's ischaemic contracture
This is shortening of the long flexor muscles of the forearm due to ischaemia. There may be a history of trauma, e.g. supracondylar fracture of the humerus, a tight plaster restricting blood flow, or arterial disease, e.g. embolism. Movements of the fingers are painful and limited. There may be pins and needles in the hand due to pressure on nerves. Eventually a claw hand results.

Spinal cord lesions
By the time deformity of the limb has resulted the diagnosis will usually be apparent. There may be a history of poliomyelitis.

Brachial plexus lesions
There will usually be a history of trauma, although occasionally invasion of the brachial plexus from tumours may occur.

Peripheral nerve lesions
There is usually a clear history of trauma to suggest a nerve lesion. Check for any possible causes of peripheral neuropathy, e.g. diabetes, uraemia, connective tissue disease, leprosy.

Ollier's disease
This results in deformities of the limb. There are irregularly distributed areas of cartilage and bone. The patient will complain of deformity of joints and bones and possible shortening of the limb, and will have noticed nodules along the line of bone.

EXAMINATION

Congenital

Congenital anomalies will be obvious at birth. They may be associated with congenital anomalies elsewhere.

Acquired

Trauma and burns

A variety of deformities may be seen, depending upon the degree and type of trauma. With burns, scarring of the skin will be obvious.

Dupuytren's contracture

Examination will reveal a firm nodule in the palmar fascia near the base of the ring finger. Puckering of the skin is usually present around the nodule. The MCP joint and the PIP joint are flexed, the DIP joint being extended. The ulnar digits (ring and little finger) are most commonly affected.

Rheumatoid arthritis

There is thickening of the joints, especially the MCP joint and PIP joints. The joints become fusiform in shape. There is ulnar deviation of the fingers. The wrist joint develops a fixed flexion deformity with some ulnar deviation. Swan-neck and boutonnière deformities of the fingers will be apparent. Ultimately tendon rupture occurs and this leads to a variety of deformities.

Volkmann's ischaemic contracture

The skin of the hand is pale and the hand clawed and wasted. Extension of the fingers is limited but improves if the wrist is flexed. Eventually the forearm muscles feel hard and taut due to fibrosis.

Spinal cord lesions

In the case of poliomyelitis there is usually a clear history and the limb usually looks reddish–blue, wasted and deformed. Syringomyelia may cause a variety of hand deformities. With upper motor neurone lesions there may be fixed flexion of the wrist and fingers with adduction of the thumb.

Brachial plexus injuries

Upward traction on the arm may damage the lowest root (T1) of the brachial plexus, which is the segmental supply of the intrinsic muscles of the hand. The hand becomes clawed (Klumpke's paralysis). Check for a possible associated Horner's syndrome due to traction of the cervical sympathetic chain.

Peripheral nerve lesions

With ulnar nerve lesions it is appropriate to check for damage to the medial epicondyle. Also check for any evidence of recent lacerations at the wrist. With division at the wrist all the intrinsic muscles of the fingers (except for the radial two lumbricals – median nerve) are paralysed and the hand appears clawed. The clawing is less for the index and middle fingers because the lumbricals are intact. In late cases, wasting of the interossei is clearly seen on the dorsum of the hand. There is sensory loss over the medial 1½ fingers. If the nerve is injured at the elbow the flexor digitorum profundus to the ring and little fingers is paralysed so that the clawing of these two digits is not so pronounced.

In median nerve lesions at the wrist the thenar eminence becomes wasted due to paralysis of opponens pollicis and sensation is lost over the lateral 3½ digits. Fine movements, e.g. picking up a small object, are clumsy. With lesions at the elbow, wrist flexion is weak and the forearm muscles wasted. Ulnar deviation occurs at the wrist, as the wrist flexion depends upon flexor carpi ulnaris and the medial half of flexor digitorum profundus. Often the hand is held with the medial two fingers flexed and the lateral two fingers straight.

Ollier's disease

Multiple lumps (chondromas) are located on the bones. Often associated with limb shortening. Only one limb or one bone may be involved.

GENERAL INVESTIGATIONS

Most of the conditions described above will be obvious on clinical examination.
- **FBC, ESR**
  Hb ↓ in anaemia of chronic disease, e.g. rheumatoid arthritis.
- **CRP**
  ↑ in inflammatory disease
- **Rheumatoid factor**
  Rheumatoid arthritis.
- **LFTs**
  Cirrhosis (Dupuytren's).
- **Blood glucose**
  Diabetes. Peripheral neuropathy, Dupuytren's contracture.

- **Arm X-ray**
  Local fractures, e.g. evidence of previous supracondylar fracture of the humerus with subsequent Volkmann's ischaemic contracture.
- **Hand X-ray**
  Rheumatoid arthritis. Ollier's disease – multiple translucent areas in the bones of the hand. Evidence of mal-united fracture following trauma.
- **MRI**
  Spinal lesions, e.g. syringomyelia.
- **Nerve conduction studies**
  Brachial plexus and peripheral nerve lesions.

▶ HEADACHE

When assessing a patient with headache it is important to exclude life-threatening causes first.

CAUSES

Acute headache
- Trauma
- Cerebrovascular
  - Subarachnoid haemorrhage
  - Intracranial haemorrhage/infarction
- Meningitis
- Systemic infection
- Acute angle-closure glaucoma

Chronic or recurrent headache
- Tension headache
- Migraine
- Cluster headaches
- Raised intracranial pressure
  - Tumour
  - Hydrocephalus
  - Cerebral abscess
- Temporal arteritis
- Drugs
  - Glyceryl trinitrate, Nifedipine, Substance withdrawal

HISTORY

Onset
Sudden onset of severe pain is usually due to a vascular cause, especially subarachnoid haemorrhage from a ruptured berry aneurysm. Cluster headache and migraine intensify over minutes and may last several hours, while meningitis tends to evolve over hours to days. Progressive severe headaches that develop over days or weeks should lead to the consideration of raised intracranial pressure from tumour or chronic subdural haemorrhage. The onset of headache may be preceded by an aura with migraine.

Site
Classically, headache from migraine is unilateral. More localised is the pain over the superficial temporal arteries with temporal arteritis

that can be accompanied by jaw claudication. Ocular pain is experienced with glaucoma, and retro-orbital pain with cluster headaches.

Character

The intensity of pain contributes little when discriminating between the causes; however, the character of the pain may be useful. Patients with tension headache often complain of a tight band-like sensation; this is in contrast to the pain experienced with raised intracranial pressure, which is often reported to have a bursting quality. Migraine-related headaches have a throbbing character.

Precipitating factors

Headache originating from raised intracranial pressure is precipitated by changes in posture, coughing or sneezing, and is often worse in the mornings. Photophobia may be experienced by patients suffering with migraine, meningitis or glaucoma. They may prefer to lie in a darkened room when headaches arise. Certain food such as cheese is known to precipitate migraine. It is very common for headache to be precipitated by systemic illnesses such as a cold or influenza. Headache precipitated by touch occurs with superficial temporal artery inflammation from temporal arteritis. A drug history may elucidate the relationship between the administration of drugs with headache as a side-effect, such as glyceryl trinitrate and nifedipine. Alternatively, headache can also result from substance withdrawal in substance-dependent patients.

Associated symptoms

Neck stiffness (meningism) is experienced with both meningitis and subarachnoid haemorrhages. Visual disturbances in the form of haloes occur with glaucoma. Flashing lights and alternations in perception of size may be reported by patients suffering with migraine, and this may be accompanied by photophobia, nausea and vomiting. Transient neurological deficits may also occur. However, progressive neurology associated with headache is more suggestive of an intracranial space-occupying lesion, such as haemorrhage, abscess and tumour. Unilateral visual loss may result as a complication of temporal arteritis, and this may be accompanied by proximal muscle weakness or tenderness. Conjunctival injection is experienced with both glaucoma and cluster headaches, along with lacrimation, which is a feature of the latter. With normal pressure hydrocephalus in adults, headaches are associated with dementia, drowsiness, vomiting and ataxia.

EXAMINATION

Temperature
Pyrexia may indicate the presence of systemic infection or meningitis.

Inspection
An assessment of the conscious state should be undertaken and quantified on the GCS. Impairment of consciousness is a sign of a serious underlying aetiology, such as meningitis, subarachnoid haemorrhage and raised intracranial pressure. Inspection of the eyes may reveal conjunctival injection with glaucoma and cluster headaches during an acute attack. With acute angle-closure glaucoma the cornea is hazy and the pupil fixed and semidilated. Petechial haemorrhages on the skin are visible classically with meningococcal meningitis.

Palpation
Tenderness along the course of the superficial temporal artery, with absent pulsation, is consistent with temporal arteritis.

Neurological examination
A detailed neurological examination is performed to identify the site of any structural lesion. Unilateral total visual loss can be precipitated by temporal arteritis due to ischaemic optic neuritis. Visual field defects (hemianopia) can be caused by contralateral lesions in the cerebral cortex. Fundoscopy is performed to identify papilloedema from raised intracranial pressure.

Transient hemiplegia can occur with migraine, but progressive hemiplegia is more indicative of a space-occupying lesion, such as a tumour or intracranial haemorrhage. Neck stiffness is a feature of both meningitis and subarachnoid haemorrhage. With meningitis, Kernig's sign (pain on extending the knee with the hip in a flexed position) may be present.

GENERAL INVESTIGATIONS

- **FBC**
  WCC ↑ meningitis, cerebral abscess and systemic infection.
- **ESR**
  ↑ temporal arteritis, infection, intracranial bleeding.
- **U&Es**
  Hypertensive headaches with renal disease.

SPECIFIC INVESTIGATIONS

In most cases, the diagnosis can be made on clinical assessment. Features in the history and examination may guide specific investigations.

- **Blood cultures**
  With meningitis, systemic infection.

- **CT/MRI**
  Visualisation of the anatomical structures in the cranium is very useful in the presence of neurological deficit. Cerebral tumours may be visualised as high- or low-density masses. Intracranial bleeding can be identified as areas of high density during the first 2 weeks. An extradural haematoma presents as a lens-shaped opacity, and subdural haematoma presents as a crescent-shaped opacity. After 2 weeks, intracranial haematomas become isodense and more difficult to visualise. Following subarachnoid haemorrhage, blood may be visualised in the subarachnoid space. Occasionally the offending aneurysm or arteriovenous malformation may be imaged. Enlargement of the ventricles may be an indication of hydrocephalus. Contrast-enhanced CT scanning will increase the sensitivity to diagnose cerebral abscesses.

- **Lumbar puncture**
  A lumbar puncture may be undertaken following the exclusion of raised intracranial pressure when there is suspicion of meningitis or subarachnoid haemorrhage. The CSF obtained is inspected for consistency and colour. The consistency of the CSF is turbid with meningitis, and yellow staining of the CSF (known as xanthochromia) occurs with subarachnoid haemorrhage, owing to breakdown of haemoglobin from red blood cells. The CSF is then sent for microscopy, culture, cytology and biochemical analysis for glucose and protein. An abnormal increase in white cells may be seen on microscopy with meningitis. With bacterial or tuberculous meningitis, the glucose is low and protein content high. With viral meningitis the glucose content is normal and protein content mildly elevated.

- **Temporal artery biopsy**
  Inflammation and giant cells may be seen with temporal arteritis. A normal biopsy does not, however, exclude the disease, as there may be segmental involvement of the temporal artery.

- **Intraocular pressure measurements**
  Tonometry will reveal high intraocular pressures with glaucoma.

▶ HEMIPLEGIA

Hemiplegia is paralysis of one side of the body; it usually arises from unilateral lesions above the midcervical spinal cord.

CAUSES

Vascular
- Cerebrovascular ischaemia
- Cerebral or spinal infarction
- Intracerebral haemorrhage
- Cerebral vasculitis

Traumatic
- Subdural haematoma
- Extradural haematoma

Other
- Epilepsy
- Brain tumour
- Cerebral abscess
- Multiple sclerosis

HISTORY

Onset
The speed of onset of hemiplegia is useful when trying to determine the underlying aetiology. Sudden onset of hemiplegia is usually due to a cerebrovascular event such as a TIA, infarct or intracerebral haemorrhage. Developing hemiplegia over minutes or hours after trauma can be due to an evolving extradural or subdural haemorrhage. Although a history of trauma is usually evident, chronic subdural haematomas in the elderly may result from tearing of bridging veins without apparent trauma. Subacute hemiplegia may also result as part of a spectrum of neurological deficits caused by demyelination from multiple sclerosis. Gradual onset of hemiplegia is usually due to a tumour, although a cerebral abscess or chronic subdural haemorrhage may pursue a similar time course.

Precipitating factors
A history of trauma may be evident with extradural and subdural haemorrhages. Cerebral abscesses may result from

haematogenous dissemination of bacteria from a distant site of infection, such as the lung, or more commonly from adjacent infections, such as middle ear, mastoid and paranasal sinus infections. Transient hemiplegia may also result from an epileptic seizure and this phenomenon is known as Todd's paralysis. Unfortunately the precipitating factor for the seizure may be underlying structural abnormalities such as a cerebral abscess or tumour.

Associated symptoms

Due to the multifocal nature of demyelination, patients with multiple sclerosis may present with a host of associated symptoms, such as areas of motor deficits, sensory deficits, diplopia and monocular blindness from optic neuritis. Space-occupying lesions such as extradural haematoma, brain tumour and cerebral abscesses may also present with symptoms of raised intracranial pressure, such as headaches, classically worse in the morning, and with coughing or sneezing, nausea, vomiting and drowsiness.

EXAMINATION

The neurological examination is the key to determining the location of the lesion. Cortical lesions impinging on the motor area of the frontal lobe produce total contralateral paralysis. Similar effects can result from lesions of the internal capsule. Midbrain lesions tend to produce ipsilateral neurological deficits of the face and contralateral deficits of the limbs. Multifocal neurological deficits may be produced by demyelination or cerebral metastasis.

After determining the site of the lesion, the examination should be continued to determine the cause. A pyrexia should alert the clinician to the presence of infection, which may be caused by a cerebral abscess. The presence of facial myokymia, which is rippling of the muscles on one side of the face, is reported to be very suggestive of multiple sclerosis; cervical involvement may produce Lhermitte's sign, which is paraesthesia of the hands and feet on flexion of the neck.

Examination of the ear, mastoid and sinuses is useful to locate the site of primary infection, which may give rise to a cerebral abscess. Distant sites of infection that may precipitate cerebral abscesses are the lungs and emboli from infective endocarditis. The fingers are examined for nailfold infarcts with endocarditis and the precordium is auscultated for new or changing murmurs. The pulse is assessed for irregularity from atrial fibrillation, which is a predisposing factor for cerebral emboli. The blood pressure is measured, as hypertension is an additional risk factor for stroke. Carotid bruits from artherosclerotic plaques may be the only examination feature present with TIAs.

GENERAL INVESTIGATIONS

- **FBC**
  WCC ↑ infection, infarction.
- **ESR**
  ↑ infection, infarction, vasculitis.
- **U&Es, magnesium, calcium and glucose**
  Abnormal electrolytes may precipitate a seizure.

SPECIFIC INVESTIGATIONS

- **Blood cultures**
  For suspected cerebral abscess.
- **CT head**
  Intracerebral haemorrhage, stroke, head injuries, tumour and abscess.
- **MRI head and cervical spine**
  Abscess, tumours, focal demyelination and periventricular plaques with multiple sclerosis.
- **EEG**
  Epilepsy.
- **Lumbar puncture**
  Exclude raised intracranial pressure first. With multiple sclerosis, there is raised CSF IgG, and oligoclonal bands are present on electrophoresis.

HEPATOMEGALY

Hepatomegaly is enlargement of the liver. The most common causes in the UK are cirrhosis, cardiac failure and secondary malignancy.

CAUSES

Hepatitis/infection

Acute
- Viruses
- Bacteria
- Protozoans
- Parasites
- Alcohol

Chronic
- Chronic active hepatitis

Congestion
- Congestive cardiac failure
- Constrictive pericarditis
- Budd–Chiari syndrome

Infiltration
- Fatty liver
- Amyloid

Biliary tract disease
- Extrahepatic obstruction, e.g. carcinoma of the pancreas, bile duct stricture
- Sclerosing cholangitis
- Primary biliary cirrhosis

Malignancy
- Metastases
- Hepatoma
- Myeloproliferative disorders
- Myelofibrosis
- Leukaemia

Metabolic
- Glycogen storage diseases
- Haemochromatosis
- Wilson's disease (hepatolenticular degeneration)

Others
- Cryptogenic cirrhosis
- Riedel's lobe

HISTORY

Hepatitis/infection
Contact with hepatitis. Blood transfusion. Drug abuse. Homosexuals. Haemophiliacs. Health workers. The institutionalised, e.g. homes, prison. Travel abroad. Amoebiasis – worldwide. Hepatitis B – tropics and Mediterranean areas. Hydatid disease – sheep-rearing countries, e.g. Australia, Africa, Wales. Leptospirosis – swimming in rat-infested waters. History of alcohol abuse. Chronic active hepatitis – history of alcohol, hepatitis B or hepatitis C. In the majority of hepatitis/infection cases, the patient presents with general malaise, pyrexia, weight loss and jaundice.

Congestion
History of congestive cardiac failure. The patient often complains of upper abdominal pain caused by a tender liver due to stretching of the liver capsule. With constrictive pericarditis there is often a history of TB but it may follow any cause of pericarditis, e.g. acute renal failure. Budd–Chiari syndrome is hepatic vein thrombosis. A history of taking the contraceptive pill may be contributory. Tumour may also cause Budd–Chiari syndrome. It presents insidiously with portal hypertension, jaundice and cirrhosis.

Infiltration
There is usually a history of alcohol abuse with fatty infiltration. Secondary amyloidosis follows chronic infection, e.g. rheumatoid arthritis, bronchiectasis, inflammatory bowel disease.

Biliary tract disease
There may be a history of biliary tract obstruction, e.g. carcinoma of the pancreas or stricture of the common bile duct. Sclerosing cholangitis causes jaundice and fevers and is associated with inflammatory bowel disease. Primary biliary cirrhosis is of unknown aetiology. Ninety per cent of the patients are female. It presents with obstructive jaundice, pruritus and hepatosplenomegaly. The patient will complain of dark urine and pale stools.

Malignancy
The chief cause is metastases from a known malignancy, which may have been treated, e.g. gastrointestinal tract or bronchus.

Hepatoma is rare. With hepatoma there may be a past history of hepatitis B infection, use of the contraceptive pill, aflatoxin exposure, or use of anabolic steroids. Myeloproliferative disease presents with tiredness, lethargy and spontaneous bruising.

Metabolic

Glycogen storage disease is rare. There is usually hepatomegaly from birth. The early features of haemochromatosis include fatigue, arthralgia and hepatomegaly. Skin pigmentation, diabetes and cardiac failure occur later.

Others

Cryptogenic cirrhosis presents with hepatomegaly without an obvious cause. Riedel's lobe is usually an incidental finding and asymptomatic. Riedel's lobe is an extension of the right lobe of the liver below the costal margin. It is a normal anatomical variation.

EXAMINATION

Remember that a liver edge that is palpable is not always enlarged and may have been pushed down by pulmonary hyperinflation, e.g. emphysema. The upper border of the liver should therefore be identified by percussion and is usually at the level of the eighth rib in the midaxillary line. The edge of the liver can be sharp or rounded and its surface smooth or nodular.

Regular generalised enlargement without jaundice
Cirrhosis
Congestive cardiac failure
Reticulosis
Budd–Chiari syndrome
Amyloid.

Regular generalised enlargement with jaundice
Viral hepatitis
Biliary tract obstruction
Cholangitis.

Irregular generalised enlargement without jaundice
Secondary tumours
Macronodular cirrhosis
Polycystic disease of the liver
Primary tumours.

Irregular generalised enlargement with jaundice
Cirrhosis
Widespread liver secondaries.

Localised swellings
Riedel's lobe
Hydatid disease
Amoebic abscess
Primary carcinoma.

General

Carry out a general examination of the patient. Look for signs
of liver failure: jaundice, flapping tremor, ascites, spider naevi,
liver palms, clubbing, gynaecomastia, testicular atrophy, caput
medusae, peripheral oedema, leuconychia, Dupuytren's
contracture, xanthoma, mental changes, coma, bruising. Look
for Kayser–Fleischer rings (Wilson's disease).

Congestion
Signs of CCF. Peripheral oedema. Tense tender liver. JVP ↑. With
Budd–Chiari syndrome there will be acute ascites and right upper
quadrant pain. In constrictive pericarditis there will be right heart
failure associated with ascites. The JVP rises paradoxically with
inspiration. Pulsus paradoxus. Hypotension.

Biliary tract disease
Deep jaundice. There may be a palpable mass associated with
the primary malignancy. The gall bladder may be palpable
with carcinoma of the head of the pancreas (Courvoisier's law).
With primary biliary cirrhosis there will be clubbing, xanthomata,
arthralgia, hirsutism, portal hypertension and skin pigmentation.

Storage disease
With haemochromatosis there will be signs of portal hypertension
and skin pigmentation.

Malignancy
Jaundice and ascites may be present. There may be an abdominal
mass representing the primary malignancy. With myeloproliferative
disorders, in addition to hepatomegaly, there will be splenomegaly
and lymphadenopathy.

GENERAL INVESTIGATIONS

- **FBC, ESR**
  Hb ↓ malignancy, myeloproliferative disorders. WCC ↑ infection,
  leukaemia. Platelets ↓ leukaemia. ESR ↑ infection and
  malignancy.
- **U&Es**
  Creatinine. Often deranged in liver failure. Renal failure may
  occur with amyloidosis.
- **LFTs**
  Liver enzymes deranged in hepatitis. Alkaline phosphatase
  grossly raised in obstruction. The pattern varies according to
  the cause of hepatomegaly.
- **Clotting screen**
  PT ↑ absence of clotting factors.
- **Hepatitis serology**
  Raised according to cause.

SPECIFIC INVESTIGATIONS

- **Serum iron, TIBC and serum ferritin**
  Abnormal in haemochromatosis.
- **Blood, urine, CSF culture**
  Positive in leptospirosis.
- **Antibody screen**
  Antimicrosomal antibodies raised in primary biliary cirrhosis.
- **Bone marrow aspiration**
  Myelofibrosis. Leukaemia.
- **US**
  Cirrhosis. Secondaries. Amoebic abscess. Hydatid cyst. Riedel's
  lobe.
- **CT**
  Pancreatic lesions. Cirrhosis. Liver cysts.
- **MRCP**
  Ductal abnormalities e.g. stricture, stone.
- **Liver biopsy**
  Establish cause, e.g. malignancy, amyloid.

▶ HICCUPS

Hiccups are the characteristic sounds produced by the involuntary contractions of the diaphragm terminated by sudden closure of the glottis. In the majority, it is a self-limiting condition. The most common cause of hiccups is thought to be gastric distension after rapid ingestion of food, fluid or air. The causes of intractable hiccups are listed below.

CAUSES

Phrenic nerve irritation
- Oesophageal carcinoma
- Lung tumour
- Thoracic surgery

Diaphragmatic irritation
- Lower lobe pneumonia
- Empyema
- Subphrenic abscess
- Diaphragmatic hernia
- Gastric distension

CNS conditions
- Encephalitis
- Meningitis
- Tumours
- Intracranial haemorrhage
- Brainstem stroke

Others
- Hysterical
- Uraemic
- Toxic

HISTORY

The causes of hiccups predominantly originate in the respiratory, abdominal and nervous systems, therefore the history is structured similarly.

Respiratory history

The presence of cough with purulent sputum production implies respiratory tract infection. However, patients with pneumonia tend to be more unwell and may complain of rigors with high temperatures. Following pneumonia or thoracic surgery, chronic pyrexia and pleuritic chest pains with failure of resolution of symptoms of the original infection may herald the onset of an empyema. Hiccups may (rarely) complicate routine thoracic surgery. When a chronic cough is associated with haemoptysis and weight loss in a smoker, bronchial tumour is the most likely diagnosis.

Abdominal history

Symptoms of rapid progressive painless dysphagia (page 111) may be due to oesophageal carcinoma. At birth, a diaphragmatic hernia may present with respiratory distress; adults with diaphragmatic hernias may, however, be completely asymptomatic, the hernia being detected incidentally on a chest X-ray. Unremitting pyrexia and malaise in patients after abdominal surgery, or following localised inflammatory conditions such as appendicitis and cholecystitis, may have developed an intra-abdominal abscess. The subphrenic region is the most common site of a collection of pus. This is associated with intractable hiccups and pain referred to the shoulder, scapula or neck. A pleural effusion may be an accompanying feature.

Neurological history

Pyrexia, headache, photophobia and neck stiffness are associated with meningitis. Patients with encephalitis tend to present with confusion, alterations in consciousness and seizures. The brainstem is a very anatomically complex structure, therefore symptoms of infarction or tumour may be very variable, depending on distribution of involvement of the lower cranial nerves. The presenting features may be diplopia, difficulty swallowing, dysarthria and facial sensory loss. Cortical lesions arising from infarction or haemorrhage may present with aphasia, visual field defects and hemiplegia. The principal differentiating feature between infarction and tumour is the speed of onset; in general, stroke presents suddenly and tumours progressively.

Others

Amelioration of hiccups by sleep, bizarre accompanying symptoms and inconsistencies in the history are suggestive of hysterical hiccups. Uraemia may be responsible for hiccups.

EXAMINATION

A substantial number of causes of intractable hiccups are associated with pyrexia. High swinging fevers are suggestive of collections of pus, such as empyema and subphrenic abscesses.

An abdominal examination should be performed. Areas of tenderness may suggest appendicitis or cholecystitis as a predisposing cause for a subphrenic abscess. More specifically, an abdominal abscess may point to the skin surface, or present with tenderness over the lower chest wall.

Respiratory examination may reveal tracheal deviation with a large empyema or pleural effusion from carcinoma. Areas of percussion dullness correspond to consolidation, effusion and empyema. A large diaphragmatic hernia may elevate the diaphragm sufficiently to produces clinical signs suggestive of an effusion. Localised coarse crepitations may be auscultated, corresponding to areas of consolidation by pneumonia. Vocal resonance is increased with consolidation but attenuated with effusion and empyema.

A neurological examination is performed to identify the presence of and define the anatomical territory of any deficit. Specialised tests should be performed for meningitis. This will include Kernig's sign (pain on extension of the knee from a flexed hip and knee position) and Brudzinski's sign (flexion of the neck produces flexion of the hip and knee).

GENERAL INVESTIGATIONS

In the absence of features in the history to guide specific investigations, the following general investigations should be performed.

- **FBC**
  WCC ↑ with infection, malignancy.
- **ESR**
  ↑ infection, malignancy.
- **U&Es**
  ↑ urea, ↑ creatinine with renal failure.
- **CXR**
  Peripheral shadow or cavitation, hilar mass, collapse of a lobe may suggest carcinoma. Consolidation is seen with pneumonia. Fluid with a meniscus may be due to empyema, effusion from malignancy, or as a result of a subphrenic abscess. Elevation of a hemidiaphragm may be due to phrenic nerve palsy from carcinomatous infiltration or apparent elevation due to the presence of a diaphragmatic hernia.

SPECIFIC INVESTIGATIONS

- **Upper GI endoscopy and biopsy**
  Oesophageal carcinoma.
- **Bronchoscopy and mediastinoscopy**
  Biopsy for bronchial carcinoma.
- **CT thorax**
  Biopsy for bronchial carcinoma, definition and identification of loculations with empyema.
- **US abdomen**
  Subphrenic abscess; aspiration and drainage may also be performed.
- **CT/MRI head**
  Infarction and tumour may be appreciated as low-density areas. Mass effects may be produced by tumour or bleeding causing midline shifts. Intracranial bleeding may be identified as a high-density area. Cortical swelling may be seen with encephalitis. Raised intracranial pressure can be identified and is a contraindication to lumbar puncture.
- **EEG**
  Encephalitis – periodic complex formation and slowing of the background rhythm.
- **Lumbar puncture**
  Meningitis. Encephalitis – high lymphocyte count as the majority are due to viral aetiology.

▶ HIRSUTISM

Hirsutism is the presence of male-pattern hair growth in women. This is not synonymous with virilism, which, in addition to hirsutism, is associated with the development of male secondary sexual characteristics in women. Hypertrichosis refers to the excessive growth of hair and may occur in either sex.

CAUSES

Physiological
- Familial
- Senility

Pathological

Drugs
- Progestogens
- Testosterone
- Cyclosporin
- Antiepileptic drugs, e.g. phenytoin
- Minoxidil

Pituitary
- Prolactinoma
- Acromegaly

Ovarian
- Polycystic ovarian syndrome
- Androgen-producing ovarian tumour

Adrenal
- Cushing's syndrome
- Androgen-producing adrenal tumours
- Congenital adrenal hyperplasia

HISTORY

General
The onset and duration of hirsutism are useful features in the history to help determine the aetiology. Onset in childhood is suggestive of congenital adrenal hyperplasia, whereas sudden onset of hirsutism in adult females raises concerns of androgen-producing tumours of the ovaries or adrenal glands. Enquiries

should be undertaken as to whether any relatives have similar problems as the aetiology may be familial. However, beware of family cancer syndromes, such as BRCA gene mutation, which is associated with familial ovarian carcinoma. Excessive androgens may result in virilisation, producing symptoms such as acne and deepening of the voice.

Menstrual history

A detailed history regarding the onset, periodicity and regularity of the menstrual cycle should be taken, as amenorrhoea is a feature of polycystic ovarian syndrome, congenital adrenal hyperplasia and prolactinomas. In addition, galactorrhoea may also be an accompanying feature of prolactinomas.

Drug history

A drug history may identify the use of progestogen-containing hormone replacement therapy or oral contraceptive pills. Hirsutism may also result as a side-effect of anabolic steroid use by body builders; phenytoin for epilepsy; minoxidil for hypertension; and cyclosporin as an immunosuppressive agent in organ transplantation.

Associated symptoms

Weight gain may result from Cushing's syndrome, but is also a common complaint with polycystic orvarian syndrome. Symptoms such as headaches, vomiting and visual field loss is suggestive of a pituitary adenoma, which can result in acromegaly, Cushing's disease or hyperprolactinaemia (prolacintoma). Additional symptoms that may accompany Cushing's disease are easy bruising of the skin, abdominal striae and proximal muscle weakness. Patients with acromegaly may also complain of muscle weakness, joint pains, enlarging features of the face, jaw, hands and feet, with corresponding increases in hat, glove and shoe sizes. Paraesthesia may also result as a consequence of entrapment neuropathies. Infertility may result from hyperprolactinaemia and polycystic ovarian syndrome.

EXAMINATION

An assessment should be made regarding the pattern of hair distribution. With a degree of normal variation, the distribution of hair growth with hirsutism is on the face, chin, chest and extremities. The pubic hair may adopt a male pattern, and male type frontal balding can also be present. Careful inspection for virilism may identify increased shoulder-girdle muscle mass and enlargement of the clitoris. Truncal obesity is a feature of Cushing's syndrome, and generalised obesity occurs with polycystic ovarian syndrome. This may also be accompanied by acanthosis nigricans.

Inspection is then continued to identify coexisting endocrine disease. Features of acromegaly are thick greasy skin, prominent supraorbital ridging, broad nose, prognathism, tongue enlargement, poor jaw occlusion, wide interdental separation, enlarged hands and feet. Features of Cushing's syndrome are moon-like facies, truncal obesity, buffalo hump, skin bruising, striae and proximal muscle weakness. Hypertension, diabetes and visual field defects (bitemporal hemianopia) are associated with both Cushing's disease and acromegaly. In addition, visual field defects may also result from a prolactinoma. Hypertension is also associated with congenital adrenal hyperplasia.

Following this, an abdominal and pelvic examination should be performed to exclude a mass, which may be suggestive of a large adrenal or ovarian tumour.

GENERAL INVESTIGATIONS

- **Urine dipstick**
  The presence of glucose may be due to diabetes, which is a feature of Cushing's syndrome and acromegaly. In addition, polycystic ovarian disease is also associated with insulin resistance.
- **U&Es**
  ↓ sodium and ↓ potassium with salt-losing congenital adrenal hyperplasia.
- **Serum glucose**
  Diabetes or insulin resistance with Cushing's syndrome, acromegaly and polycystic ovarian disease.
- **Serum testosterone and DHEA**
  ↑↑ suggests an excess of androgens from a neoplastic origin and warrants detailed investigation.

SPECIFIC INVESTIGATIONS

- **24-hour free urinary cortisol**
  ↑ with Cushing's syndrome.
- **Low-dose dexamethasone suppression test**
  Failure of suppression occurs with Cushing's syndrome.

- **Oral glucose tolerance test with serial growth hormone estimations**
  Failure of suppression or increasing growth hormone concentrations occur with acromegaly.
- **IGF-1**
  ↑ with acromegaly.
- **Plasma prolactin**
  ↑ with prolactinomas.
- **Plasma 17-hydroxyprogesterone**
  ↑ with congenital adrenal hyperplasia.
- **CA 125**
  ↑ with ovarian carcinoma.
- **US abdomen and pelvis**
  Polycystic ovaries, ovarian carcinoma.
- **CT abdomen and pelvis**
  Adrenal carcinoma, ovarian carcinoma.
- **CT head**
  Pituitary tumour.

▶ HYPERTENSION

Hypertension is the elevation of blood pressure. An individual is classified as hypertensive when there is a sustained rise in blood pressure to more than 140/90 mmHg on three or more readings, each at least a week apart. Most patients have essential hypertension and an underlying cause is identified in less than 10%.

CAUSES

Renal
- Renal parenchymal diseases, e.g. glomerulonephritis
- Renal artery stenosis
- Chronic pyelonephritis
- Polycystic kidney disease
- Connective tissue disease (especially systemic sclerosis)
- Diabetic nephropathy

Endocrine
- Adrenal
  - Conn's syndrome
  - Phaeocromocytoma
- Cushing's syndrome
- Acromegaly

Drugs
- Oestrogen-containing oral contraceptives
- Glucocorticoids – corticosteroids
- Mineralocorticoids – liquorice
- Monoamine oxidase inhibitors and tyramine
- Sympathetomimetics – nebulised salbutamol

Cardiovascular
- Coarctation of the aorta

HISTORY

Patients with uncomplicated essential hypertension are asymptomatic and are identified only in the course of routine physical examination; however, patients with secondary hypertension may complain of symptoms from the underlying disorder.

Patients with chronic pyelonephritis may have experienced recurrent urinary tract infections, with loin pain, pyrexia and rigors, or have a history of childhood urinary tract infections or prolonged enuresis. Hypertension can also complicate glomerular disease; in particular it is associated with acute nephritic syndrome. Patients with nephritic syndrome may have experienced an acute illness with fatigue, malaise, haematuria, oliguria and oedema.

With Conn's syndrome, patients may complain of muscle weakness and fatigue due to hypokalaemia and polyuria from impaired urine-concentrating ability. Paroxysms of headache, sweating, palpitations with flushing may be experienced by patients with phaeochromocytoma. Classically these patients have attacks of hypertension; however, in the majority the hypertension is sustained.

Weight gain, hair growth, acne, abdominal striae, muscle weakness, back pain and depression may be some of the symptoms experienced by patients with Cushing's syndrome. With acromegaly, patients may complain of headaches, galactorrhoea, deepening of the voice, muscle weakness and joint pains. Hats and rings may no longer fit due to increasing size of the cranium and hands.

A complete drug history will identify offending drugs that may precipitate hypertension.

EXAMINATION

Inspection

On inspection, patients with acromegaly may have thick greasy skin, large hands, feet and tongue. Prominent supraorbital ridging with a large nose and protruding jaw accompanied by interdental separation may be noted on close inspection of the face and teeth. Confrontational testing of the visual fields may reveal bitemporal hemianopia, which may also be present with Cushing's syndrome owing to compression of the optic chiasma by a pituitary adenoma. Additional features of Cushing's disease include truncal obesity, acne, moon-like facies, bruising, striae, kyphosis and proximal muscle weakness.

Palpation and auscultation

In coarctation of the aorta, radiofemoral delay may be appreciated with simultaneous palpation of the radial and femoral arteries;

bruits may be auscultated across collateral blood vessels along the axilla, chest wall and scapula. A systolic bruit may also be auscultated over the fourth left posterior intercostal space. Wide discrepancy of measured blood pressure may exist between the arm and leg.

Palpation of the abdomen may reveal bilateral ballotable masses due to enlarged polycystic kidneys, and bruits may be auscultated over stenosed renal arteries.

GENERAL INVESTIGATIONS

- **Urinalysis**
  Dipstick may indicate the presence of blood and protein. Urine microscopy is necessary to confirm the presence of red blood cells and also casts.
- **U&Es**
  Levels of serum potassium may be reduced with Conn's syndrome due to hyperaldosteronism. High levels of creatinine and urea are found with renal failure.
- **Blood glucose**
  Atherosclerosis, renal vascular disease and nephropathy may be associated with diabetes. All of these may contribute to hypertension. Moreover conditions such as Cushing's syndrome, acromegaly and phaeochromocytoma are associated with hyperglycaemia.
- **Serum cholesterol**
  Serum cholesterol estimation is used as a screening for risk factors for atherosclerosis, and therapy may be initiated for the prevention of cerebrovascular and ischaemic heart disease.
- **ECG**
  A 12-lead ECG is recommended for all patients to provide a baseline and screen for left ventricular hypertrophy which may result as a complication of hypertension.

SPECIFIC INVESTIGATIONS

- **Autoantibodies**
  Anti-GBM and ANCA may be positive with glomerulonephritis.
- **Plasma catecholamines**
  Elevated in phaeochromocytoma.

- **Urinary catecholamines, metanephrines and vanillylmandelic acid**
  Elevated in phaeochromocytoma.
- **24-hour urinary free cortisol**
  Excess cortisol in Cushing's syndrome.
- **Low-dose dexamethasone suppression test**
  Failure of suppression of cortisol occurs in Cushing's syndrome.
- **Oral glucose tolerance test**
  Failure of suppression of serum growth hormone occurs in acromegalics.
- **Plasma renin and aldosterone**
  Hypersecretion of aldosterone in the presence of low plasma renin levels confirms autonomous secretion in Conn's syndrome.
- **US abdomen**
  Polycystic kidneys. Duplex Doppler can screen for renal artery stenosis.
- **Renal angiography**
  Renal artery stenosis.
- **Renal biopsy**
  Renal causes of hypertension.
- **MRI**
  This is increasingly useful in the diagnosis of renal artery stenosis and avoids the need for potentially nephrotoxic radiocontrast administration.
- **Cardiac catheterisation**
  Coarctation of the aorta.

▶ IMPOTENCE

Impotence is failure in the adult male to sustain an adequate erection for vaginal penetration. Impotence leads to psychological problems, often with marital breakdown. Psychological causes of impotence are common but the most common organic disease is diabetes mellitus.

CAUSES

Vascular
- Aortoiliac disease (Leriche's syndrome)
- Diabetic vascular disease

Neurological
- Spina bifida
- Spinal lesions
- Neuropathies, e.g. diabetes
- Pelvic surgery (damage to nervi erigentes)

Endocrine
- Diabetes mellitus
- Hypogonadism
- Hypothyroidism
- Addison's disease
- Cushing's syndrome

Drugs
- Antihypertensives
- Antidepressants
- Oestrogens
- Alcohol
- Cocaine

Local painful conditions
- Phimosis
- Peyronie's disease
- Short frenulum

Systemic disease
- Malignancy
- Chronic renal failure
- Cirrhosis

Psychogenic

HISTORY

Is there a clear history of stress to account for the onset of impotence? Does the patient experience erections at any time, especially during the night? History of peripheral vascular disease, especially buttock claudication (Leriche's syndrome). History of neurological disease. Take a full drugs history, including any recreational drugs. Check for a history of diabetes, hypothyroidism, Addison's disease or Cushing's disease. Pelvic surgery, e.g. abdominoperineal resection of the rectum with damage to the nervi erigentes. Check for any local, painful conditions of the penis. History of malignant disease. History of chronic renal failure: nausea, lethargy, nocturia, peripheral oedema, pulmonary oedema, dyspnoea, vomiting, hiccups, convulsions.

EXAMINATION

Vascular
Check all the pulses in the lower limb. Listen for bruits in the abdomen and pelvis.

Neurological
Carry out a full neurological examination.

Endocrine
There will usually be a clear history of diabetes. Complications may be apparent. Check for peripheral neuropathy. Check for hypothyroidism – weight gain, dislike of cold weather, hoarse voice, lethargy, constipation. Check for Cushing's syndrome – thin skin, cushingoid facies, abdominal striae, obesity, buffalo hump, hypertension. Check for Addison's disease – weakness, weight loss, pigmentation of palmar creases and buccal mucosa, hypotension. Examine the testes for hypogonadism. Check for development of male secondary sexual characteristics.

Local painful conditions
Examine the penis for phimosis, Peyronie's disease or short frenulum.

Systemic disease
Malignant disease may be obvious. Check for chronic renal failure: pallor of skin, peripheral oedema, pericarditis, pleural effusions, hypertension. Check for cirrhosis, liver palms, spider naevi, ascites, leuconychia, flapping tremor, testicular atrophy, Dupuytren's contracture.

GENERAL INVESTIGATIONS

History and examination suggests the diagnosis in most cases.

- **FBC, ESR**

  Hb ↓ anaemia, e.g. chronic renal failure and malignancy. ESR ↑ malignancy.

- **U&Es**

  Creatinine raised in chronic renal failure.

- **LFTs**

  Abnormal in cirrhosis.

- **Blood glucose**

  Diabetes.

- **TFTs**

  Hypothyroidism.

- **Doppler studies**

  Peripheral vascular disease. Penile–brachial pressure index <0.6 suggests a vascular cause.

SPECIFIC INVESTIGATIONS

- **Nocturnal penile tumescence study**

  Erection versus no erection.

- **Intracorporeal injection of papaverine**

  If no abnormality of arterial inflow, this should cause an erection. If there is excessive venous leakage the penis remains flaccid.

- **Skull X-ray**

  Pituitary abnormality.

- **CT head**

  Pituitary abnormality.

- **Arteriography**

  May show vascular lesion, especially isolated narrowings of the internal iliac arteries.

- **Serum prolactin**

  Hypoprolactinaemia.

- **Serum testosterone**

  Low in hypogonadism.

- **Serum FSH and LH**

  Low in pituitary dysfunction.

- **ACTH stimulation test**
  Addison's disease.
- **Urinary cortisol assay**
  Cushing's syndrome.
- **Plasma cortisol**
  Cushing's syndrome.

▶ INTESTINAL OBSTRUCTION

Mechanical obstruction of the bowel may be simple (one-point obstruction) or closed loop (obstruction at two points enclosing a segment of bowel). If the bowel is viable the obstruction is termed non-strangulating. If the arterial blood supply is compromised, strangulating obstruction occurs with subsequent infarction of the bowel. Intestinal obstruction is a common surgical emergency.

CAUSES

Small bowel

In the lumen
- Gallstone ileus
- Food bolus (after pylorus-destroying or bypass surgery)

In the wall
- Atresia
- Crohn's disease
- TB
- Tumour, e.g. lymphoma, carcinoma (rare)

Outside the wall
- Hernia
- Adhesions
- Volvulus
- Intussusception

Large bowel

In the lumen
- Faeces

In the wall
- Carcinoma
- Diverticular disease
- Crohn's disease
- Hirschsprung's disease

Outside the wall
- Volvulus
- Hernia
- Adhesions

Adynamic obstruction (paralytic Ileus)

- Peritonitis
- Postoperative
- Spinal and pelvic fractures
- Retroperitoneal haemorrhage
- Retroperitoneal malignancy
- Hypokalaemia
- Drugs, e.g. ganglion blockers, anticholinergics
- Immobilisation

HISTORY

Small bowel

Central abdominal colicky pain. Vomiting – food, bile, faeculent, depending upon the level of obstruction. Distension – degree depends on level of obstruction. There may be very little distension with high small bowel obstruction. It may be gross with low small bowel obstruction. Constipation. There may be a history of abdominal surgery to suggest adhesive obstruction. The patient may be aware of a hernia.

Large bowel

Central (right colon to two thirds of the way along the transverse colon) or lower abdominal colicky pain (remainder of the colon). Constipation. Vomiting is a late feature with large bowel obstruction. Abdominal distension. There may be a previous history of change in bowel habit and bleeding PR to suggest carcinoma. A long history of constipation (years) and abdominal distension suggest Hirschsprung's disease. Development of a constant severe pain suggests infarction.

Adynamic obstruction

Carefully check the drug history. Patients on anticoagulants may have retroperitoneal haemorrhage. Precipitating cause may be obvious, e.g. recent surgery or spinal fracture. The abdominal distension may be painless but uncomfortable. Vomiting, constipation. The elderly immobilised in bed are especially vulnerable.

EXAMINATION

Small bowel

Observe for scars. Exclude obstructed incisional hernia. Check hernial orifices. It is easy to miss a small femoral hernia in an obese patient. Distended tympanitic abdomen usually non-tender. High-pitched tinkling obstructed bowel sounds. Pyrexia, tachycardia and localised tenderness suggest impending infarction. A palpable mass in the right iliac fossa may suggest Crohn's disease or caecal carcinoma (obstructing the ileocaecal valve and causing small bowel obstruction). Carry out a digital rectal examination.

Large bowel

Distended tympanitic abdomen, which may be very tense. Obstructed bowel sounds. Rectum may be empty on examination PR unless obstruction is due to faecal impaction. A mass may be palpable to suggest an obstructing carcinoma. A palpable, tense, tender caecum suggests closed loop obstruction with a competent ileocaecal valve. Caecal perforation may be imminent.

Adynamic obstruction

Abdominal distension. Tense tympanitic abdomen. Absent bowel sounds. Evidence of previous surgery, trauma, retroperitoneal haemorrhage and peritonitis, fractures.

GENERAL INVESTIGATIONS

- **Hb, FBC**
  Hb $\downarrow$ malignancy. WCC $\uparrow$ infection, infarcted bowel.
- **U&Es and creatinine**
  Dehydration. Hypokalaemia leading to paralytic ileus.
- **Clotting screen**
  May be abnormal with retroperitoneal haemorrhage, especially if patient on anticoagulants.
- **AXR**
  Distended loops of bowel in central abdomen. Proximal small bowel shows lines closely together crossing completely the lumen of the bowel (valvulae conniventes). These get progressively further apart until there are none seen in the terminal ileum. Gas in the biliary tree (gallstone ileus). Large bowel obstruction – distended bowel with air–fluid levels at the periphery of the abdomen. Sigmoid volvulus – distended loop of bowel, the shape of a 'coffee bean', arising out of the pelvis on the left side.
- **Sigmoidoscopy**
  Tumour at rectosigmoid. Sigmoid volvulus may be decompressed by careful insertion of sigmoidoscope. Biopsy – carcinoma, absence of ganglion cells in Hirschsprung's disease.

SPECIFIC INVESTIGATIONS

- **Barium enema**
  Limited barium enema may show 'apple core' lesion of carcinoma. 'Bird's beak' sign of sigmoid volvulus. Intussusception.
- **Small bowel enema**
  Crohn's disease. TB of the terminal ileum. Small bowel carcinoma.
- **CT**
  Retroperitoneal haemorrhage. Retroperitoneal tumour.

▶ JAUNDICE

Jaundice is yellow discoloration of the tissues, noticed especially in the skin and sclera, due to accumulation of bilirubin. For jaundice to be clinically apparent the circulating bilirubin levels should be in excess of 35 μmol/l. Jaundice may be prehepatic (due to haemolysis), hepatic (due to intrinsic liver disease) or cholestatic (due to either intrahepatic cholestasis or posthepatic biliary tract obstruction).

CAUSES

Prehepatic (unconjugated hyperbilirubinaemia)

Congenital defects
- Gilbert's disease
- Crigler–Najjar syndrome

Haemolysis
Congenital red cell defects
- Hereditary spherocytosis (congenital acholuric jaundice)
- Sickle cell disease
- G6PD deficiency
- Thalassaemia
Acquired
- Malaria
- Incompatible blood transfusion
- Autoimmune
- Haemolytic disease of the newborn
- Absorbing large haematoma
- Hypersplenism

Hepatic

Acute hepatocellular disease
- Viral hepatitis
  - Hepatitis A, B, C
  - Epstein–Barr virus
  - CMV
- Other infections
  - Leptospirosis
- Drugs, e.g. paracetamol, halothane
- Toxins, e.g. carbon tetrachloride
- Autoimmune

Chronic hepatocellular disease
- Chronic viral hepatitis
- Chronic autoimmune hepatitis
- End-stage liver disease
  - Alcohol
  - Cirrhosis
  - Haemochromatosis
  - Wilson's disease

Cholestatic

Intrahepatic
- Drugs, e.g. chlorpromazine
- Total parenteral nutrition (TPN)
- Primary biliary cirrhosis
- Viral hepatitis
- Pregnancy

Extrahepatic (obstructive)
In the lumen
- Gallstones
- Infestation
  - Clonorchiasis (liver fluke)
  - Schistosomiasis
In the wall
- Congenital biliary atresia
- Cholangiocarcinoma
- Stricture, e.g. inflammatory, postoperative
- Cholangitis
- Sclerosing cholangitis
- Choledochal cyst
Outside the wall
- Carcinoma of the head of the pancreas
- Carcinoma of the ampulla of Vater
- Malignant nodes in the porta hepatis
- Chronic pancreatitis
- Mirizzi syndrome

HISTORY

General

Fever, malaise, weight loss, dark urine, pale stools, itching.

Newborn

Biliary atresia presents as deepening jaundice within 2–3 days of birth. Liver failure develops over 3–6 months. Physiological jaundice is common and is due to immaturity of liver function. It usually settles within the first week of life.

Prehepatic

Ask about family history, racial origin, drugs, haematuria, history of anaemia. Gilbert's disease is inherited as an autosomal dominant. There is a failure of uptake of unconjugated bilirubin by the hepatocyte. Crigler–Najjar syndrome is a failure of conjugation within the hepatocyte.

Hepatocellular

Occupation. Contact with jaundice. Travel. Alcohol. Sexual activity. Drugs (tablets, injections, anaesthetic agents, drug abuse). Exposure to industrial solvents. Previous episodes of jaundice. Infection. Influenza-like symptoms. Rashes. Joint pains. Blood transfusions.

Cholestatic

Drugs, e.g. chlorpromazine. Travel abroad. Severe upper abdominal pain preceding jaundice (biliary colic followed by impaction of stone in common bile duct). Insidious onset of painless jaundice (malignancy). Dark urine, pale stools, itching.

EXAMINATION

Prehepatic (haemolytic)

Often the jaundice is not intense, with only a mild lemon tinge. Anaemia. Splenomegaly.

Hepatic

Tender liver in hepatitis. Signs of liver failure: spider naevi, palmar erythema, leuconychia, clubbing, gynaecomastia, testicular atrophy, ascites, peripheral oedema, bruising, Dupuytren's contracture, caput medusae, liver flap. Haematemesis may have occurred from bleeding oesophageal varices.

Cholestatic

Hepatomegaly – usually smooth liver with 'sharp' edge. Palpable gall bladder (Courvoiser's law – in the presence of obstructive jaundice if the gall bladder is palpable, the cause is unlikely to be due to gallstones). Epigastric mass, e.g. carcinoma of the pancreas. Other abdominal masses, e.g. carcinoma of the stomach and carcinoma of the colon with secondary deposits in the porta hepatis. Recent surgical scars. Scratch marks on abdomen from itching.

GENERAL INVESTIGATIONS

● **FBC, ESR, blood film**
  Hb ↓ malignancy, haemolysis. WCC ↑ infection, e.g. hepatitis, cholangitis. ESR ↑ infection, malignancy. Blood film – spherocytosis.
● **Reticulocyte count**
  Haemolysis.
● **U&Es**
  Deranged renal function with hepatorenal syndrome.
● **LFTs**
  See the table below.

Urine and blood biochemistry in jaundice

Biochemical parameter	Prehepatic	Hepatic	Cholestatic
Blood			
Bilirubin			
Unconjugated	↑	N/↑	N
Conjugated	N	N/↑	↑
Alkaline phosphatase	N	N/↑	↑↑
Transaminases	N	↑	N/↑
Urine			
Bilirubin	0	↑	↑
Urobilinogen	N/↑	↑	↓↓/0

N, normal; 0, no bilirubin present in urine.

● **Clotting screen**
  PT ↑.
● **Viral antibodies**
  Hepatitis A, hepatitis B, hepatitis C, CMV, Epstein–Barr virus.

- **US**
  Gallstones. Dilated biliary tree. Level of obstruction (may not show cause of obstruction). Hepatic secondaries. Cirrhosis.
- **ERCP**
  Periampullary carcinoma. Stones in common bile duct. Tumour of common bile duct. Stricture of common bile duct. Biopsy. Brush cytology. Stenting.
- **PTC**
  Undertaken if ERCP fails.
- **MRCP**
  Bile duct anomalies. Stones.
- **CT**
  Carcinoma of the head of the pancreas – assess spread and local resectability. Liver secondaries.
- **Liver biopsy**
  Hepatocellular disease. Carcinoma.

SPECIFIC INVESTIGATIONS

- **Serum copper**
  Reduced in Wilson's disease.
- **Serum ceruloplasmin**
  Reduced in Wilson's disease.
- **Serum α_1-antitrypsin**
  α_1-Antitrypsin deficiency.
- **Serum iron and TIBC**
  Iron raised in haemochromatosis. TIBC saturation >70%.
- **Leptospirosis complement fixation test**
  Leptospirosis.
- **Blood culture**
  Septicaemia. Leptospirosis.
- **Lumbar puncture**
  Leptospirosis.

JAW PAIN AND SWELLINGS

Pain and/or swelling of the jaw results most commonly from dental conditions. In the upper jaw, pain may also result from infection of the paranasal sinuses. The latter condition is considered under facial swellings (page 135).

CAUSES

Traumatic

Infective
- Dental abscess
- Acute osteomyelitis
- Actinomycosis

Temporomandibular joint
- Temporomandibular joint pain dysfunction syndrome
- Rheumatoid arthritis
- Osteoarthritis
- Dislocation

Cystic
- Dental cysts
- Dentigerous cysts

Neoplastic

Benign
- Giant cell granuloma

Locally invasive
- Ameloblastoma

Malignant
- Osteogenic sarcoma
- Burkitt's lymphoma
- Secondary deposits

Other
- Postherpetic neuralgia
- Referred pain (e.g. myocardial ischaemia)

HISTORY

Traumatic

History of trauma, e.g. fights, road traffic accidents. Fracture of the mandible is the most common.

Infective

Dental abscess presents with a dull ache in the jaw, becoming throbbing and severe. There is often accompanying malaise and loss of appetite. Previous history of dental caries. Acute osteomyelitis of the mandible is rare. It may follow dental infection or tooth extraction. There may be a history of fractures, irradiation, leukaemia, diabetes, malnutrition, alcoholism or immunosuppression.
There is a severe, throbbing deep-seated pain. The patient has difficulty opening the mouth and swallowing due to muscle oedema. Actinomycosis presents with swelling of the jaw with persistent low-grade infection.

Temporomandibular joint

Temporomandibular joint pain dysfunction syndrome results from grinding and clenching the teeth. The patient may have had a stress-related illness. Pain arises in the region of the temporomandibular joint or ear, which may be associated with a clicking noise and is aggravated by wide opening of the mouth, as with yawning and chewing. Rheumatoid arthritis of the temporomandibular joint is rare. Other signs and symptoms of rheumatoid arthritis are usually apparent. Osteoarthritis usually causes pain, swelling and limitation of jaw movement. Temporomandibular joint dislocation may be recurrent, habitual or isolated. The condyle is displaced forwards and upwards into the temporal fossa. The patient's mouth remains open and cannot be closed following yawning, tooth extraction or general anaesthesia. The condition may be unilateral or bilateral. The patient presents with an open mouth, which he or she cannot close, and pain due to muscle spasm.

Cystic

Cysts often present as asymptomatic lucencies on radiographs. Otherwise they present as painless swellings, which may reach a large size. If the cyst becomes infected the patient presents with pain, swelling and discharge. Occasionally pathological fractures occur. A dental cyst is attached to the root of a normally erupted but decayed tooth; the swelling grows slowly. Dentigerous cysts contain an unerupted tooth.

Neoplastic

The patient presents with a jaw swelling which grows steadily and often painlessly. Giant cell granuloma may erode through bone to produce a soft tissue purplish swelling on the gum. Ameloblastomas usually occur around the age of 30–50 years and are symptomless until the swelling becomes obtrusive. Osteogenic sarcoma of the jaw is extremely rare. Initially it is painless but becomes painful as it grows. Teeth may be loosened. The patient may complain of paraesthesia due to involvement of the mental nerve. Coughing may be a symptom if lung metastases have occurred. Burkitt's tumour is associated with EBV. It is a malignant tumour of B lymphocytes. It is endemic in certain parts of Africa and New Guinea. It affects most commonly children below the age of 12 years. The child presents with a progressive painless swelling of the jaw. Secondary deposits in the jaw are uncommon but may arise from lung, breast, thyroid, prostate or kidney.

Others

With postherpetic neuralgia there is usually a history of herpes zoster in the distribution of the trigeminal nerve. The pain tends to be distributed in a division of the trigeminal nerve. Pain may involve a large area of the face rather than just the region of the jaw. Referred pain to the jaw is common with angina. The patient usually complains of associated chest pain and radiation of the pain down the left arm.

EXAMINATION

Traumatic

Check for a normal bite. Bruising, swelling, crepitus, tenderness. Bloodstained saliva. Broken teeth. Step deformities in occlusion.

Infective

With dental abscesses there is reddening of the mucosa with a firm, hot, acutely tender, boggy swelling. The dental abscess may point on the outer side of the jaw. There may be associated dental caries and gingivitis. Cervical lymphadenopathy is usually present. With acute osteomyelitis there is usually difficulty in opening the mouth and swallowing due to muscle oedema. There is a tender, red, painful swelling overlying the mandible. In actinomycosis there may be multiple discharging sinuses, usually near the angle of the jaw, on which characteristic 'sulphur granules' may be seen discharging.

Temporomandibular joint

Diagnosis of temporomandibular joint dysfunction syndrome is usually made from the history. There is usually trismus and spasm around the joint. In rheumatoid arthritis there may be tenderness and swelling over the joint. In osteoarthritis there may be swelling over the joint and limitation of movement. In temporomandibular joint dislocation the condyles are palpable anterior to the articular eminence. The mouth is gagged open.

Cystic

Often the only abnormality on examination is a swelling in the bones. Sometimes the bone is so thin that it crackles when touched, like a broken eggshell. With dentigerous cysts the tooth remains unerupted and therefore a tooth will be missing when the teeth are counted.

Neoplastic

Often the only abnormality is a bony swelling, which grows steadily, initially without pain. With giant cell granuloma it may rarely erode through the bone to produce soft-tissue purplish swelling on the gum. Osteogenic sarcoma is initially painless but as it grows it may loosen the teeth. Check for loose teeth and paraesthesia in the distribution of the mental nerve. Examine the lung for metastases. With Burkitt's lymphoma there is progressive painless swelling. The eye may be displaced and the mouth partly occluded by the swelling. Secondary deposits often present as painful lesions within the bone. Check for a previous history of malignancy and check the lungs, breast, prostate, kidney and thyroid for the site of a primary.

Other

The diagnosis of postherpetic neuralgia is usually made on the history, as is referred pain from myocardial ischaemia.

GENERAL INVESTIGATIONS

- **FBC, ESR**
  Hb ↓ malignancy. WCC ↑ infection, leukaemia (acute osteomyelitis).
- **LFTs**
  Alcoholism (acute osteomyelitis commoner).
- **Blood glucose**
  Diabetes (acute osteomyelitis).

- **Swab**
  C&S. Dental infection. Actinomycosis.
- **Temporomandibular joint X-rays**
  Dislocation. Osteoarthritis. Rheumatoid arthritis.
- **Skull X-rays with special views**
  Fractures, cysts, tumours.
- **CXR**
  Secondary deposits.

SPECIAL INVESTIGATIONS

- **Blood cultures**
  Osteomyelitis.
- **ECG**
  Myocardial ischaemia.
- **EBV serology**
  Burkitt's lymphoma.
- **Biopsy**
  Benign versus malignant lesions.

▶ JOINT DISORDERS

Disorders of joints are common problems. They may be acute, as in gout or rheumatic fever, or chronic, as in osteoarthritis. Some acute disorders go on to become chronic, e.g. rheumatoid arthritis. The first part of this section deals with causes of arthropathy in general; the second part deals with disorders of specific joints. The list of causes of arthropathies is legion and only the more common ones will be mentioned.

CAUSES

Congenital

- Achondroplasia (dwarfism)
- Ehlers–Danlos syndrome
- Marfan's syndrome
- Osteogenesis imperfecta

Acquired

Infective
- Pyogenic arthritis
- Viral
- Rheumatic fever
- Endocarditis
- Brucellosis
- Typhoid
- Tuberculosis

Inflammatory
- Rheumatoid arthritis
- Psoriatic arthropathy
- Henoch–Schönlein disease
- Reiter's disease
- Ankylosing spondylitis
- Connective tissue disease
- Polymyalgia rheumatica

Degenerative
- Osteoarthritis

Enteropathic
- Acute gastrointestinal infections
- Inflammatory bowel disease
- Gastrointestinal bypass surgery

Endocrine
- Acromegaly

Metabolic
- Gout
- Haemochromatosis

Neuropathic
- Charcot's joints

Haematological
- Haemophilia
- Leukaemia
- Sickle cell disease

Drugs
- Anticoagulants
- Steroids

Neoplastic
- Hypertrophic pulmonary osteoarthropathy

Other
- Avascular necrosis of bone
- Sarcoidosis
- Behçet's disease (rare)

HISTORY

Congenital

Premature osteoarthritis may occur in achondroplasia. In Ehlers–Danlos syndrome there is a genetic disorder of connective tissue. Patients have hypermobile joints and hyperextensible skin. They may present with joint subluxations, dislocations and swellings due to effusions. They may also present with the bleeding complications of Ehlers–Danlos syndrome. In Marfan's syndrome generalised joint laxity occurs. Patients present with joint pain and swellings due to effusions. In osteogenesis imperfecta (brittle bones) bones fracture readily.

Acquired

Infective

Septic arthritis usually presents as a monoarthritis with a red, swollen, painful, immobile joint. Spread has usually occurred by the haematogenous route but may occur from adjacent osteomyelitis.

Organisms responsible include *Staphylococcus aureus*, gonococcus, *Brucella* and *Salmonella typhi*. With TB the patient usually presents with swelling and stiffness of the joint. It is not as red or hot as with acute septic arthritis. Patients who are on steroids or who are immunosuppressed are particularly at risk from infective arthritis. Viral arthritis may occur with rubella, mumps, hepatitis and certain enteroviruses. Rheumatic fever usually follows a streptococcal infection, e.g. scarlet fever or tonsillitis. There is a migratory polyarthritis together with carditis, erythematous skin lesions and subcutaneous nodules.

Inflammatory

Rheumatoid arthritis presents initially with swollen, painful, stiff hands and feet. Eventually characteristic hand deformities with swelling of the metacarpophalangeal joints, swan-neck and boutonnière deformities, and ulnar deviation occur. Large joints are also involved eventually. The patient may complain of extra-articular manifestations, i.e. rheumatoid nodules, vascular changes, eye changes or neuropathies. Psoriatic arthropathy usually follows several years after the skin lesions. Reiter's disease may present with arthritis in a single joint or a few joints. There will be a history of sexual contact, urethritis and conjunctivitis. Ankylosing spondylitis presents in young males and initially presents with morning stiffness in the spine. The sacroiliac joints are involved. Eventually bony ankylosis occurs with a fixed kyphotic spine. The patient may also complain of symptoms in the hip and knee. Arthritis may occur in SLE. Other manifestations may be present, e.g. cutaneous, pulmonary or renal. Polymyalgia rheumatica occurs in elderly women. There is aching and morning stiffness with a mild polyarthritis. Henoch–Schönlein purpura presents with a purpuric rash often over the buttocks and extensor surfaces. There may be associated nephritis and abdominal pain. Pain, swelling and stiffness in the joints, usually the ankles and knees, is transient and lasts only a few days.

Degenerative

Osteoarthritis usually occurs after the age of 50 years unless it is secondary to previous joint pathology. The patient complains of pain on movement, worse at the end of the day, together with stiffness, swelling and instability of joints.

Enteropathic

Check for a history of Crohn's disease or ulcerative colitis. There may also be a history of gastric bypass surgery. The spine or the peripheral joints may be affected.

Endocrine

Acromegaly will lead to arthralgia. The patient will usually complain of other symptoms, namely large hands, large feet (increase in shoe size), deepening of the voice.

Metabolic

Gout usually presents with severe pain, redness and swelling in the first metatarsophalangeal joint. It may affect other joints. There may be a history of polycythaemia, leukaemia or medication with cytotoxic or immunosuppressive drugs. With haemochromatosis the diagnosis will usually be apparent when the patient presents. There will be cirrhosis, diabetes, cardiomyopathy and skin pigmentation.

Neuropathic

The patient usually complains of swollen joints, which are unstable but painless. There may be a history of diabetes, tabes dorsalis (syphilis), syringomyelia or leprosy.

Haematological

Bleeding into joints (haemarthrosis) occurs in haemophilia. The history will be apparent. Eventually crippling arthropathy occurs. Pain in bones and joints may occur both in childhood and adult leukaemia. In sickle cell disease, painful crises may occur in bones and joints. Aseptic necrosis of bone may occur, leading to subsequent osteoarthritis.

Drugs

Anticoagulants may cause bleeds into joints. Steroids may lead to septic arthritis or avascular necrosis of bone with subsequent secondary osteoarthritis.

Neoplastic

Rarely a patient will present with direct infiltration of a joint with malignant disease. However, hypertrophic pulmonary osteoarthropathy is more common, occurring usually in association with bronchial carcinoma but it may occur in association with congenital heart disease.

Other

Avascular necrosis of bone may lead to secondary arthritis. The most common sites are the head of the femur, proximal scaphoid, talus and lunate. Check for a history of steroid drugs. Avascular necrosis of the scaphoid will follow scaphoid fractures, and avascular necrosis of the head of the femur may follow fractures of the neck of the femur or slipped upper femoral epiphysis. Arthralgia may occur in sarcoidosis. The patient presents with fever, malaise and lymphadenopathy. Behçet's disease may present with arthritis. Usually there are eye signs, mouth ulcers and genital ulcers. CNS involvement with meningoencephalitis may occur.

EXAMINATION

Congenital

Achondroplasia is obvious. In Ehlers–Danlos syndrome there will be hypermobile joints and hyperextensible skin. There may be evidence of dislocation or subluxation of joints. In Marfan's syndrome the patient will be tall with long extremities, long fingers (arachnodactyly), high-arched palate, lens dislocation and aortic incompetence. Diagnosis of osteogenesis imperfecta will usually be obvious. There is stunted growth due to repeated fractures with deformities. The patient has blue sclerae and often hypotonia.

Acquired

Infective

With infective arthritis there is usually a red, painful, swollen, tender joint which has virtually no active or passive movement. The patient will be pyrexial. Usually a single joint is involved. With viral infections there may be signs of childhood illnesses, e.g. mumps (swollen salivary glands), rubella (rash), hepatitis (jaundice). With rheumatic fever there will be carditis with changing murmurs, migratory polyarthritis, subcutaneous nodules, erythema marginatum and occasionally chorea (Sydenham's).

Inflammatory

With rheumatoid arthritis there will be swelling of the metacarpophalangeal joints. Swan-neck and boutonnière deformities will be apparent, as will ulnar deviation. There may be subluxation at the wrist. Tendon ruptures may occur. Eventually large joint involvement occurs and there may be atlantoaxial subluxation with myelopathy. General signs include anaemia, lymphadenopathy, splenomegaly, vasculitis and eye signs. With psoriatic arthropathy there is usually obvious psoriasis of the skin. Polyarthritis occurs but the sacroiliac joints are often affected. With Reiter's disease there may be urethritis, conjunctivitis, keratoderma blenorrhagica, circinate balanitis, plantar fasciitis and Achilles tendonitis. With ankylosing spondylitis there may be minimal signs initially, the first sign usually being reduced respiratory excursion, but eventually there will be involvement of the sacroiliac joints together with a fixed kyphotic spine and a hyperextended neck. SLE presents with malaise, arthralgia, myalgia, a butterfly rash on the face, Raynaud's syndrome, splenomegaly, pleurisy, pleural effusion, pericarditis. Polymyalgia rheumatica is associated with tender muscles, mild polyarthritis and there may be associated temporal arteritis.

Degenerative

Osteoarthritis usually involves the distal interphalangeal joints, the metacarpophalangeal joint of the thumb, the first metatarsophalangeal joint, the cervical spine, the lumbar spine, the hips and knees. There will be joint tenderness and thickening, limitation of movements, Heberden's nodes and often effusions into joints.

Enteropathic

There is normally spondyloarthritis with sacroiliitis. Large joint monoarthropathies and peripheral arthritis may occur.

Endocrine

With acromegaly there will be large hands and feet, a large tongue, prognathism, arthralgia, kyphosis, deep voice and heart failure. There may be signs of the pituitary tumour, i.e. bilateral hemianopia due to local pressure on the optic chiasma.

Metabolic

There is an acutely painful, red, swollen joint with gout. The first metatarsophalangeal joint is most often involved but any joint may be affected. There may be evidence of gouty tophi, e.g. pinna, tendons, joints. With haemochromatosis, in addition to arthropathy there may be evidence of hepatomegaly, cirrhosis, diabetes, cardiomyopathy and skin pigmentation.

Neuropathic

Deformed, painless joints with subluxation may occur. There is usually no warmth or tenderness in relation to the joint. Abnormal movements may occur. Neurological examination may reveal dorsal column signs. If the condition is due to syphilis (tabes dorsalis) there may be Argyll Robertson pupils.

Haematological

With haemophiliacs the patient will present with an acute, painful, immobile joint with an acute bleed. Eventually there will be deformed joints. Joints may be involved in leukaemia and acute sickle cell crises.

Drugs

Steroids may cause avascular necrosis, especially of the hips. There will be pain and limitation of movement. Osteoarthritis develops eventually. Patients on anticoagulants may have acute haemarthroses.

Neoplastic

Hypertrophic pulmonary osteoarthropathy usually occurs in association with bronchial carcinoma. The ends of long bones are affected by symmetrical but irregular widespread thickening. Clubbing usually occurs. Pain from local tumours is constant and may progress to a pathological fracture.

Other

With avascular necrosis of bone there is usually pain, tenderness and limitation of movement in relation to the avascular bone. Ultimately osteoarthritis develops. With sarcoidosis there is usually fever, lymphadenopathy, hepatosplenomegaly, eye signs, cardiac signs and CNS involvement. With Behçet's disease there will be arthritis, keratitis, uveitis, mouth ulcers, genital ulcers and occasionally CNS involvement.

GENERAL INVESTIGATIONS

- **FBC, ESR**
  Hb ↓ anaemia of chronic disease, e.g. rheumatoid arthritis, SLE. WCC ↑ infective causes. Leukaemia. ESR ↑ chronic infection, rheumatoid arthritis, ankylosing spondylitis, rheumatic fever.
- **CRP**
  ↑ infective causes ↑ inflammatory causes.
- **U&Es**
  Renal involvement, e.g. SLE.
- **LFTs**
  Hepatic involvement, e.g. haemochromatosis.
- **Serum uric acid**
  Gout.
- **Rheumatoid factor**
  Rheumatoid arthritis.
- **PSA**
  Prostatic carcinoma.
- **Sickling test**
  Sickle cell disease.
- **Joint X-ray**
  Osteoarthritis – loss of joint space, subchondral sclerosis and

cyst, osteophytes. Rheumatoid arthritis – soft-tissue thickening, juxta-articular thinning of bone, loss of joint space, erosion of bone, subluxations. Avascular necrosis – avascular bone is more dense than adjacent bone. Gout – soft-tissue swelling initially then 'punched-out' lesions in juxta-articular bone. Ankylosing spondylitis – bamboo spine, obliteration of sacroiliac joints.

- **CXR**
  Bronchial carcinoma – hypertrophic pulmonary osteoarthropathy.

SPECIFIC INVESTIGATIONS

- **Antistreptolysin O titre**
  Rheumatic fever.
- **Blood culture**
  Septic arthritis – *Staphylococcus aureus*, *Brucella*, *Salmonella*.
- **Antibody screen**
  ANA positive. Anti-double-stranded DNA ↑ SLE.
- **Brucella serology**
  Brucellosis.
- **Viral titres**
  Viral infections.
- **Hepatitis screen**
  Hepatitis B-associated arthralgia.
- **Sickling test**
  Sickle cell disease.
- **Coagulation screen**
  Anticoagulant therapy. Haemophilia.
- **Mantoux test**
  TB.
- **Skeletal survey**
  Tumours are usually visible only when more than 50% of bone mineral is lost. Acromegaly – pituitary fossa changes, hand and skull changes.
- **Bone scan**
  Metastatic disease. Primary bone tumours. Paget's disease. Inflammatory bone lesions. Osteoarthritis. Rheumatoid arthritis. Bone fractures.
- **MRI**
  Soft tissue injuries. Meniscal injuries. Ligamentus injuries.
- **Joint aspirate**
  Microscopy and culture and sensitivity. Crystals in gout.
- **Synovial biopsy**
  Confirms type of arthritis in rare cases.

INDIVIDUAL JOINTS

The following section covers individual joints. It must be appreciated that the conditions covered in joint disorders (above) can involve almost any joint; however, the conditions described under the individual joints (below) will refer to those conditions that normally affect, or cause pain in, the region of the particular joint.

SHOULDER

CAUSES

Congenital
- Klippel–Feil syndrome

Acquired

Traumatic
- Dislocation
- Fracture of the neck of the humerus
- Fracture of the clavicle
- Fracture of the scapula

Degenerative
- Supraspinatus tendinitis
- Impingement syndromes
- Rotator cuff tears
- Frozen shoulder (adhesive capsulitis)
- Osteoarthritis
  - Acromioclavicular
  - Glenohumeral

Inflammatory
- Rheumatoid arthritis

Infective
- Septic arthritis (rare)
- Tuberculous arthritis (rare)

Neoplastic
- Metastases in the upper end of the humerus/ribs/neck

Referred pain
- Cervical spondylosis
- Diaphragmatic irritation
- Pancoast's tumour

Neurological
- Winged scapula

HISTORY

Congenital

In Klippel–Feil syndrome, the neck is short and there are anomalies of the cervical vertebrae; the scapula is also highly placed.

Acquired

Traumatic

With dislocation of the shoulder there is usually a history of a fall on the outstretched hand. Recurrent dislocation may occur. The patient presents in pain supporting the arm, which is abducted. Anterior dislocation is the most common but posterior dislocation is often missed and can occur after trauma such as fits or electric shocks. With dislocation of the acromioclavicular joint there is usually a history of a fall on the shoulder (common in rugby players). Fracture of the surgical neck of the humerus occurs with a fall on the shoulder. The patient presents with pain, deformity and inability to move the shoulder. Clavicular fracture is usually caused by a fall on the outstretched hand or point of the shoulder. Scapular fractures are usually high-energy injuries often due to RTAs.

Degenerative

Supraspinatus tendinitis causes inflammation of the tendon due to either degeneration, ischaemia or calcification. There may be sudden pain or there may be just a painful arc at the initiation of movement. With impingement syndromes the rotator cuff becomes compressed under the acromion, or acromioclavicular joint, resulting in pain on abducting the arm. A painful arc between 30 and 60° suggests supraspinatus tendinitis; between 60 and 120° it suggests subacromial bursitis, when the greater tuberosity passes under the acromion. Rotator cuff tears often occur in older patients and probably relate to degeneration of the cuff. In the younger, fit patient, the rotator cuff tear may be due to violent trauma with rupture of supraspinatus. The patient is unable to initiate abduction of the arm but passive movement is normal. Frozen shoulder (adhesive capsulitis) is a response of the shoulder to local painful conditions or immobility. The middle-aged are usually affected. There may be a history of minor injury. There is pain and limitation of both active and passive movement of the shoulder. The pain is often severe and disturbs sleep. It may occur in the elderly following immobilisation of the arm, e.g. following a Colles' fracture. Osteoarthritis of the acromioclavicular joint presents as pain associated with overhead movement and a high painful arc greater than a 140°. Osteoarthritis of the glenohumeral joint may be idiopathic or follow avascular necrosis, or radionecrosis following radiotherapy for carcinoma of the breast. The patient complains of pain on shoulder movement and night pain.

Inflammatory

Rheumatoid arthritis is more common than osteoarthritis in the shoulder joint. There is usually a history of rheumatoid arthritis elsewhere.

Infective

These are rare. The patient presents with a painful, red, swollen joint with limited movement. TB of the shoulder is extremely rare in the UK. There are systemic symptoms of malaise and fever and there is usually wasting of the muscle around the shoulder joint.

Neoplastic

Secondary deposits may occur in the upper end of the humerus, giving rise to pain. Pathological fractures may occur. Check for a history of carcinoma of the bronchus, breast, thyroid, prostate or kidney.

Referred pain

This is an extremely common cause of shoulder pain. Cervical spondylosis often results in referred pain to the upper part of the shoulder. Check for a history of neck pain with limitation of movement of the neck. Irritation of the diaphragm may refer pain to the dermatome C4 at the shoulder tip. This may be due to peritonitis below the diaphragm or pleurisy above. The symptoms of peritonitis will be obvious. A history of chest problems should be sought if Pancoast's tumour is suspected, especially if Horner's syndrome is present.

Neurological

Winged scapula may cause difficulty with shoulder movements. Check for recent surgery to the neck or axilla, e.g. axillary clearance in breast carcinoma which may damage the long thoracic nerve. Carrying heavy loads on the shoulders over a prolonged period of time may also be responsible.

EXAMINATION

Congenital

Klippel–Feil syndrome. The patient will present with a short neck and a highly placed scapula. Other congenital conditions may be present.

Acquired

Traumatic

With dislocation of the shoulder the patient supports the arm. The normal contour of the shoulder is lost. Check for axillary nerve damage (anaesthesia over the 'badge' area). With acromioclavicular dislocation there will be a palpable lump at the site of dislocation. With fracture of the surgical neck of the humerus there will be pain and tenderness, and inability to abduct the arm due to pain. Check for axillary nerve damage. With fractures of the clavicle the patient supports the weight of the arm with the other hand. The site of the break is usually palpable.

Degenerative

There will be limitation of movement. Check for a painful arc. Check for the ability to initiate abduction (supraspinatus tendon tears). With frozen shoulder there is a limitation of active and passive movements of the shoulder. With osteoarthritis there will be limitation of movement. Check for mastectomy scars or signs of radiotherapy. With osteoarthritis of the acromioclavicular joint there is usually obvious prominence of the joint with localised tenderness and a high painful arc.

Inflammatory

With rheumatoid arthritis there are often signs elsewhere. There may be fever, malaise and heat in the joint. Glenohumeral movements may cause crepitus.

Infective

There will be a red, hot, swollen, tender joint. There may be a focus of infection elsewhere in the body.

Neoplastic

There may be little to find on examination or there may be a pathological fracture with pain, local tenderness and limitation of movement.

Referred pain

Check for movements of the cervical spine. Carry out a full neurological examination. With referred pain from the diaphragm, examine the abdomen for tenderness, guarding and rigidity. Examine the chest for signs of pneumonia, pleurisy or tumour.

Neurological

Check for scars in the neck or axilla. Note the winging of the scapula when the patient pushes the hand against a wall with the arm forward flexed to 90° (protraction of the scapula).

GENERAL INVESTIGATIONS

- **FBC, ESR**
  Hb ↓ anaemia of chronic disease, e.g. rheumatoid arthritis. WCC ↑ infection. ESR ↑ rheumatoid arthritis. CRP ↑ infection/inflammatory disease.
- **X-ray**
  X-rays in two planes. Arthritis. Dislocation. Fracture. Secondary deposits.

SPECIFIC INVESTIGATIONS

- **Blood culture**
  Septic arthritis.
- **Mantoux test**
  TB.
- **Bone scan**
  Secondary deposits.
- **Aspiration**
  Gram stain. C&S. Septic arthritis.
- **Arthroscopy**
  Cause of arthritis.
- **CT/MRI**
  Painful arc syndrome. Rotator cuff tears.

ELBOW

CAUSES

Traumatic
- Supracondylar fracture of the humerus
- Dislocation of the elbow
- Pulled elbow
- Fracture of the radial head
- Fractured olecranon
- Fractured epicondyle/condyle
- Myositis ossificans

Degenerative
- Osteoarthritis
- Osteochrondritis dissecans

Inflammatory
- Rheumatoid arthritis

Neurological
- Nerve entrapment, e.g. ulnar, posterior interosseous and median

Other
- Olecranon bursitis
- Tennis elbow
- Golfer's elbow
- Cubitus varus/valgus

HISTORY

Traumatic
Supracondylar fracture is chiefly a fracture of childhood. There is a history of a fall on the outstretched hand followed by pain and swelling around the elbow. This is a serious injury with several serious complications. Dislocation of the elbow may occur in children or adults. The symptoms are similar to those of supracondylar fracture. Pulled elbow occurs in children aged 2–6 years. The radial head slips out of the annular ligament. The child may have been 'swinging' with the parents holding the hands. Fractures of the olecranon may result as a fall on the point of the elbow or by sudden contraction of the triceps. Condylar and

epicondylar fractures are rare and easily missed. With myositis ossificans there will be a history of a supracondylar fracture or dislocation of the elbow. A calcified haematoma forms in front of the joint. Movement of the joint, especially flexion, is affected. It may follow ill-advised physiotherapy with passive stretching of the joints after trauma or after surgery.

Degenerative

Osteoarthritis of the elbow may occur in heavy manual workers or following complicated fractures involving the joint. Osteochondritis dissecans may cause elbow pain and restrict movement because of a loose body in the joint.

Inflammatory

Rheumatoid arthritis may affect the elbow joint. There will usually be signs of rheumatoid arthritis elsewhere. If there is gross disorganisation of the joint with deformity, the ulnar nerve may be involved and there may be symptoms of ulnar nerve palsy.

Neurological

Various nerve entrapment syndromes can occur around the elbow. Symptoms may present in the distribution of ulnar, median or posterior interosseous nerves.

Other

Olecranon bursitis results in a painless swelling over the olecranon. It is common in carpet layers and students (students rest their heads in their elbows while studying late into the night with their elbows resting on the desk). The bursa may become infected with a red, tender, hot swelling. Tennis elbow is common between the ages of 30 and 50 years. It presents with pain on the lateral side of the elbow. It affects tennis players and anyone whose job involves extending and twisting the forearm. The pain is often worse on gripping. Golfer's elbow is similar to tennis elbow but affects the medial epicondyle. The patient complains of pain and tenderness over the medial epicondyle and also of pain on hyperextending the fingers and wrists. Cubitus valgus/varus may follow fractures around the elbow in childhood. Cubitus valgus may progressively stretch the ulnar nerve, with a slowly developing ulnar nerve palsy.

EXAMINATION

Traumatic

With supracondylar fractures there will be swelling around the elbow joint and limitation of movement. The olecranon, medial epicondyle and lateral epicondyle preserve their normal relationship with one another in an equilateral triangle. Damage to the brachial artery and median or radial nerve may occur. With posterior dislocation at the elbow, the triangular relationship referred to above is lost. Otherwise the findings are similar. It is important to check the distal circulation and to assess for median and radial nerve palsies. With a fracture of the olecranon there is swelling and tenderness directly over the olecranon. With damage to the medial epicondyle it is important to test the integrity of the ulnar nerve. With myositis ossificans a calcified mass occurs in front of the elbow joint and there will be limitation of flexion. With radial head fractures the patient will be focally tender over the radial head and there will be lack of full extension.

Degenerative

With osteoarthritis there are often few signs. There may be thickening of the joint with loss of movement and crepitus. With osteochondritis dissecans there may be restriction in movement, crepitus and locking of the joint due to a loose body.

Inflammatory

With rheumatoid arthritis there will often by signs elsewhere. In long-standing arthritis there will be a swollen, disrupted joint with deformity. Check the integrity of the ulnar nerve.

Neurological

Examine carefully in the distribution of the median, ulnar and radial nerve.

Other

With olecranon bursitis there will be a swelling over the olecranon. This is fluid-filled and exhibits fluctuation and transilluminates. With infection it may become red and tender. With tennis elbow there is tenderness over the lateral epicondyle. Pronating the forearm while extending the elbow exacerbates the pain. With golfer's elbow there is tenderness over the medial epicondyle. With cubitus valgus/ varus the deformity is usually obvious. With cubitus valgus it is important to check the integrity of the ulnar nerve.

GENERAL INVESTIGATIONS

- **FBC, ESR**
  Hb ↓ anaemia of chronic disease, e.g. rheumatoid arthritis. WCC ↑ septic arthritis. ESR ↑ rheumatoid arthritis. CRP ↑ infection/ inflammatory disease.

- **Rheumatoid factor**
  Rheumatoid arthritis.
- **X-ray**
  Fractures around the elbow. Fracture of the radial head – anterior fat pad sign ('Sail' sign). Dislocation of the elbow. Osteoarthritis. Rheumatoid arthritis. Osteochondritis dissecans with loose body. Myositis ossificans.

SPECIFIC INVESTIGATIONS

- **US**
  Olecranon bursitis (diagnosis should be obvious on clinical examination).
- **Aspiration**
  Gram stain. C&S – infection. Crystals – gout.

WRIST

CAUSES

Traumatic
- Distal radial fracture, e.g. Colles', Smith's
- Dislocations
- Scaphoid fracture
- Carpal dislocations

Degenerative
- Osteoarthritis

Inflammatory
- Rheumatoid arthritis

Other
- Ganglion
- Tenosynovitis
  - de Quervain's
  - Extensor tenosynovitis
- Carpal tunnel syndrome
- Avascular necrosis of the lunate (Kienböck's disease)

HISTORY

Traumatic

The patient with a Colles' fracture is usually an elderly osteoporotic female. There is a history of a fall on the outstretched hand. The patient presents with pain and deformity. A Smith's fracture is the reverse of a Colles'. Again there is pain and deformity. Dislocations of the carpus are rare, the most common being dislocation of the lunate. This is usually due to a fall on the dorsiflexed hand. There may be involvement of the median nerve. Fracture of the scaphoid results from a fall on the outstretched hand or a blow to the palm of the hand. The patient presents with a painful, swollen wrist.

Degenerative

Osteoarthritis of the wrist is uncommon and usually a sequel to injury, e.g. a fracture of the scaphoid. The patient complains of pain and stiffness in the wrist.

Inflammatory

The wrist is commonly affected in rheumatoid arthritis. In the early stages there will be swelling, heat, pain and stiffness. Ultimately, ulnar deviation of the wrist and palmar subluxation occur.

Other

A ganglion is a painless lump, usually on the dorsum of the wrist. de Quervain's tenosynovitis usually occurs in the middle-aged. It involves the abductor pollicis longus and extensor pollicis brevis. The patient complains of pain on movement of the wrist and a weakness of the grip. Extensor 'tenosynovitis crepitans' follows excess activity and may affect all or only one of the extensor tendons. The patient usually complains of pain and tenderness over the dorsum of the wrist occurring with activity. With carpal tunnel syndrome there is usually a history of pregnancy, rheumatoid arthritis, myxoedema, osteoarthritis, anterior dislocation of the lunate or an arteriovenous fistula created for dialysis. Middle-aged women are most affected with carpal tunnel syndrome. There is pain in the distribution of the median nerve in the hand, worse in bed at night. It is relieved by hanging the hand out of bed. The patient often complains of clumsiness with fine movements due to median nerve involvement. With avascular necrosis of the lunate there may be a history of trauma. The patient is usually a young adult who complains of ache and stiffness.

EXAMINATION

Traumatic

With a Colles' fracture there is a classical 'dinner fork' deformity. The distal fragment is displaced backwards and radially. With Smith's fracture there is forward angulation of the distal fragment. Pain, limitation of movement and swelling occur. With dislocation there is a swollen wrist. Test the median nerve. Scaphoid fractures result in swelling around the wrist, with localised tenderness in the anatomical snuff box.

Degenerative

With osteoarthritis, the wrist may appear normal. There may be limited painful movement with crepitus.

Inflammatory

With rheumatoid arthritis there may be gross swelling with increased local heat, pain and stiffness. Ultimately, ulnar deviation occurs and there may be palmar subluxation.

Other

A ganglion is a well-defined cystic non-tender lump. It transilluminates. With tenosynovitis there is usually localised tenderness and occasionally swelling. Often there is little else to find except for a weak grip. Look for a precipitating cause for carpal tunnel syndrome, e.g. pregnancy, myxoedema. The diagnosis is often made on the history. There may be wasting of the thenar eminence and sensory abnormalities in the distribution of the median nerve. Tinel's sign may be positive, i.e. percussion over the median nerve in the carpal tunnel causes paraesthesia in the median nerve distribution. With Kienböck's disease there will be localised tenderness and limited dorsiflexion.

GENERAL INVESTIGATIONS

- **FBC, ESR**
  Hb ↓ anaemia of chronic disease, e.g. rheumatoid arthritis. WCC ↑ infection. ESR ↑ inflammatory disease, e.g. rheumatoid arthritis. CRP ↑ infection/inflammatory disease.
- **Rheumatoid factor**
  Rheumatoid arthritis.
- **X-ray**
  Fractures. Dislocation. Scaphoid views for suspected scaphoid fractures. Increased density of bone in avascular necrosis. Osteoarthritis. Rheumatoid arthritis.

SPECIFIC INVESTIGATIONS

- **Blood culture**
  Septic arthritis.
- **Aspiration**
  Infection – Gram stain, C&S. Crystals in gout.
- **Nerve conduction studies**
  Carpal tunnel syndrome (if the presentation is not classical).

HIP

CAUSES

Congenital

- Developmental dysplasia of the hip (DDH) (formerly congenital dislocation of the hip)

Acquired

Traumatic
- Fractured neck of femur
- Dislocation of the hip
- Fracture of the pubic ramus
- Acetabular fracture

Infective
- Acute pyogenic arthritis
- TB

Inflammatory
- Reiter's syndrome
- Rheumatoid arthritis
- Ankylosing spondylitis

Degenerative
- Neoplastic
  - Metastases
  - Leukaemia in childhood
- Osteoarthritis
  - Primary
  - Secondary
- Avascular necrosis

Ot her
- Transient synovitis
- Perthes' disease
- Slipped upper femoral epiphysis

HISTORY

Congenital

CDH is usually picked up on routine examination of the neonate with Ortolani's test and confirmed by US scan. If the diagnosis is missed on routine testing, the child may present with a limp and waddling gait (Trendelenburg gait). There is an increased risk of CDH if one parent has a history of the disease. Commoner with breech delivery, primagravida and female infants. Check for other congenital anomalies.

Acquired

Traumatic

Fracture of the neck of the femur usually occurs in an elderly female. The trauma may be minor, e.g. tripping over the carpet. The patient presents with pain in the hip with painful movements and weight-bearing is often impossible. In the young patient there is usually a history of major trauma. Dislocation of the hip, which is usually posterior, is associated with other severe injuries. It often occurs with road traffic accidents, the knee striking the dashboard. Pelvic fractures (usually pubic rami) are usually a result of a fall in the elderly. The patient feels deep-seated pain in the region of the hip. Walking is painful. Acetabular fractures usually result from direct violence, e.g. a fall on the side, or indirect, such as a fall on the feet or from impact of the knee on a car dashboard.

Infective

The infection is usually blood-borne. It may occur in children where the metaphysis is intracapsular, as in the hip. Check for a history of steroid medication or other immunosuppression. The patient presents with a hot, painful, tender joint. There is limitation of movement and weight-bearing is painful. With TB there is usually a history of contact. The patient presents with malaise, weight loss and night sweats. There is local pain and swelling with limitation of movement and local muscle atrophy.

Inflammatory

Reiter's disease presents with a history of urethritis and conjunctivitis. There will usually be a history of sexual contact or dysentery. Rheumatoid arthritis usually presents with a systemic illness with malaise and weight loss. There is pain in the hip, which may be held in flexion. Ankylosing spondylitis may affect the hips. Initially there is usually stiffness in the spine as a presenting symptom.

Degenerative

Osteoarthritis presents with pain, stiffness and deformity. The patient has difficulty in walking. There may be a joint effusion and loss of movement. Secondary osteoarthritis may follow a history of fractures, Perthes' disease, slipped upper femoral epiphysis, avascular necrosis, gout, haemophilia. Avascular necrosis of the head of the femur may occur following intracapsular fractures of the neck of the femur. It may also occur in patients on steroid therapy.

Neoplastic

The upper end of the femur near the neck is a common site for metastases. Hip pain in children may be due to leukaemic infiltration.

Other

Transient synovitis gives rise to an irritable hip with a limp, pain and restriction of movement. Perthes' usually occurs with a maximum incidence around 7–8 years. There is pain in the hip and a limp. The patient is otherwise well. The pain may be referred to the knee joint. Slipped upper femoral epiphysis usually presents between 11 and 16 years. It occurs more commonly in boys. There is usually pain in the hip and a limp. It may present with referred pain to the knee.

EXAMINATION

Congenital

Ortolani's test is carried out after birth. The hips and knees are flexed to a right angle and the thighs are abducted. There is a 'clunk' as the head of the femur slips into the joint over the acetabulum (Ortolani's test). In Barlow's test the surgeon holds the upper femur between the middle finger on the great trochanter and the thumb in the groin and levers the femoral head in and out of the acetabulum, readily demonstrating dislocation.

Acquired

Traumatic

The patient with a fractured neck of femur classically shows shortening, adduction and external rotation of the leg. If the fracture is undisplaced, limb alignment may be normal. Movements are painful. With dislocation the patient is usually shocked with other injuries. With posterior dislocation the thigh is flexed, adducted and internally rotated. Check for sciatic nerve injury. There may be associated injury to femur or patella. With isolated fractures of the pubic ramus there may be little to find on examination, although a second fracture/joint injury is common at the back of the pelvic ring.

Infective

Acute pyogenic arthritis presents with a hot, tender, painful swollen hip. All movements are painful. There is spasm in the surrounding muscles. The patient usually has a high fever. TB presents with local tenderness, swelling and effusion. There is muscle wasting and spasm. There is usually a constitutional upset with malaise and fever.

Inflammatory

With Reiter's disease there is usually associated urethritis and conjunctivitis. With rheumatoid arthritis there is usually malaise, fever and joint swelling. The hip is often held in flexion. Movements are painful. There is a decreased range of movements. Ankylosing spondylitis usually presents with a stiff spine with a limited range of movement, although the hips may be stiff. Small joints are unaffected.

Degenerative

Osteoarthritis usually presents with a limp. The leg lies externally rotated and appears shortened because of fixed adduction. There is usually a degree of fixed flexion. Restriction in movement occurs: abduction, extension and internal rotation loss occurring early and being most restrictive. There is apparent shortening. Avascular necrosis results in distortion of joint shape with stiffness, limitation of movement and ultimately secondary osteoarthritis.

Neoplastic

Check for localised pain over the hip joint. Check for any tumour of breast, bronchus, thyroid, prostate or kidney. In children with leukaemic infiltration there may be other signs, e.g. spontaneous bruising, lymphadenopathy, splenomegaly.

Other

Transient synovitis presents with a limp. There is no systemic upset. There is limitation of movement at the joint. Perthes' disease presents with a limp and a decreased range of joint movement.

With slipped upper femoral epiphysis the leg lies in external
rotation and passive internal rotation is diminished.

GENERAL INVESTIGATIONS

- **FBC, ESR**
  Hb ↓ anaemia of chronic disease, e.g. rheumatoid arthritis. WCC ↑
  infection. ESR ↑ inflammatory disease, e.g. rheumatoid arthritis,
  ankylosing spondylitis. CRP ↑ infection/inflammatory disease.

- **Hip X-ray**
  AP and lateral. Fractures, osteoarthritis, rheumatoid arthritis,
  dislocation, Perthes' disease, slipped upper femoral epiphysis,
  tuberculosis, avascular necrosis.

SPECIFIC INVESTIGATIONS

- **Blood culture**
  Septic arthritis.
- **Aspiration**
  Infection – Gram stain, C&S. Crystals in gout.
- **US**
  Developmental dysplasia of the hip.
- **Bone scan**
  Avascular necrosis. Occult fracture.

KNEE

CAUSES

Traumatic

Bones
- Patellar fractures
- Supracondylar fractures of the femur
- Tibial fractures involving the joint

Ligaments
- Medial and lateral collateral ligament damage
- Cruciate ligament damage
- Rupture of quadriceps tendon
- Rupture of the patellar tendon

Menisci
● Meniscal tears

Infective
● Pyogenic arthritis

Inflammatory
● Rheumatoid arthritis
● Reiter's syndrome
● Ankylosing spondylitis

Degenerative
● Osteoarthritis

Metabolic
● Gout
● Pseudogout

Neuropathic
● Charcot's joint

Neoplastic
● Osteogenic sarcoma

Other
● Bursitis
  ● Prepatellar bursitis (housemaid's knee)
  ● Infrapatellar bursitis (clergyman's knee)
  ● Semimembranosus bursitis
● Baker's cyst
● Osteochondritis dissecans
● Disorders of alignment
  ● Genu varum (bow legs)
  ● Genu valgum (knock knee)
● Patellofemoral instability
● Osgood–Schlatter's disease (osteochondritis of the tibial tuberosity)
● Chondromalacia patellae
● Referred pain from the hip/back

HISTORY

Traumatic

With fractures around the knee joint there will usually be an obvious history of trauma. Fractures of the patella may arise because of violent contraction of quadriceps or because of direct blows to the patella. With ligamentous tears there is often a history of damage during sport, e.g. footballers. The patient will present with a painful, swollen knee joint. Posterior cruciate ligament injury is usually due to a force drawing the tibia backwards on the femur with the knee flexed, e.g. in a car accident when the upper tibia strikes the dashboard. Meniscal tears often occur in sportsmen and coal miners. The knee is twisted while it is flexed and weight is being taken on it. The patient presents with a swollen knee with pain and tenderness on the side on which the meniscus is torn. The knee may be 'locked', i.e. lacks the last 10–15° of extension. Very rapid swelling indicates bleeding into the joint, and hence fracture or cruciate damage or peripheral meniscal detachment.

Infective

Usually blood-borne. More common in children. May occur in adults on steroids or who are immunosuppressed. The patient presents with a hot, painful, tender joint with malaise and fever. The patient is reluctant to move the joint.

Inflammatory

In rheumatoid arthritis the patient complains of pain and swelling together with constitutional upset. Symptoms of rheumatoid arthritis may be present elsewhere. Reiter's syndrome may present with swelling and discomfort in the knee. There is often a history of urethritis, conjunctivitis or dysentery. Ankylosing spondylitis may present with discomfort in the knee joint. Usually the patient also complains of stiffness of the spine.

Degenerative

Osteoarthritis is common in the knee. The patient may be overweight and elderly. There is pain on movement, stiffness and deformity. There may be a history of previous joint pathology, e.g. septic arthritis, meniscal tear, mensical surgery or osteochondritis dissecans.

Metabolic

Gout may present with pain and swelling of the knee. Pseudogout (pyrophosphate deposition disease) may also present in the knee joint. The condition is associated with chondrocalcinosis, i.e. there is calcification visible in hyaline and fibrocartilage.

Neuropathic

The patient presents with a painless joint, which is grossly deformed and hypermobile. There may be a history of diabetes, syphilis or leprosy.

Neoplastic

The lower end of the femur and the upper end of the tibia are common sites of osteogenic sarcoma. The patient is usually male and under the age of 30 years. There is pain, swelling and deformity around the knee. The patient may also complain of cough due to lung metastases.

Other

Bursitis presents with swelling, either in front of or behind the knee. The swelling may be painless. Patients who work on their knees leaning forwards, e.g. carpet fitters, may get prepatellar bursitis. Infrapatellar bursitis occurs in those who sit back on their heels (e.g. vicars praying, hence the name clergyman's knee). A semimembranosus bursa presents behind the knee on the medial side. A bursa may become infected, in which case the patient will present with a tender, red, hot swelling. Baker's cyst presents in the midline of the popliteal fossa. The patient will notice a lump. There may also be pain associated with concurrent osteoarthritis of the joint.

Osteochondritis dissecans

This occurs most commonly in the second decade of life. A segment of bone undergoes avascular necrosis, separates and forms a loose body in the joint. The patient complains of pain, swelling and intermittent 'locking' of the joint.

Disorders of alignment

With genu varum the patient presents with bow legs. In children this is usually associated with a disorder of growth, often with a bony injury to the area of epiphyses. In adults there may be a history of rickets, Paget's disease, or rheumatoid arthritis. In genu valgum (knock knee), the patient is often a child who has flat feet. In adults there may be a history of rheumatoid arthritis.

Patellofemoral instability

Dislocation of the patella may occur. In the acute form there may be a history of a blow to one side of the knee. Recurrent dislocation of the patella affects adolescent girls. It is usually associated with flattening of the lateral condyle, a high-riding patella or genu valgum.

Osgood–Schlatter's disease

The patient is usually a boy aged between 10 and 14 years. There is a history of physical activity, e.g. football. Pain and swelling occur, accurately located to the area of the tibial tuberosity.

Chondromalacia patellae

The patient presents with ill-localised pain in front of the knee. It is most common in females in the 15–35 years age group. There may be a history of injury. There is usually some swelling, and pain occurs especially when climbing stairs. The knee tends to give way.

Referred pain

It is very common for pain to be referred from the hip or the back to the knee. Always enquire about hip symptoms and back symptoms.

EXAMINATION

Traumatic

Fractures will usually be obvious. There will be pain, tenderness, deformity and crepitus. With supracondylar fractures it is important to check the distal circulation. With ligamentous injuries, test for joint stability, effusions, tenderness over the affected ligament. Testing for active straight leg raising will exclude injury to the extensor mechanism (rupture of quadriceps, rupture of patellar tendon, patellar fracture). Valgus and varus strain testing may be necessary to diagnose ligamentous injury. Test for anterior and posterior drawer signs and carry out Lachman's test. With meniscal injuries there is tenderness, swelling and effusion in the acute phase. The joint may be locked, i.e. loss of the last 10–15° of extension. In the chronic phase there will be wasted quadriceps, effusion, tenderness over the meniscus in the joint line. McMurray's test will be positive with medial meniscus injury, although it is rarely carried out these days.

In acute knee injuries, often little examination can be formed at the time of injury due to pain and re-assessment at 10 days is often appropriate.

Infective

The patient will be febrile with a hot, red, tender, painful, swollen joint. There will be spasm in the surrounding muscles and no active or passive movement will be possible (occasionally, movements are possible in diabetics and patients on steroids and immunosuppressive drugs).

Inflammatory

With rheumatoid arthritis there will be fever, pain and swelling with decreased range of movements and synovial thickening. There will often be signs of rheumatoid in other joints. With Reiter's syndrome there will be swelling and reduced movements. Urethritis and conjunctivitis may be apparent. Ankylosing spondylitis may affect the knee joints, in which case there will be swelling and stiffness. There is usually reduced movement of the spine.

Degenerative

With osteoarthritis there will be swelling due to osteophytes, a thickened synovium or effusion. There will be wasting of quadriceps. There will be reduced movement, with pain at the limits of movement. Gait will be disturbed. Alignment may be distorted if one side of the joint only is affected.

Metabolic

With gout the joint is red, hot and swollen and there is limitation of movement. A similar appearance occurs in pseudogout.

Neuropathic

The joint will be grossly swollen and deformed. There will be abnormal mobility, which is painless. Test for abnormality of dorsal column sensation (joint position sense).

Other

Bursitis – soft, fluctuant swelling in front of the patella (prepatellar bursitis) or below the patella (infrapatellar bursitis). Semimembranosus bursitis presents as a cystic swelling on the medial aspect of the popliteal fossa. If the bursa becomes infected then the swelling becomes hot, red and tender. With osteochondritis dissecans there will be joint swelling due to effusion, and intermittent locking of the joint. Genu valgum and genu varum will be apparent on examination. Patellofemoral instability may result from acute or chronic dislocation. With acute dislocation the patella is visibly displaced laterally with the knee flexed. There will be localised tenderness and swelling. With chronic dislocation the knee locks in semiflexion. Spontaneous reduction often occurs. The patella may feel too high or too small. With Osgood–Schlatter's disease there is tenderness and swelling over the tibial tuberosity. With chondromalacia patellae there is slight swelling and pain when the patella is pressed and moved against the femur. Always remember to examine the hip joint and spine. Pain in the knee may be referred from the hip or spine. Baker's cyst is a soft, diffuse swelling in the popliteal fossa. Pain occurs if the cyst ruptures.

GENERAL INVESTIGATIONS

- **FBC, ESR**
  Hb ↓ anaemia of chronic disease, e.g. rheumatoid arthritis. WCC ↑
  infection, e.g. pyogenic arthritis. ESR ↑ rheumatoid arthritis,
  ankylosing spondylitis. CRP ↑ infection/inflammatory disease.
- **Rheumatoid factor**
  Rheumatoid arthritis.
- **Serum uric acid**
  Gout.
- **Knee X-ray (AP, lateral, tunnel and sky line' views)**
  Fractures. Osteoarthritis. Rheumatoid arthritis. Loose bodies.
  Osteogenic sarcoma. X-ray stressing the joints may be
  necessary to diagnose ligamentous injuries.
- **CXR**
  Secondary deposits in osteogenic sarcoma.

SPECIFIC INVESTIGATIONS

- **Blood culture**
  Pyogenic arthritis.
- **Joint aspiration**
  Gram stain and culture and sensitivity – infection. Microscopy
  shows crystals in gout and pseudogout.
- **Isotope scan**
  Tumour. Infections. Acute arthritis.
- **MRI**
  Meniscal injuries. Ligamentous injuries e.g. cruciates
- **Arthroscopy**
  Loose bodies. Effusion. Meniscal injuries.
- **Synovial biopsy**
  Confirmation of diagnosis.

ANKLE

CAUSES

Traumatic
- Sprains (lateral ligaments)
- Fractures around the ankle
- Rupture of the Achilles tendon

Infective
- Pyogenic arthritis (rare)
- TB (rare)

Inflammatory
- Rheumatoid arthritis
- Degenerative
- Osteoarthritis

Others
- Tenosynovitis
- Footballer's ankle
- Osteochondritis of the talus
- Tarsal tunnel syndrome

HISTORY

Traumatic

History of recent injury. Sprains usually affect the lateral ligament. With fractures there will be swelling, deformity, bruising and crepitus around the ankle. With tibiofibular diastasis there may be a high fibular fracture. Rupture of the Achilles tendon often occurs during sport (occasionally in bed!), particularly in middle-aged men. Patients feel as though they have been kicked in the back of the heel.

Infective

Pyogenic arthritis will result in a red, hot, tender joint. Tuberculous arthritis is rare. There will be pain on walking. There is usually a history of TB elsewhere.

Inflammatory

Rheumatoid arthritis is the commonest cause of chronic pain and swelling at the ankle joint. There will invariably be other symptoms of rheumatoid arthritis. Fever and malaise may also be present.

Degenerative

Primary osteoarthritis of the ankle is rare. Osteoarthritis is often a sequel to an imperfectly reduced fracture, or avascular necrosis of the talus. Symptoms are often minimal.

Others

Tenosynovitis may occur in the tendons behind either the lateral or medial malleolus. Pain is present on either side of the ankle, particularly during inversion or eversion. Footballer's ankle, as the name implies, occurs in those who play football. The patient presents with poorly localised pain in front of the ankle. Osteochondritis of the talus is rare. It occurs in teenagers and young men. There is often severe pain in the ankle. In tarsal tunnel syndrome the tibial nerve may be compressed as it passes beneath the flexor retinaculum, giving rise to paraesthesia and a burning pain in the sole of the foot and the toes.

EXAMINATION

Traumatic
In fractures there will be deformity, a palpable swelling, tenderness and crepitus. With ruptures of the Achilles tendon there is usually an obvious gap in the Achilles tendon, and a weakness of plantar flexion of the foot against resistance. Apply the Thomson squeeze test. Normally when the calf is squeezed the foot plantar flexes. This does not occur with rupture of the Achilles tendon.

Infective
In pyogenic arthritis there will be a hot, tender, swollen, painful ankle. With TB the ankle will be swollen, with wasting of calf muscles.

Inflammatory
Rheumatoid arthritis seldom affects the ankle only. It presents with a swollen, tender ankle but there will be signs of arthritis elsewhere in the foot.

Degenerative
In osteoarthritis there is swelling, with a decreased range of movements of the ankle with crepitus.

Others
With tenosynovitis there is a puffy swelling and tenderness along the tendons. There is pain on forced eversion and inversion if the tibialis posterior and peroneus longus are involved. With footballer's ankle there is tearing of the anterior capsule of the joint with subsequent calcification. Examination often reveals restriction in dorsiflexion. With osteochondritis of the talus there is ankle swelling and tenderness. Loose bodies may present in the joint.

GENERAL INVESTIGATIONS

- **FBC, ESR**
  Hb ↓ anaemia of chronic disease, e.g. rheumatoid arthritis. WCC ↑
  infection, e.g. pyogenic arthritis. ESR ↑ rheumatoid arthritis. CRP
  ↑ infection/inflammatory disease.
- **Ankle X-ray**
  Fractures. Stress X-rays may be required to delineate the type
  of fracture. Always include the upper fibula in the X-ray, as in
  diastasis of the joint there may be a fracture of the upper part
  of the shaft of the fibula. Rheumatoid arthritis. Osteoarthritis.
  Osteochondritis of the talus. Calcification of the anterior part
  of the capsule in footballer's ankle.

SPECIFIC INVESTIGATIONS

- **Blood culture**
  Pyogenic arthritis.
- **Joint aspiration**
  Gram stain and C&S in infection. Crystals in the fluid in gout.
- **Bone scan**
  Infections. Acute arthritis.
- **MRI**
  Osteochondritis of the talus.

KIDNEY SWELLINGS

Kidney swellings are not uncommon. They may present silently or may be associated with haematuria, urinary tract infections and pyrexia.

CAUSES

Congenital
- Polycystic kidney

Acquired

Infective
- Perinephric abscess
- TB

Obstructive
- Hydronephrosis
- Pyonephrosis

Degenerative
- Solitary cyst

Neoplastic
- Hypernephroma
- Nephroblastoma

HISTORY

Congenital

There will often be a family history with adult polycystic kidney disease; however, it does not usually present until the third or fourth decade, when the patient may present with an abdominal mass, haematuria, loin pain (infection or bleeding into a cyst) or chronic renal failure. Hypertension may be a presenting symptom. Rarely, hydronephrosis may present at birth. Hydronephrosis in infants may be a cause of failure to thrive.

Acquired

There may be a history of TB. The patient may present with haematuria, dysuria or pyuria. With perinephric abscess there may be a history of diabetes. Nephroblastoma presents with an abdominal mass, pain, haematuria, pyrexia and weight loss within the first 3 years of life.

EXAMINATION

A mass may be palpated in either the right or the left loin. This
moves with respiration and is palpable bimanually and ballotable.
Generally, a kidney swelling is dull to percussion, but there may
be a strip of resonance across the swelling due to the gas-filled
overlying transverse colon. A solitary cyst may be large, tense and
smooth. Polycystic kidneys may be very large and extend down to
the groin. They are smooth and embossed with many cysts. They
may be tender if the cysts are infected or tense following bleeding.
Hydronephrotic kidneys may be very large, smooth and tense.
Perinephric abscesses may be associated with redness, swelling
and oedema in the loin. Occasionally they may point in the loin, but
this is rare nowadays. Hypernephromas are usually firm, irregular,
nodular, and may be fixed. A nephroblastoma presents with a large
mass in the loin and abdomen.

GENERAL INVESTIGATIONS

- **FBC, ESR**
  Hb ↑ (hypernephroma may be associated with polycythaemia).
  Hb ↓ blood loss due to haematuria. WCC ↑ pyonephrosis,
  perinephric abscess. ESR ↑ hypernephroma, nephroblastoma,
  TB, infection.
- **U&Es**
  Urea and creatinine raised if bilateral disease.
- **Blood glucose**
  Perinephric abscess in diabetes.
- **KUB**
  Hydronephrosis due to renal or ureteric stones. Renal outline.
- **CXR**
  Metastases – hypernephroma (cannonball metastases),
  nephroblastoma. TB.
- **Urinalysis**
  Blood, pus cells, organisms, EMSUs for TB.
- **US**
  Cystic versus solid. Biopsy.

SPECIFIC INVESTIGATIONS

- **IVU**
  Absent function. Hydronephrosis. Distortion of calyces (hypernephroma).
- **CT**
  Solid versus cystic. Spread of tumour. Biopsy.
- **Cystoscopy**
  Bladder tumour obstructing ureters. TB. Bladder outlet obstruction.
- **Antegrade pyelography**
  Site of obstruction.
- **Retrograde pyelography**
  Site of obstruction.
- **Angiography**
  Tumour circulation (rarely used).
- **MRI**
  Renal parenchymal lesions. Vascular lesions.

▶ LEG PAIN

This section deals with causes of pain arising from local lesions within the leg, or referred into the leg. Pain in the leg is a common complaint and the majority of cases are of vascular or orthopaedic origin. Joint problems are dealt with in the section on joint disorders (page 250).

CAUSES

Traumatic
- Fractures
- Dislocations
- Crush injuries

Inflammatory
- Rheumatoid arthritis
- Reiter's disease
- Ankylosing spondylitis

Infective
- Cellulitis
- Myositis (rare)
- Osteomyelitis (rare)
- Septic arthritis

Degenerative
- Osteoarthritis
- Baker's cyst
- Meniscal lesions

Vascular
- Deep venous thrombosis
- Acute arterial occlusion
- Intermittent claudication

Neurological
- Sciatica
- Peripheral neuropathy
- Neurogenic claudication

Metabolic
- Gout

Neoplastic
- Osteogenic sarcoma
- Secondary deposits

Other
- Polymyalgia rheumatica
- Cramp
- Strenuous exercise

HISTORY

Traumatic
Obvious history of trauma.

Inflammatory
History of joint swelling, stiffness, limitation of movement. Pain on walking. There may be an obvious history of rheumatoid arthritis with signs elsewhere, e.g. the hands. Reiter's disease – conjunctivitis, urethritis. Ankylosing spondylitis – stiffness of the spine, especially in the morning; hip and knee involvement.

Infective
Cellulitis may arise from puncture wounds, e.g. insect bites, or in a lymphoedematous leg. The patient presents with pain, redness, tenderness, malaise and fever. Myositis may occur in association with collagen diseases, e.g. scleroderma, dermatomyositis. Osteomyelitis is rare but more common in childhood. History of immunosuppression or diabetes. Recent history of infection elsewhere. Pain aggravated by movement. Swelling and redness of the affected area. Septic arthritis presents with a red, hot, tender, painful joint. More common in children. In adults, enquire about a history of steroid therapy or diabetes.

Degenerative
Osteoarthritis presents with pain, stiffness and deformity. The pain is often worse on starting walking and then improves. Baker's cyst presents with a lump behind the knee. The patient may complain of pain and swelling of the calf if the cyst ruptures. With meniscal lesions there is usually a history of twisting the knee, e.g. playing football. The knee may lock.

Vascular
Deep venous thrombosis presents with painful swelling of the leg. There may be a history of the contraceptive pill, prolonged immobilisation, recent surgery, malignancy. Acute arterial occlusion

results in sudden onset of severe pain in the affected limb. The patient is unable to move the leg and complains that the leg feels cold. With intermittent claudication there is a pain on walking, relieved by rest. It may affect the calf, thigh or buttock. Rest pain in the foot may occur with advanced arterial disease. The pain is often worse in bed at night and the patient obtains relief by hanging the foot out of bed.

Neurological

Pain down the back of the leg (sciatica) often made worse by coughing, movement or straining. The patient may also complain of backache with painful spasm in the back muscles. There are restricted movements of the spine. Neurogenic claudication results from central spinal canal stenosis. Symptoms improve with flexion as this increases the diameter of the canal. Therefore, patients find it easier to cycle than walk and easier to walk upstairs than downstairs. With neurogenic claudication, the claudication distance becomes progressively shorter with each bout of pain during one walk but not with vascular claudication. It also takes the pain of neurogenic claudication longer to settle than the pain of vascular claudication. The two forms of claudication may co-exist, making diagnosis difficult.

Metabolic

Gout presents as acute severe pain with redness and swelling of a joint. There may be a history of previous episodes. History of trauma, surgery, infection, diuretics, polycythaemia, leukaemia, cytotoxic therapy or immunosuppressive therapy.

Neoplastic

Osteogenic sarcoma usually presents in males between 20 and 40 years old. There is usually swelling around the knee, the commonest sites of the tumour being the lower femur or upper tibia. The patient often complains of bone pain, swelling or cough due to lung secondaries. Pain or pathological fractures may be due to secondary deposits. These may occur from the breast, lung, thyroid, prostate or kidney. Check for symptoms related to these or previous surgery for malignancy.

Other

Polymyalgia rheumatica usually occurs in elderly females. There is aching, morning stiffness in proximal muscles and often associated arthritis. Cramp is painful muscle spasm. The patient often complains of severe pain in the legs, especially at night or after exercise. It may occur with salt depletion, myopathy or muscle ischaemia. It is common in chronic renal failure.

EXAMINATION

Traumatic

Pain, loss of function, tenderness, deformity, crepitus, abnormal mobility. Check for associated nerve and vascular injuries.

Inflammatory

Pain in joints, swelling, tenderness, loss of movement, fixed deformities, disturbances of gait. Signs of rheumatoid arthritis elsewhere. Reiter's disease – conjunctivitis, urethritis. Ankylosing spondylitis – stiffness of the spine, reduced thoracic excursion, fixed kyphotic spine, hyperextended neck.

Infective

In acute cellulitis there is redness and tenderness over the affected area. Inguinal lymphadenopathy may be present. With acute osteomyelitis there is tenderness and heat over the site of infection. With myositis there is tenderness and wasting of the muscles. There may be other signs of collagen diseases, e.g. polyarteritis nodosa, SLE, scleroderma or dermatomyositis. In septic arthritis there is a hot, tender, painful, swollen joint and all movements are painful. Surrounding muscle spasm is present.

Degenerative

In osteoarthritis there is deformity, synovial thickening, bony enlargement due to osteophytes, effusion, loss of movement and fixed deformities. Baker's cyst presents as a swelling in the popliteal fossa. If it has ruptured there is pain and swelling of the calf. Meniscal lesions present with swelling of the knee and tenderness over the joint line in the early phase. Later there may be a continued effusion with wasted quadriceps and a positive McMurray sign.

Vascular

Deep vein thrombosis presents with pain, tenderness, swelling and heat, usually over the calf. There is ankle oedema. Homans' sign is positive. With iliofemoral thrombosis there may be phlegmasia alba dolans (white leg) or phlegmasia cerulea dolans (painful blue leg). Acute ischaemia presents with pain, pallor, pulselessness, paraesthesia and paralysis. Check for atrial fibrillation. With intermittent claudication, examine for absent pulses. Buerger's test.

Neoplastic

There is usually a hot, tender swelling around the knee joint in either the lower femur or upper tibia. Examine the chest for lung metastases. With secondary deposits, check the lung, breast, thyroid, prostate and kidney.

Neurological
Lordosis, limited straight leg raising, restricted back movements. Reduced reflexes in the lower limb. Areas of absent sensation.

Metabolic
With gout there will be a tender, red, swollen joint with limitation of movement. Check for gouty tophi elsewhere.

Other
Polymyalgia rheumatica presents with tenderness over muscles and arthritis. Occasionally there is associated giant cell arteritis. Examine the temporal artery for tenderness. With cramp there may be signs of chronic renal failure.

GENERAL INVESTIGATIONS

- **FBC, ESR**
  Hb ↓ anaemia of chronic disease, e.g. rheumatoid arthritis, collagen disease. WCC ↑ infection, e.g. osteomyelitis, septic arthritis. ESR ↑ inflammation, e.g. rheumatoid arthritis, malignancy, polymyalgia rheumatica.
- **CRP**
  ↑ infection/inflammatory disease.
- **U&Es**
  Chronic renal failure. Renal involvement in collagen disease.
- **LFTs**
  Alkaline phosphatase ↑ in liver secondaries.
- **Rheumatoid factor**
  Rheumatoid arthritis.
- **Blood glucose**
  Diabetes – neuropathy, peripheral vascular disease.
- **Serum uric acid**
  Gout.
- **Local X-rays**
  Fractures. Osteoarthritis. Rheumatoid arthritis. Chronic osteomyelitis. Tumours.
- **Lumbosacral spine X-ray**
  Disc lesions. Osteophytes. Narrowing of joint spaces. Lordosis.
- **CXR**
  Secondary deposits in osteogenic sarcoma.

SPECIFIC INVESTIGATIONS

- **CT**
  Local lesion. Spine, e.g. disc lesion, tumour, neurogenic claudication – narrowing of canal.
- **MRI**
  Spine, disc lesion, tumour.
- **Duplex Doppler**
  DVT. Arterial disease.
- **Arteriography**
  Vascular disease.
- **Venography**
  DVT.
- **Nerve conduction studies**
  Nerve lesions, peripheral neuropathy.

▶ LEG SWELLINGS

Swelling of the lower limb may be unilateral or bilateral. Bilateral swellings are usually due to medical conditions such as cardiac, renal or hepatic failure. Unilateral swellings are commonly due to trauma, venous disease or lymphatic disease.

CAUSES

Local

Acute swelling
- Trauma
- DVT
- Cellulitis
- Allergy
- Rheumatoid arthritis

Chronic swelling
- Venous
  - Varicose veins
  - Obstruction to venous return, e.g. pregnancy, pelvic tumours, IVC, obstruction, postphlebitic limb
- Lymphoedema
- Congenital malformations, e.g. arteriovenous fistulae
- Paralysis (failure of muscle pump)
- Dependency

General
- Congestive cardiac failure
- Hypoproteinaemia, e.g. liver failure, nephrotic syndrome, malnutrition
- Renal failure
- Fluid overload
- Myxoedema

HISTORY

Pain will be associated with trauma, DVT, infection or complications of varicose veins. Other causes of swelling of the lower limb may be painless, although the limb may be uncomfortable if the oedema becomes tense. Evidence of the following should be sought in the past medical history: trauma to the limb, recent pregnancy (DVT), abdominal or pelvic malignancy, previous surgery or radiotherapy to lymph nodes, thyroid disease, congestive cardiac failure, renal failure, liver failure, malnutrition, poliomyelitis in childhood, nerve lesions. With primary lymphoedema the leg may have been swollen since birth or oedema may have developed at puberty (lymphoedema praecox) or in the third decade (lymphoedema tarda).

EXAMINATION

The presence of fracture, contusion or haematoma should be obvious. With cellulitis the limb will be red, swollen, hot and tender. A puncture wound may be visible. DVT may be suspected if the limb is tender and swollen, particularly the calf with a positive Homans' sign, i.e. pain in the calf on dorsiflexion of the foot. Tenderness may be present over the femoral vein with femoral vein thrombosis. The limb may be pale and swollen to the groin (phlegmasia alba dolens) or tense and purplish and extremely painful (phlegmasia cerulea dolens) with iliofemoral thrombosis. Bilateral swelling with dilated collateral veins on the abdominal wall suggests IVC thrombosis. Swelling and tenderness over the joints may suggest rheumatoid arthritis. Lymphoedema pits in the early stages but in the later stage it becomes non-pitting, when the skin and subcutaneous tissue become thick and eventually hyperkeratotic and warty. Previous scars in the groin, a mass of malignant nodes or signs of previous radiotherapy will suggest lymphoedema as a possible cause.

In the presence of an arteriovenous fistula there will be dilated veins which do not collapse on elevation of the limb. The limb will be warmer than the opposite limb; palpation will reveal a thrill and auscultation will reveal a continuous machinery bruit.

Localised swelling of the limb may be due to a tumour. There may be also associated distal swelling due to venous or lymphatic obstruction.

Swelling due to neurological damage, e.g. nerve lesions or poliomyelitis, will result in wasting, which should be apparent. Examination of the abdomen may reveal hepatomegaly or an abdominal mass, which could obstruct the venous outflow. It is appropriate to carry out a rectal examination for a pelvic tumour, which may be causing back pressure on the venous and lymphatic system or may have resulted in a 'frozen' pelvis.

GENERAL INVESTIGATIONS

- **FBC, ESR**
  A large haematoma associated with trauma or fracture may result in a low Hb. WCC ↑ will suggest infection. Haematoma may be associated with a reduced platelet count.
- **Urinalysis**
  Proteinuria may suggest a renal cause.
- **U&Es and creatinine**
  Raised urea and creatinine will be associated with renal failure.
- **LFTs**
  May indicate impaired liver function with associated hypoalbuminaemia.
- **Blood glucose**
  Cellulitis or other infections of the leg may be associated with diabetes.
- **CXR**
  Findings suggestive of cardiac failure are cardiomegaly, pulmonary oedema and pleural effusions. Pulmonary oedema may be associated with fluid overload associated with renal failure. Secondary deposits may be seen in association with sarcoma of the limb.
- **Limb X-ray**
  May show fracture, tumour or gas in the tissues associated with gas gangrene.

SPECIFIC INVESTIGATIONS

- **Clotting screen**
  There may be abnormal clotting associated with coagulopathy, resulting in spontaneous haematoma.
- **US**
  Haematoma or soft tissue sarcoma.
- **CT**
  Haematoma or tumour.
- **MRI**
  Soft tissue sarcoma.
- **US or CT pelvis**
  May show an abdominal or pelvic mass causing extrinsic pressure on the veins.
- **Duplex Doppler**
  Will show DVT or arteriovenous fistula.

- **Venography**
  Will confirm DVT.
- **Arteriography**
  Will confirm the presence of an arteriovenous fistula.
- **Lymphangiography**
  May demonstrate the cause of lymphoedema, e.g. hypoplasia or obstruction.
- **Lymph node biopsy**
  Infection or tumour.

▶ LEG ULCERS

An ulcer is a discontinuity of an epithelial surface. Leg ulcers are common and the site of an ulcer on the leg may provide a clue to its aetiology.

CAUSES

Infective
- Syphilis (rare)
- TB (rare)

Neoplastic
- Squamous cell carcinoma
- Malignant melanoma
- Basal cell carcinoma (rare on the leg)

Vascular
- Venous stasis ulcers
- Arterial (ischaemic) ulcers
- Arteriovenous fistulae

Neuropathic
- Diabetes
- Leprosy (rare)
- Tabes dorsalis (syphilis – rare)

Autoimmune/vasculitic
- Rheumatoid arthritis (rare)
- SLE (rare)

Haematological
- Sickle cell anaemia
- Polycythaemia rubra vera
- Thrombotic thrombocytopenic purpura

Other
- Dermatitis artefacta (self-inflicted)
- Pyoderma gangrenosum

HISTORY

A history of trauma may be apparent. In self-inflicted injury it may not. Pain suggests trauma, ischaemia or infection. Lack of pain suggests a neuropathic cause, e.g. diabetes mellitus or tabes dorsalis. A history of varicose veins or DVT suggests a venous stasis ulcer. A prior history of intermittent claudication suggests ischaemic ulcers, as does a history of atrial fibrillation or subacute bacterial endocarditis (embolic). The presence of a long-standing venous ulcer with recent change in the shape of the ulcer suggests development of a squamous cell carcinoma (Marjolin's ulcer). A history of rheumatoid arthritis or collagen disease may suggest a vasculitic lesion. A pigmented ulcerating lesion arising at the site of a previous mole or de novo may suggest a malignant melanoma, especially if there is a history of prolonged exposure to the sun or sunburn. A history of any haematological conditions should be sought. Pyoderma gangrenosum may occur in association with Crohn's disease or ulcerative colitis.

EXAMINATION

Site

The site of an ulcer may give a clue to the aetiology. Venous stasis ulcers usually occur on the medial aspect of the lower third of the leg, usually over the medial malleolus. Arterial ulcers occur over the metatarsal heads, tips of the toes, lateral aspect of the head or the fifth metatarsal, around the heel, in between the toes, and on the tips of the toes. Diabetic ischaemic ulcers occur at the same sites. Diabetic neuropathic ulcers usually occur at pressure points, e.g. under the heel, under the heads of the first and fifth metatarsals and under the toes. They are often associated with callosities.

Edge

Classically, five types are described. A sloping edge suggests a healing ulcer, e.g. venous stasis ulcer. A punched-out edge suggests an ischaemic ulcer or a syphilitic gummatous ulcer (rare). An undermined edge suggests a tuberculous ulcer (rare). A rolled edge is characteristic of a rodent ulcer, while an everted edge is suggestive of a malignant ulcer, e.g. squamous cell carcinoma.

Base

This may contain slough or granulation tissue. Ischaemic ulcers may contain no granulation tissue but have black necrotic tissue, or tendon or bone visible in the base. Syphilitic ulcers have a classical appearance of slough in the base which resembles a wash leather.

Surrounding tissues

Is the surrounding skin pink and healthy with normal innervation? Are there black satellite lesions associated with malignant melanoma?

Examine the regional lymph nodes for sites of secondary infection or metastases. Examine for varicose veins, changes following DVT, or the absence of pulses and the presence of bruits. Examine the whole patient, e.g. signs of rheumatoid arthritis.

Remember that although the initial lesion may have been caused by trauma, other abnormalities may be present to prevent healing, e.g. poor circulation, malnutrition or steroid therapy. Ulcers over the shin in elderly women with thin skin may have been due to minor trauma. However, the fact that the skin here is poorly supported on the periosteum of the underlying bone means that they may be extremely slow to heal. Ulcers occurring in inflammatory bowel disease may be due to pyoderma gangrenosum. The ulcers may be multiple and may have started as pustules.

GENERAL INVESTIGATIONS

- **FBC, ESR**
  Hb ↓ suggests haematological disease. WCC ↑ infection. ESR ↑ collagen diseases (vasculitis), syphilis, TB.
- **U&Es**
  Renal involvement may suggest autoimmune disease.
- **Blood glucose**
  Diabetes mellitus.
- **Swab of ulcer**
  C&S.

SPECIFIC INVESTIGATIONS

- **Rheumatoid factor**
  Rheumatoid arthritis.
- **Antibody screen**
  e.g. ANCA (SLE).
- **VDRL**
  Syphilis.
- **Doppler studies**
  Venous disease. Arterial disease.

- **Biopsy**
  Incision biopsy for possible squamous cell carcinoma or diagnosis of the cause of an obscure ulcer. Excision biopsy is required for suspected malignant melanoma.
- **Venography**
  Assess varicose veins. Deep venous patency.
- **Arteriography**
  Assess arterial tree.

▶ LIP LESIONS

Lip lesions are common. They may be extremely painful and interfere with speech and feeding. They may be socially embarrassing for the patient. They may also prevent appropriate contact with a partner, leading to emotional problems. In the elderly, carcinoma is a common cause of a lump on the lip, especially in those with outdoor occupations.

CAUSES

Congenital
- Cleft lip (hare lip)

Acquired

Flat lesions
- Junctional naevus
- Peutz–Jeghers syndrome
- Telangiectasia (hereditary haemorrhagic telangiectasia)

Raised lesions
- Mucous retention cysts
- Warts
- Pyogenic granuloma
- Squamous cell carcinoma
- Malignant melanoma
- Syphilitic chancre (rare)
- Vascular malformations (rare)

Erosions
- Herpes simplex
- Impetigo
- Pemphigus

Swelling
- Trauma, e.g. burns, bites, assault
- Angioneurotic oedema
- Drug reactions
- Crohn's disease

Cheilitis
- Infection, e.g. candidiasis
- Contact dermatitis, e.g. lipstick, pen-sucking
- Lip-licking (especially in children)

HISTORY

Congenital

Cleft lip occurs due to failure of fusion of the nasal and maxillary processes which form the upper lip and the maxilla. The only abnormality may be a slight indentation in the outer part of the middle third of the upper lip. However, it may extend to the anterior nares. It may be associated with a cleft palate. The condition may be unilateral or bilateral. Abnormal phonation occurs.

Acquired

Flat lesions

Junctional naevi develop at or before puberty. Ensure that there has been no change in a junctional naevus to suggest development of malignant melanoma. In Peutz–Jeghers syndrome pigmentation will be on the gums as well as the lips. There will usually be a family history (autosomal dominant). These pigmented lip lesions do not become malignant. There may be associated history of bowel problems, e.g. bleeding or intussusception. In hereditary telangiectasia, the patient may also have noticed lesions in the mouth and on the skin, especially the fingertips.

Raised lesions

Mucous retention cysts may occur at any age. The patient complains of a lump on the inner aspect of the lip which interferes with eating. With warts, pyogenic granuloma and squamous cell carcinoma, the patient's only complaint is usually of a lump on the lip. With carcinoma there may be a history of leukoplakia, betel-nut chewing or pipe smoking. Classically it used to relate to clay-pipe smoking. There may also be a history of exposure to sunlight, and carcinoma is common in outdoor workers, e.g. sailors, farmers, fisherman and fair-skinned people in sunny climates. Ulcerating and bleeding of the lesion may be a presenting complaint. Syphilitic lesions are now extremely rare. A primary chancre may present on the lip. They are highly contagious. A gummatous lesion on the lip is extremely rare. Malignant melanoma may present as a black, ulcerating or raised lesion at the site of a junctional naevus.

Erosions

The commonest are herpes simplex lesions. Small painful ulcers, which itch, may present on the lips. They are common in immunocompromised patients. Impetigo is common around the mouth and face of children but may affect any age. Pemphigus is a blistering disorder which affects the mucosa and skin.

Swelling

Swelling of the lips may be due to a variety of causes. Trauma is probably the most common, usually following assault, but may arise as a result of burns (hot fluids), sun rays or angioneurotic oedema, which is rare and may affect the tongue and other parts of the body. Drug reactions may cause oedema when associated with urticaria. They usually affect the whole face rather than just the lips. Crohn's disease may also cause swelling of the lips. Other symptoms and signs of Crohn's disease, e.g. diarrhoea, abdominal pain or perianal sepsis, may be present.

Cheilitis

This usually refers to inflammation of the lips and may occur at the angles of the mouth, i.e. angular cheilitis or angular stomatitis. Contact dermatitis may be apparent from either lipstick or pen-sucking. A history of lip-licking should be sought, especially in children. Candida may cause cheilitis in the immunocompromised, infants, those with dentures, and iron-deficiency anaemia.

EXAMINATION

Congenital

Cleft lip is obvious at birth. Cleft palate is discovered on routine inspection soon after birth or may be discovered when difficulties occur with feeding. Beware missing a submucous cleft in which the palate initially appears intact. Late presentation may occur with speech and hearing difficulties.

Acquired

Flat lesions

Junctional naevi are flat, pigmented lesions. The lesions of Peutz–Jeghers syndrome are also flat lesions but, in addition to occurring on the lips, occur also on the gums. In hereditary telangiectasia, telangiectasia may also be present in the mouth, on the palate and on the skin, especially the fingertips.

Raised lesions

Mucous retention cysts tend to occur on the inner aspects of the lips. They are generally pale pink with a grey glairy appearance when the cyst contents show through the stretched overlying mucosa. They are usually smooth, well localised and rarely get bigger than 2 cm in diameter. A warty lesion is usually obvious, with a rough hyperkeratotic surface. Warts may be pedunculated. A pyogenic granuloma is a firm, small, cherry-red nodule consisting of hyperplastic granulation tissue. A squamous cell carcinoma is usually a hard ulcerated lesion with a raised everted edge. The regional lymph nodes may be palpable due to metastases. Malignant melanoma may arise *de novo* or in a preexisting junctional naevus. The lesion is usually raised, pigmented, occasionally friable, and bleeds easily. There may be satellite nodules and regional nodes may be palpable due to metastases. Syphilitic lesions are rare nowadays. A chancre associated with primary syphilis may occur on the lips. The initial lesion is elevated, flat, hard and painless. Eventually, however, ulceration may occur, to give a slightly painful ulcer which crusts over. The regional lymph nodes become enlarged and tender, usually 7–10 days after the appearance of the chancre.

Erosions

Herpetic lesions begin as a patch of painful, itchy erythema. Vesicles form subsequently, which dry up and crust over after 4–5 days, the crust eventually separating, leaving tiny scars. Impetigo causes golden-coloured crusts, usually on the faces of children. In pemphigus, blisters erode quickly and become painful erosions on the mucous membrane and skin.

Swellings and cheilitis

These are usually diagnosed from the history. They usually cause reddening and inflammation of the lips.

GENERAL INVESTIGATIONS

- **FBC, ESR**
  Hb ↓ iron-deficiency anaemia (associated with cheilitis). WCC ↑ infection. WCC ↓ immunosuppression. ESR ↑ Crohn's disease, syphilis, malignancy.

- **Swab**
  C&S. Dark-ground illumination of fluid from syphilitic chancre (spirochaetes visible).

SPECIFIC INVESTIGATIONS

- **VDRL**
  Syphilis.

- **Biopsy**
  Benign versus malignant. Pyogenic granuloma. Squamous cell carcinoma. Malignant melanoma (excision biopsy). Crohn's disease.

- **FNAC**
  May be diagnostic when lymph node enlargement is associated with lip lesion.
- **Gastroscopy**
  Peutz–Jeghers. Mucosal lesions.
- **Colonoscopy**
  Peutz–Jeghers. Mucosal lesions.

LYMPHADENOPATHY

Lymphadenopathy is a common presenting condition. It may be
localised or generalised. The causes are multiple but a careful history
and clinical examination will often simplify the diagnosis.
Lymphadenopathy, especially cervical, is extremely common in
children who are otherwise healthy. Painful tender nodes are usually
associated with infection. Firm or hard, painless nodes are commonly
the seat of malignancy. Only the commoner causes, which the
student would be expected to know, are described in this section.

CAUSES

Primary infection

Viral
- Infectious mononucleosis
- HIV
- CMV
- Rubella
- Measles

Bacterial
- TB
- Syphilis
- Brucellosis
- Cat scratch disease
- Septicaemia

Protozoal
- Toxoplasmosis

Parasitic
- Filariasis

Secondary infection
- E.g. tonsillitis with cervical lymphadenitis, abscess with
  regional lymphadenitis

Primary malignancy
- Acute lymphoblastic leukaemia
- Chronic lymphatic leukaemia
- Hodgkin's disease
- Non-Hodgkin's lymphoma
- Myeloproliferative disorders

Secondary malignancy
- Metastases from local malignancy
- Metastases from distant malignancy

Others
- Sarcoidosis
- SLE
- Rheumatoid arthritis

HISTORY

Infection
Local infections will be usually obvious, e.g. dental abscess with cervical lymphadenopathy. With generalised lymphadenopathy there may be a history of malaise, lethargy and fever. Check for exposure to TB, which may be a cause of lymphadenopathy in the immunocompromised patient. Check for visits abroad. Check if there are animals in the household, e.g. cats (cat scratch fever) or dogs (toxoplasmosis). In the case of cat scratch fever the scratches are often healed before the patient presents. Note any history of local trauma.

Primary malignancy
There will normally be a history of malaise, fever or night sweats. The patient may have noticed lumps at several sites. Spontaneous bruising and bleeding associated with thrombocytopenia may also be present.

Secondary malignancy
The primary may be obvious or may be very small and have not been noticed by the patient (e.g. a malignant melanoma in an inaccessible site). There may be a history of malignancy that has been treated several years previously with metastases presenting late (e.g. axillary lymphadenopathy or cervical lymphadenopathy occurring several years after an apparently curative operation for carcinoma of the breast). Occasionally the lymph node swelling is distant from the primary e.g. cervical lymphadenoapthy (left supraclavicular fossa) from testicular cancer; Virchow's node in gastric cancer.

Other conditions
Sarcoidosis causes bilateral hilar lymphadenopathy but may present with lymphadenopathy at other sites. Check for a history of SLE or rheumatoid arthritis.

EXAMINATION

Examine the enlarged lymph nodes. Are they painful and tender, suggesting infection, or are they firm and painless, suggesting malignancy? Check the sites draining to these nodes for a site of infection or primary malignancy. Check for linear scratches suggestive of cat scratch disease. Examine for bruising. Examine all other sites of potential lymphadenopathy: cervical, axillary, inguinal, popliteal and epitrochlear nodes. Check for splenomegaly and hepatomegaly. Carry out a full general examination.

GENERAL INVESTIGATIONS

- **FBC, ESR**
  Hb ↓ blood dyscrasias. Platelets ↓ dyscrasias. WCC ↑ infection, leukaemia. ESR ↑ tumour, infection. Blood film. Leukaemia.
- **LFTs**
  Malignant infiltration of the liver.
- **Clotting screen**
  Blood dyscrasias.
- **Viral titres**
  Viral infections, e.g. Epstein–Barr, HIV.
- **CXR**
  Hilar glands in sarcoidosis. TB. Secondary deposits.
- **Mantoux test**
  TB.
- **Swab**
  Local infection. C&S.

SPECIFIC INVESTIGATIONS

- **Antibody screen**
  SLE, rheumatoid arthritis.
- **Blood cultures**
  Septicaemia.
- **VDRL**
  Syphilis.
- **Kveim test**
  Sarcoidosis.
- **Toxoplasma screen**
  Toxoplasmosis.

- **CT**
  Nodal distribution. Staging of Hodgkin's disease.
- **FNAC of lymph node**
  Malignancy versus other conditions.
- **Biopsy**
  Lymph node, e.g. Hodgkin's disease, secondary deposit. Biopsy of local lesion, e.g. infective versus malignant.

MELAENA

Melaena is the passage of altered blood PR. A melaena stool is black and tarry and has a characteristic smell. The blood is degraded by hydrochloric acid and intestinal enzymes high in the gastrointestinal tract. Melaena is unlikely to occur if bleeding comes from lower than the jejunum, although occasionally melaena may result from a bleeding Meckel's diverticulum.

CAUSES

Swallowed blood
- Epistaxis
- Haemoptysis

Oesophagus
- Oesophageal varices
- Reflux oesophagitis
- Oesophageal carcinoma

Stomach
- Peptic ulceration
- Mallory–Weiss syndrome
- Acute gastric erosions
- Carcinoma
- Leiomyoma (rare)
- Hereditary haemorrhagic telangiectasia (rare)
- Vascular malformations (rare)

Duodenum
- Peptic ulceration
- Duodenal diverticulae
- Aortoduodenal fistulae
- Invasive pancreatic tumours (rare)
- Haemobilia (rare)

Small intestine
- Leiomyoma (rare)
- Meckel's diverticulum (rare)

Bleeding disorders
- Liver disease-associated
- Thrombocytopenia
- Haemophilia

Drugs
- Anticoagulants
- Aspirin
- NSAIDs
- Steroids

Others
- Uraemia
- Connective tissue disorders

Other causes of dark stools
- Iron therapy
- Bismuth preparations
- Liquorice
- Charcoal biscuits
- Red wine (large quantities)

HISTORY

Swallowed blood
Check for a recent history of epistaxis or haemoptysis.

Oesophagus
There may be a history of excess alcohol consumption or a history of other liver disease to suggest oesophageal varices. Check for retrosternal burning pain and heartburn, which would suggest oesophagitis. Check for a history of dysphagia. The bleeding associated with varices is often torrential. That associated with oesophagitis is minor.

Stomach
History of epigastric pain to suggest peptic ulceration. There may be a history of steroid or NSAID medication. Mallory–Weiss syndrome usually occurs in the younger patient who has had a large meal with much alcohol and has a forceful vomit. The first vomit contains food, the second contains blood. Acute gastric erosions may occur with stressful illnesses, e.g. major surgery, acute pancreatitis, burns (Curling's ulcer), head injuries (Cushing's ulcer). It is unusual to get a large bleed with a carcinoma. Anaemia is a common presentation, and there may be 'coffee ground' vomit. Leiomyoma causes a moderate haematemesis. There is usually no preceding history. There will also be no preceding history with vascular malformations. Hereditary haemorrhagic telangiectasia is rare. The patient may present with a history of the condition, or it

may be apparent from the telangiectasia around the lips and oral cavity.

Duodenum

Melaena tends to be a more common symptom than haematemesis with duodenal lesions. There may be a history of chronic duodenal ulceration, although often presentation may be acute with little background history. Bleeding from invasive pancreatic tumours is rare. The patient will present with malaise, lethargy, weight loss and vomiting. Haemobilia is rare. Aortoduodenal fistula is rare and usually follows repair of an aneurysm with subsequent infection of the graft. There is massive haematemesis and malaise.

Small intestine

Leiomyomas are rare but may bleed, resulting in melaena. Bleeding from a Meckel's diverticulum, if it occurs fast enough, usually causes dark-red bleeding rather than characteristic melaena.

Other causes of dark stools

Take a full dietary and drug history.

EXAMINATION

Depending upon the severity of the bleed, there may be shock. The patient will be cold, clammy, with peripheral vasoconstriction; there will be a tachycardia and hypotension.

Swallowed blood

Check for blood around the nose. Examine the chest for a possible cause of haemoptysis.

Oesophagus

There may be little to find on examination except clinical signs of anaemia and weight loss unless the cause is oesophageal varices, in which case there may be jaundice, abdominal distension due to ascites, spider naevi, liver palms, clubbing, gynaecomastia, testicular atrophy, caput medusae, splenomegaly or hepatomegaly.

Stomach

There may be little to find on examination. There may be an epigastric mass with a carcinoma, or a palpable left supraclavicular node (Virchow's nodes). There may be epigastric tenderness. With hereditary haemorrhagic telangiectasia there may be telangiectasia on the lips and mucous membrane of the mouth.

Duodenum

Again, there may be little to find on examination other than epigastric tenderness. In the rare case where duodenal bleeding comes from an invasive pancreatic carcinoma, there may be a palpable mass in the region of the pancreas.

Small intestine

Often there is little to find. Leiomyomas may be palpable.

Bleeding disorders

There may be sites of bruising or bleeding from other orifices.

GENERAL INVESTIGATIONS

- **FBC, ESR**
  Hb ↓ anaemia due to chronic bleeding, e.g. from carcinoma. ESR ↑ connective tissue disease.
- **U&Es**
  Urea and creatinine will be raised in uraemia. Urea may be raised due to absorption of blood from the bowel.
- **LFTs**
  Liver failure, oesophageal varices, haemobilia.
- **Clotting screen**
  Liver disease. Bleeding diatheses. Anticoagulants.

SPECIFIC INVESTIGATIONS

- **OGD**
  Will demonstrate most lesions, e.g. varices, oesophagitis, peptic ulcer, gastric erosions, Mallory–Weiss tear, carcinoma and rarer causes of bleeding. Biopsy may be carried out where necessary.
- **Angiography**
  Vascular malformations. Also may diagnose rarer distal duodenal causes, e.g. aortoduodenal fistulae.
- **Technetium scan**
  Meckel's diverticulum containing gastric mucosa.
- **Labelled red cell scan**
  Rare small bowel causes of bleeding.
- **Small bowel enema**
  Leiomyoma. Meckel's diverticulum

MOUTH ULCERS

Ulceration in the mouth is common. It is important to be able to distinguish between simple benign ulcers, e.g. traumatic or aphthous, from those that are malignant. Tongue lesions are dealt with on page 426.

CAUSES

Traumatic

Aphthous

Inflammatory
● Crohn's disease

Infective

Bacterial
● Acute ulcerative gingivitis
● Syphilis

Viral
● Herpes simplex

Fungal
● Candidiasis

Neoplastic
● Squamous cell carcinoma
● Blood dyscrasias
● Agranulocytosis
● Leukaemia

Skin disease-associated
● Lichen planus
● Pemphigus
● Pemphigoid
● Bullous erythema multiforme

Connective tissue disease
● SLE

Other
● Behçet's syndrome
● Reiter's disease

HISTORY

Traumatic
Diagnosis usually obvious. Ill-fitting dentures. Sharp teeth. Ulcers heal when precipitating cause is removed.

Aphthous
Patient presents with small, painful ulcers, usually inside the cheeks or lips. They heal in about 1 week but others may occur while the initial ulcers are healing. A number of patients will have a history of gastrointestinal disease, e.g. coeliac disease or Crohn's disease. They may also arise in patients with debilitating disease.

Inflammatory
Chronic granulomatous disease (Crohn's) may affect the oral cavity. The patient may complain of painful ulcers, swelling of the lips or gum swelling.

Infective
Vincent's angina (acute ulcerative stomatitis) presents with swollen gums with small ulcers, which may spread to the buccal mucosa. The patient will complain of bleeding gums, together with constitutional upset with fever and malaise. Syphilis is now rarely seen but chancres, snail-track ulcers and gummas may occur within the mouth. Candida is not uncommon in the oral cavity. There may be a history of debilitating disease, diabetes or immunosuppressive therapy. Herpes simplex presents as painful vesicles, which ulcerate. The patient may be immunocompromised. Herpes zoster may occur on the palate in the distribution of the maxillary division of the trigeminal nerve. There will be severe pain and ulceration.

Neoplastic
Squamous cell carcinomas occur as ulcers with hard edges, which bleed. They tend to occur in the older patient. There may be a history of leucoplakia or the six 'Ss', i.e. syphilis, smoking, sharp tooth, spirits, spices, sepsis.

Blood dyscrasias
Agranulocytosis may be due to drugs or marrow infiltration. Take a careful drug history. The ulceration may be due to bacterial infection consequent on the low white cell count. Leukaemia may also present with mouth ulcers.

Skin disease-associated
These include lichen planus, pemphigus pemphigoid and bullous erythema multiforme. The reader is referred to a textbook of dermatology for the characteristics of these conditions.

Connective tissue disease
Oral ulceration may be associated with SLE. The patient may present with other features of this disease, e.g. skin lesions, joint pains or renal failure.

Other
Although Behçet's disease may present with mouth ulcers, the patient may also complain of arthritis, eye disease, scrotal or labial ulcers. With Reiter's disease the patient will complain also of urethritis, conjunctivitis and arthritis. There will usually be a history of sexual contact.

EXAMINATION

Traumatic
There will be ulceration related to ill-fitting dentures or sharp teeth. Observe for healing when the precipitating cause has been removed.

Aphthous
Small, white, circular, deep, painful ulcers with surrounding erythema. There may be signs and symptoms of gastrointestinal disease or other debilitating disease, or they may occur in otherwise healthy patients.

Inflammatory
With Crohn's disease, there may be lip swelling, nodular thickening of the buccal mucosa, diffuse granular ginigival swelling or painful linea oral ulcers.

Infective
Vincent's angina presents with red, swollen, bleeding gums covered with yellowish ulcers. The ulcers may also be seen on the buccal mucosa and occasionally on the tonsils. There is usually tender lymphadenopathy. With syphilis there may be either a chancre, snail-track ulcers or gummas. Herpes simplex presents with small 2 mm vesicles which ulcerate and coalesce and produce erosions with surrounding erythema. Herpes zoster shows small ulcers surrounded with erythema in the distribution of the maxillary nerve on the palate. There will usually be skin lesions in the

distribution of the nerve. Candidiasis appears as red patches on the buccal mucosa, which are covered with white patches of desquamated epithelium mixed with fungus.

Neoplastic

There will be an ulcer with hard, everted edges which bleeds on touching. Cervical lymphadenopathy may be present.

Blood dyscrasias

These present with bleeding gums and ulceration.

Skin disease-associated

The reader is referred to a textbook of dermatology for the characteristic features of these.

Connective tissue disorders

Oral ulceration may occur with SLE. Other features may be present on examination, e.g. skin, joint or renal disease.

Other

Behçet's disease presents with painful ulcers. Other features may be apparent on examination, e.g. arthritis, keratitis, iritis, scrotal or labial ulcers. With Reiter's syndrome there will be urethritis, conjunctivitis and balanitis, as well as mouth ulcers.

GENERAL INVESTIGATIONS

- **FBC, ESR**
  Hb ↓ malignancy, debilitating disease. WCC ↑ infection, leukaemia. ESR ↑ malignancy, connective tissue disease, chronic infection, e.g. syphilis.
- **U&Es**
  Renal disease – SLE.
- **Swab**
  C&S. Infections – *Borrelia vincentii* (Vincent's angina), candidiasis.
- **Antibody screen**
  SLE – ANA positive. Anti-double-stranded DNA ↑.
- **VDRL**
  Syphilis.
- **Viral antibodies**
  Herpes simplex. Herpes zoster.
- **Biopsy**
  Squamous cell carcinoma. Crohn's disease.

MUSCLE WASTING

Muscle wasting may occur as a manifestation of cachexia and by definition with lower motor neurone lesions. With upper motor neurone lesions, a degree of wasting may also develop as a result of disuse atrophy.

CAUSES

Localised
- Peripheral nerve lesions
  - Peripheral nerve compression
  - Peripheral nerve transection
  - Motor neuropathy
- Anterior horn cell lesions
  - Previous polio
- Disuse atrophy

Generalised
- Nutritional deficiency
- Systemic disease
  - Malignancy
  - Cardiac cachexia
  - Thyrotoxicosis
  - Cushing's disease
- Muscle and motor end plate disorders
  - Motor neurone disease
  - Myasthenia gravis
  - Muscular dystrophies
  - Myotonic dystrophy
  - Polymyositis
- Drugs and toxins
  - Alcohol
  - Statins
  - Cyclosporin
  - Steroids

HISTORY

Onset
Muscle wasting in childhood is often due to congenital disease such as inherited muscular dystrophies (e.g. Duchenne's muscular

dystrophy) a diagnosis further supported by a positive family history of a first-degree relative with similar problems. With myotonic dystrophy, first symptoms occur around the age of 15 to 30 years while with motor neurone disease the peak age of onset is in the fifties.

Site

The distribution of muscle wasting may characterise the disease. Atrophy may be confined to the motor supply of a single nerve, such as the thenar eminence with the median nerve affected by carpal tunnel syndrome. It may also occur with a group of muscles such as the leg with polio. And finally the distribution may be generalised in conditions such as motor neurone disease.

Precipitating factors

Precipitating factors such as trauma may result in transection of a peripheral nerve such as the ulnar nerve, commonly at the wrist.

Past medical history

The presence of carcinoma or chronic cardiorespiratory disease may give rise to peripheral muscle wasting from cachexia. Previous infection with polio is significant because, in a minority of affected individuals, degeneration of anterior horn cells with subsequent paralysis and muscle wasting occurs. Disuse atrophy can be localised or generalised. Conditions that result in immobility such as a long bone fracture will cause disuse atrophy of the surrounding muscles; this is commonly seen upon removal of plaster casts. Localised disuse atrophy may also result from joint pains such as quadriceps wasting with painful knee disorders. Prolonged immobility will result in generalised muscle wasting. Conditions such as diabetes and renal failure are associated with neuropathy.

Associated symptoms

Most of the causes are associated with weakness of the affected muscles. Diplopia, ptosis and fatigability are associated features suggestive of myasthenia gravis. Motor neurone disease may present with progressive weakness and wasting of the hand or leg accompanied with dysarthria and dysphasia. Cushing's disease may be associated with weight gain, hair growth, acne, abdominal striae, muscle weakness, back pain and depression.

EXAMINATION

Inspection will identify the areas of muscle wasting. Central obesity with limb wasting occurs with Cushing's disease. Generalised uniform muscle wasting should lead to a careful examination of the organ systems for malignancy and organ failure. Muscle tenderness is associated with polymyositis.

Characteristic features of myotonic dystrophy are frontal balding, ptosis, temporal and facial muscle wasting. Cataracts may be seen with inspection of the eyes. Ptosis may also be a feature of myasthenia gravis; this is accompanied with diplopia, facial weakness and a weak nasal voice. Muscle wasting with fasiculations occur with motor neurone disease, no sensory loss is experienced and mixed upper and lower motor neurone signs may be present.

Assessment of tone, reflexes and pattern of weakness will determine whether it is an upper or lower motor neurone lesion. Delayed relaxation of muscle contraction occurs with myotonic dystrophy and proximal muscle weakness occurs with Cushing's disease. With localised muscle wasting, examination of each muscle will allow you to determine whether the lesion arises from a single nerve or a nerve root.

The joint surrounding wasted muscles should be examined for deformity or pain that may restrict movement. Measurements of circumference can be obtained to assess asymmetrical muscle wasting of the limbs.

GENERAL INVESTIGATIONS

- **FBC**
  Anaemia with nutritional disorders and chronic disease.
- **ESR**
  ↑ with malignancy, polymyositis.
- **U&Es**
  ↑ urea and ↑ creatinine with renal failure.
- **Glucose**
  ↑ with diabetes.
- **LFTs**
  ↓ Albumin with malnutrition.
- **Creatine phosphokinase**
  ↑ with myopathies.
- **TFTs**
  ↓ TSH ↑ T_4 with thyrotoxicosis
- **Electromyography (EMG)**
  Allows assessment for denervation of muscle, myopathies and myotonic dystrophy, motor neurone disease.

- **Nerve conduction studies**
  Radiculopathies, peripheral neuropathy, peripheral nerve compression.

SPECIFIC INVESTIGATIONS

- **Tensilon test**
  Injection of edrophonium reverses symptoms of myasthenia gravis.
- **Muscle biopsies**
  Diagnosis of muscle dystrophies.

NASAL DISCHARGE

Nasal discharges are common. The commonest causes are the common cold and allergic rhinitis. Persistent bloodstained nasal discharge is a serious symptom requiring urgent investigation.

CAUSES

Congenital
- Choanal atresia

Acquired

Infective
- Common cold (coryza)
- Chronic rhinitis
- Sinusitis
- Adenoiditis (large adenoids)
- Fungal infections (rare)
- Chronic infection
  - Syphilis
- Viral infections
  - AIDS

Allergic
- Allergic rhinitis

Inflammatory
- Eosinophilic vasomotor rhinitis
- Nasal polyps
- Non-eosinophilic vasomotor rhinitis

Neoplastic
- Carcinoma
  - Nasopharynx
  - Sinuses
- Lymphoma (malignant granuloma)

Granulomatous disease
- Wegener's granulomatosis

Traumatic
- Foreign body
- Fracture of the anterior fossa
- Irritant gases, e.g. chlorine, tobacco smoke

Degenerative
- Senile rhinorrhoea

HISTORY

Congenital

Choanal atresia is rare. Check for other congenital abnormalities. Bilateral choanal atresia is a life-threatening condition in newborn infants. Unilateral atresia may not be picked up until 5–10 years of age when it becomes apparent that one nostril is blocked and there is a thick mucus discharge.

Acquired

Infective

The patient will often have a common cold. There is a mucoid nasal discharge, which settles rapidly once the cold has settled. With chronic rhinitis there may be a chronic purulent discharge. This is often thick and mucoid. There may be a history of immunological deficiency or cystic fibrosis. With sinusitis there may be pain or discomfort over the maxillary sinuses or a headache with pain over the frontal sinuses. With large adenoids there may be a complaint of mouth breathing, recurrent pharyngeal infections, snoring and recurrent ear infections. Fungal infections of the nose are rare, occurring in immunosuppressed patients. *Candida albicans* and *Aspergillus* spp are the most common organisms. Chronic infective lesions include syphilis. Secondary syphilis can affect the nose and cause a catarrhal rhinitis. Usually other lesions of syphilis will be present. AIDS may be associated with a watery nasal discharge. Check the sexual lifestyle of the patient. Other symptoms of AIDS may be present.

Allergic

Allergic rhinitis There may be a history of infantile eczema, allergic asthma or nasal or conjunctival allergy. It may be seasonal with allergy to pollen or perennial with exposure to animal dander (cats) or house dust mites. The patient complains of watery rhinorrhoea, sneezing attacks, nasal obstruction, and conjunctival irritation and lacrimation. There is usually a family history.

Inflammatory

Vasomotor rhinitis Eosinophilic vasomotor rhinitis presents with a watery nasal discharge and sneezing. No type I allergic reaction is involved in this condition. The condition is associated with nasal polyps and aspirin sensitivity and asthma.

Nasal polyps These occur in non-allergic eosinophilic vasomotor rhinitis. The patient will complain of nasal obstruction and discharge.

Non-eosinophilic vasomotor rhinitis The patient presents with watery nasal discharge, nasal obstruction and sneezing attacks. This condition may be associated with: (1) certain antihypertensive drugs, particularly ganglion blockers and vasodilators; (2) hormonal disturbances; (3) congestive cardiac failure; (4) anxiety states; (5) occupational irritants, e.g. ammonia, smoke.

Neoplastic

Nasopharyngeal carcinoma Nasopharyngeal carcinoma is rare in Europe but is common in South China. The patient presents with nasal obstruction and bloodstained discharge. Unilateral otitis media may occur from eustachian tube blockage. Nerve palsies may occur due to invasion of the base of the skull. The patient may complain only of a swelling in the neck due to lymphadenopathy, lymphatic spread occurring at an early stage. With this disease, unilateral deafness, cervical lymphadenopathy and cranial nerve palsies are often diagnostic.

Carcinoma of the maxillary sinus This is often diagnosed late. Early presenting symptoms include bloodstained nasal discharge and unilateral nasal obstruction. Later, swelling of the cheek occurs, with ulceration of the palate. Epiphora may occur due to invasion of the nasolacrimal duct. Erosion into the orbit results in proptosis and diplopia. Pain may be referred to the ear.

Malignant granuloma Malignant granuloma (now thought to be lymphomatous) presents with slowly progressive ulceration starting in the region of the nose. The chronic inflammatory reaction causes a nasal discharge.

Granulomatous disease

Wegener's granulomatosis affects the nose and is associated with disease of the kidneys, lungs and respiratory tract. The patient may present with either lung manifestations or chronic renal failure.

Traumatic

The commonest trauma causing a nasal discharge is a foreign body. The patient is usually a child aged between 1 and 5 years, or rarely a psychiatrically disturbed adult. The child is usually miserable with a smelly, bloodstained nasal discharge. In adults, rhinolith may occur. This results in unilateral obstruction and discharge. There is usually a large concretion blocking the nose, which may have a foreign body at the centre, with calcium and magnesium laid down round it. Following fracture of the anterior fossa, sustained during head injury, the patient may complain of a clear nasal discharge (CSF rhinorrhoea) or a bloodstained nasal discharge. Irritant gases, e.g. chlorine, which may be industrial or in excess in swimming pools, may cause irritation of the nasal mucosa, with discharge.

Degenerative

Senile rhinorrhoea occurs in the elderly. It is thought to be due to failure of vasomotor control.

EXAMINATION

Choanal atresia

Pass a probe or catheter into the nasal cavity. It will not pass. Posterior rhinoscopy under general anaesthetic will confirm the diagnosis.

Infective

With a common cold there will be oedematous nasal mucosa with clear mucus in the nose. With chronic rhinitis there will be thick mucus or a purulent nasal discharge. With enlarged adenoids, mirror examination will reveal the diagnosis, which will be confirmed by a lateral soft-tissue X-ray.

Allergic

Allergic rhinitis reveals an oedematous nasal mucosa with clear mucus in the nose.

Inflammatory

The appearance of eosinophilic vasomotor rhinitis is similar to that of allergic rhinitis except that nasal polyps may be seen. Nasal polyps are usually pink and smooth or a yellowish–grey and pedunculated. With non-eosinophilic vasomotor rhinitis excessive secretions will be noted on examination, with engorgement of the inferior turbinates. Often the signs are not as severe as the symptoms would suggest.

Neoplastic

Examination should include visualisation of the postnasal space, under general anaesthetic if necessary. A full examination of the cranial nerves must be made. With carcinoma of the maxillary sinus there may be swelling of the cheek with ulceration of the palate. Epiphora may occur due to invasion of the nasolacrimal duct. Check for proptosis and diplopia due to invasion into the orbit. Examine the neck for cervical nodes. With malignant granuloma there is slowly progressive ulceration of the face, starting in the region of the nose.

Granulomatous disease

With Wegener's granulomatosis, necrotic mucosal ulceration occurs. Erosions through the skin of the face or nose, or perforation of the palate, do not occur with Wegener's granulomatosis; if any of these are seen, malignant granuloma or neoplasm should be suspected. There may be coexisting otitis media, ulceration of the mouth or involvement of the trachea or larynx. There may be lung involvement, eye involvement and renal involvement.

Traumatic

Examination with a nasal speculum will usually reveal the foreign body. With CSF rhinorrhoea it may be difficult to distinguish bleeding from blood mixed with CSF. Place a drop of the bloodstained discharge on a clean white gauze. If CSF is present, there will be a spreading yellowish ring around the central stain of blood (halo sign). With irritant gases there will be redness and oedema of the nasal mucosa. There will almost certainly be eye irritation and a skin reaction accompanying it.

Degenerative

With senile rhinorrhoea there are usually no physical signs apart from the nasal drip.

GENERAL INVESTIGATIONS

- **FBC, ESR**
  Hb ↓ malignancy, Wegener's granulomatosis. WCC ↑ infection, e.g. adenoiditis. ESR ↑ infection, malignancy.
- **Swab**
  Culture and sensitivity. Bacterial versus fungal.
- **Skull X-ray**
  Anterior cranial fossa fracture involving ethmoid bone – CSF rhinorrhoea. Carcinoma of the maxillary antrum.

SPECIFIC INVESTIGATIONS

- **Biopsy**
- **Carcinoma. Wegener's granulomatosis. Malignant granuloma.**
- **RAST**
  Measures allergen-specific IgE.
- **CT**
  Nasopharyngeal carcinoma. Assessment of extent of disease.
  Carcinoma of the maxillary antrum. Assessment of extent of disease.

NECK LUMPS

A lump in the neck is a common problem in surgical practice. It is necessary to be able to distinguish the different causes, which may vary from a simple benign swelling to part of a generalised malignant condition.

CAUSES

Superficial
- Sebaceous cyst
- Lipoma
- Dermoid cyst
- Abscess

Lymph nodes

Deep

Anterior triangle
Move on swallowing
- Thyroid
- Thyroglossal cyst

Do not move on swallowing
- Salivary glands
- Branchial cyst
- Carotid body tumour
- Carotid aneurysm
- Sternomastoid 'tumour'

Posterior triangle
- Cervical rib
- Subclavian artery aneurysm
- Pharyngeal pouch
- Cystic hygroma

HISTORY

Symptoms
The diagnosis of superficial swellings of the neck should be obvious. A sebaceous cyst will usually have grown slowly and may have been painful and red if infected. Lipomas tend to grow slowly. An abscess will be obvious from pain and tenderness.

Lymphadenopathy may be associated with a recent pyrexial illness, local lesions in the head and neck, generalised infection or generalised malignancy. Swelling during mastication suggests a salivary gland origin. Blackouts or dizziness may suggest a carotid body tumour. A lump in the lower part of the posterior triangle, increasing in size after eating and gurgling when full, suggests a pharyngeal pouch. The patient may experience bouts of coughing or choking when lying down as the pouch empties itself and aspiration occurs. Neurological or vascular symptoms in the upper limb may be associated with a cervical rib. Sternomastoid tumours are rare and occur in the neonate. Cystic hygromas are rare and occur in infancy.

Past medical history

A history of HIV infection, TB and malignancy is relevant. Breech or forceps delivery may be relevant to the development of a sternomastoid tumour.

EXAMINATION

Decide whether the swelling is superficial or deep. Decide whether it is likely to be due to lymphadenopathy. If the swelling is deep, decide whether it is in the anterior triangle of the neck or the posterior triangle. If it is in the anterior triangle, decide whether it moves on swallowing (thyroid-associated) or not.

Sebaceous cyst

This is usually obvious, being in the skin and having a punctum.

Lipoma

May occur anywhere in the neck but often occurs in the midline posteriorly. Lipomas are soft and lobulated and not fixed to the skin.

Dermoid cyst

These may be congenital or acquired. The congenital ones are most common in the head and neck and occur where skin dermatomes fuse. They are not unlike sebaceous cysts on examination but lack a punctum. Acquired implantation dermoids usually occur in relation to scars.

Abscess

The diagnosis will usually be obvious. There will be a tender, red, inflamed swelling. They may occur in relation to lymph nodes or salivary glands.

Lymphadenopathy

Depending upon the cause of the condition, lymph nodes will be either enlarged and tender; non-tender and firm or rubbery; or small, hard and matted together. A check should be made for enlarged lymph nodes elsewhere in the body and for hepatosplenomegaly. Generalised lymphadenopathy and splenomegaly will occur with blood dyscrasias.

Thyroid

Thyroid swellings move on swallowing. Associated lymphadenopathy will suggest malignancy. The thyroid status of the patient should be checked on clinical examination.

Thyroglossal cyst

This is a painless cystic swelling in the midline of the neck that moves on swallowing. It also moves on protrusion of the tongue. It is commonly attached to the body of the hyoid bone. Occasionally it may become infected, with pain, tenderness and increased swelling.

Salivary gland

Swelling of the submandibular salivary gland is most frequently due to obstruction of the submandibular duct. Swelling will be noted on mastication. A stone may be palpated in the submandibular duct in the floor of the mouth. Swelling of the parotid gland may be due to duct obstruction, although tumour is more common with this gland. Malignant tumours of the parotid gland may be associated with facial nerve palsy.

Branchial cyst

A branchial cyst feels soft and putty-like and abuts from the anterior border of sternocleidomastoid at the junction between its upper and middle thirds.

Carotid body tumour

This feels firm and is located at the bifurcation of the common carotid artery.

Carotid aneurysm

These are extremely rare. False ones may follow surgery or trauma to the neck. A tortuous carotid artery may be mistaken for a carotid aneurysm.

Sternomastoid 'tumour'

This appears only in babies and is a result of birth trauma. There is a swelling in the middle third of the sternomastoid. The head becomes turned to the opposite side and tilted towards the shoulder on the side of the lesion.

Cervical rib

A bony, hard swelling may be palpable in the posterior triangle of the neck.

Subclavian artery aneurysm

Obvious as a pulsatile, expansile swelling in the lower part of the posterior triangle. Often associated with a cervical rib.

Pharyngeal pouch

Presents behind the lower border of sternomastoid in the posterior triangle. It may fill after a meal and empty after lying down. Signs of aspiration pneumonitis may be present.

Cystic hygromas

This is a collection of dilated lymphatics which presents in infancy. It is soft, lobulated, fluctuant, compressible and brilliantly transilluminable.

GENERAL INVESTIGATIONS

- **FBC, ESR**
  Hb ↓ malignancy. WCC ↑ infection and leukaemia. ESR ↑ infection and malignancy.
- **CXR**
  May show tuberculosis or primary or secondary tumour. Tracheal deviation may be associated with thyroid swellings. A cervical rib may be seen. Count the ribs. If there are 13 it is likely that there is a cervical rib.
- **US**
  This may be helpful in almost any lump in the neck. It will also distinguish between solid and cystic swellings, e.g. in the thyroid.

SPECIFIC INVESTIGATIONS

A detailed history and examination may suggest the aetiology of the swelling. Further confirmatory investigations may be required for specific cases.

- **Paul–Bunnell test**
  For glandular fever.

- **Toxoplasma screen**
  Toxoplasmosis.
- **Mantoux test**
  For TB.
- **Viral titres**
  For any viral infection that may cause cervical lymphadenopathy.
- **HIV screen**
  AIDS.
- **TFTs**
  If clinical examination reveals a swelling to be a goitre.
- **FNAC**
  Especially useful for swellings of lymph nodes, thyroid or salivary glands.
- **CT**
  Helpful with the diagnosis of almost any mass but particularly helpful with confirming the diagnosis of carotid body tumours.
- **Duplex Doppler**
  For suspected carotid artery aneurysm or subclavian artery aneurysm.
- **Floor of mouth X-ray**
  Will identify a calculus in the submandibular duct.
- **Sialography**
  Contrast study of salivary duct to locate possible cause and site of obstruction, e.g. stone or stricture.
- **Barium swallow**
  To confirm the presence of a pharyngeal pouch. Never perform an endoscopy if a pouch is suspected, as perforation of the pouch may result.
- **OGD**
  To check for a primary oesophageal or gastric carcinoma causing cervical lymphadenopathy.
- **Bronchoscopy**
  Check for carcinoma of the lung associated with cervical gland metastases.

▶ NECK PAIN

Neck pain is a common problem. The majority of cases are due to poor posture or cervical spondylosis. If there has been a history of trauma, extreme care must be exercised in examination of the neck and any X-rays must be strictly supervised.

CAUSES

Congenital
- Torticollis
- Klippel–Feil syndrome

Acquired

Traumatic
- Fractures
- Dislocations
- Whiplash injury

Inflammatory
- Traumatic
- Rheumatoid arthritis

Infective
- Tuberculosis

Degenerative
- Cervical spondylosis
- Cervical disc lesion

Neoplastic
- Secondary deposits

Other
- Postural
- Exposure to cold
- Meningitis
- Subarachnoid haemorrhage

HISTORY

Congenital

Torticollis may be congenital and present at birth due to sternomastoid 'tumour'. This is a rare condition often associated with breech delivery. Klippel–Feil syndrome is rare and is characterised by developmental abnormalities of the cervical vertebrae and a high-riding scapula.

Acquired

Traumatic

History of trauma. Are there any neurological sequelae, e.g. arm pain or weakness, bladder symptoms? Whiplash injuries are common. These occur in road traffic accidents where the car is struck from behind. The neck extends with sudden acceleration and flexes forward with sudden deceleration.

Inflammatory

Rheumatoid arthritis frequently affects the neck, particularly the atlantoaxial joints, which may undergo subluxation. There will usually be a history of rheumatoid arthritis elsewhere. The patient complains of pain in the neck, difficulty in walking and there may be progressive bladder involvement.

Infective

TB of the cervical spine is rare in the UK. There is usually a history of TB elsewhere.

Degenerative

Cervical spondylosis is the commonest condition involving the neck. The patient complains of neck pain and stiffness with radiation of pain into the occiput, shoulder or arms. There may be complaints of weakness of grip and wasting of the hand. Acute cervical disc lesions may cause acute neck pain, with referred pain to the arm with weakness. Central disc protrusion may cause bladder problems or even paraplegia.

Neoplastic

Primary tumours of the cervical vertebrae are extremely rare. Secondary deposits may occur from breast, bronchus, lung, prostate or kidney. The patient may have had surgery for carcinoma of one of these organs. If not, check for a history suggesting a lesion. The patient will present with pain and collapse of a vertebra, perhaps with neurological symptoms.

Other

Postural neck pain is common and relates to changes in neck posture, the patient often complaining of sleeping in an 'awkward' position. The pain is usually across the neck and shoulders. The patient may also complain of exposure to cold, e.g. 'sitting in a draught'. Meningitis may cause a stiff neck with pain, as does subarachnoid haemorrhage. The diagnosis of these will be usually obvious from the history. The headache radiates into the neck and causes neck stiffness.

EXAMINATION

Congenital

Torticollis – the head is pulled down to the affected side and often rotated to the opposite side. Klippel–Feil syndrome presents with a short neck and a high-riding scapula.

Acquired

Traumatic

Treat the patient as for spinal injury, with stabilisation of the neck. Carry out a full neurological examination. Any X-ray examination should be strictly supervised by an experienced orthopaedic surgeon. With whiplash injuries there is usually only ligamentous and soft-tissue damage. Localised tenderness may be present. Check for pain and paraesthesia in the arms and hands.

Inflammatory

Rheumatoid arthritis will be apparent elsewhere, e.g. hand deformities, ulnar deviation. Carry out a full neurological examination.

Infective

With TB the patient will be generally unwell with spasm in the neck muscles. There may be evidence of paravertebral abscess. Carry out a full neurological examination.

Degenerative

There will be reduced neck movements. Carry out a full neurological examination. There will be weakness of grip, muscle wasting and reduced reflexes. Acute disc lesions result in pain and spasm of the neck muscles. There may be weakness of the arm and reduced reflexes. Carry out a full neurological examination.

Neoplastic

Examine the possible sites of primary, e.g. breast, bronchus, prostate, thyroid, kidney. Carry out a full neurological examination.

Other

With postural neck pain or cold exposure there is usually little to find on examination. There may be some localised muscular tenderness. With meningitis the patient is usually ill, with photophobia, headache, stiff neck and a positive Kernig's sign. Subarachnoid haemorrhage is usually diagnosed from the history.

GENERAL INVESTIGATIONS

- **FBC, ESR**
  Hb ↓ anaemia of chronic disease, e.g. rheumatoid arthritis.
  WCC ↑ infection. ESR ↑ rheumatoid arthritis, TB, malignancy.
- **Rheumatoid factor**
  Rheumatoid arthritis.
- **X-ray**
  Fractures (supervised X-rays), cervical spondylosis – narrowing of joint spaces, osteophytes. Rheumatoid arthritis – atlantoaxial subluxation. Secondary deposits. Congenital anomalies.

SPECIFIC INVESTIGATIONS

- **CT**
  Disc lesion. TB. Subarachnoid haemorrhage.
- **MRI**
  Disc lesions – cord compression.
- **Bone scan**
  Secondary deposits. Acute arthritis.
- **Lumbar puncture**
  Meningitis. Subarachnoid haemorrahge.

▶ NIPPLE DISCHARGE

This is a not uncommon problem. It is embarrassing for the patient as discharge may leak through and stain the clothing. Bloodstained nipple discharge may be due to an underlying carcinoma.

CAUSES

Serous
- Early pregnancy
- Fibroadenosis

Milky
- Late pregnancy
- Lactation
- Lactorrhoea of the newborn (witch's milk)
- Puberty
- Prolactinoma (tumour of the anterior pituitary gland)

Coloured

Yellow, brown, green
- Fibroadenosis

Thick and creamy
- Duct ectasia

Purulent
- Breast abscess (rare)
- Retroareolar abscess
- TB

Bloodstained
- Intraduct carcinoma
- Intraduct papilloma
- Paget's disease of the nipple

HISTORY

Pregnancy or lactation will be apparent. Discharge may occur from the nipples of newborn babies of either sex (witches' milk). It is due to passage of female hormones across the placenta. Discharge, either serous or milky, may occur at puberty. Cyclical mastalgia with a coloured discharge, especially greenish, suggests fibroadenosis. A patient in the fifth decade with a history of retroareolar pain and a thick creamy discharge may have duct ectasia. A bloodstained discharge must be taken seriously and fully investigated. The patient may describe this as frank, red blood or altered blood, which may be darkish brown. It is important to know whether it has come from one duct or several. Does the patient have an underlying lump? Profuse milky discharge associated with amenorrhoea will suggest the possibility of prolactinoma of the anterior pituitary gland.

EXAMINATION

Is the discharge obvious? It may have stained the clothes and the colour of it may be apparent. Is it associated with a painful and lumpy breast to suggest fibroadenosis? Is it possible to express the discharge by manual pressure? Occasionally it is possible, by manual pressure on specific areas of the breast, to express blood from one particular duct. Is there an underlying discrete lump suggestive of a carcinoma? Is there retroareolar tenderness, lumpiness and nipple retraction suggestive of duct ectasia? Are there any signs of infection or abscess? Has the nipple been destroyed, as in Paget's disease? If prolactinoma is suspected (galactorrhoea, amenorrhoea, infertility), the visual fields should be checked, as a macroadenoma of the anterior pituitary gland may impinge on the optic chiasma.

GENERAL INVESTIGATIONS

- **FBC, ESR**
  WCC ↑ in infection. ESR ↑ in tumour and TB.
- **Swab**
  C&S. Infection, abscess, TB.
- **FNAC**
  Carcinoma.
- **Dipstick testing**
  Blood versus other fluid.

SPECIFIC INVESTIGATIONS

- **Mammography**
  Carcinoma, duct ectasia.

- **Microdochectomy**
  If bleeding is localised to an individual duct, this is an appropriate surgical investigation. It may demonstrate intraduct papilloma or intraduct carcinoma.
- **CT head**
  Prolactinoma of the pituitary gland.

OEDEMA

Oedema is the accumulation of excessive fluid in the subcutaneous tissue. When oedema results from lymphatic stasis, the term lymphoedema is used.

CAUSES

Generalised

Increased plasma hydrostatic pressure
- Congestive cardiac failure
- Vasodilatory drugs – nifedipine

Decreased plasma oncotic pressure
- Liver disease
- Renal disease, e.g. nephrotic syndrome
- Malnutrition/malabsorption

*Impairment of lymphatic drainage**
- Congenital deficiency of lymphatics

Increased capillary permeability
- Angio-oedema – anaphylaxis

Localised

Increased plasma hydrostatic pressure
- Venous obstruction

*Impairment of lymphatic drainage**
Congenital
- Milroy's disease
- Lymphoedema praecox
- Lymphoedema tarda

Acquired
- Malignant infiltration
- Infection, e.g. elephantiasis
- Radiation
- Surgical damage

Increased capillary permeability
- Local infection
- Trauma

*Indicates the causes of lymphoedema.

- Mechanical trauma
- Burns
- Animal bites/stings

HISTORY

Site and distribution

Enquiries should be made regarding the site of oedema, as localised and demarcated sites of oedema are usually due to trauma or infection. Oedema may be confined to both lower limbs, for example with IVC obstruction and pregnancy, or affect only a single limb, such as the leg with unilateral DVT, or arm following axillary lymph node clearance.

Precipitating factors

Precipitating factors such as trauma and infection may be obvious from the history, and should be excluded. Angio-oedema may be precipitated by a known allergen. Lymphoedema may result as a complication of infection with filarial nematodes while travelling in endemic areas such as Africa, Asia and Australia. Lymphoedema may also be congenital, occurring shortly after birth (Milroy's disease) or at puberty (lymphoedema praecox) or in the third decade (lymphoedema tarda).

Past medical and drug history

Interruption to lymphatic drainage may result as a complication of irradiation or surgery, especially in the region of the axilla and groin. Obstruction of lymphatic flow can also result from direct involvement of the lymph nodes by lymphoma, or secondary to metastatic lymphatic infiltration from tumours. A detailed drug history will identify any offending drug.

Associated symptoms

If there is no obvious precipitating factor in the history, then specific enquiries should be undertaken for each system. Symptoms suggestive of malignancy, in particular, should be sought. In addition, it is important to exclude the following conditions.

Cardiac failure

Lethargy, dyspnoea, orthopnoea, paroxysmal nocturnal dyspnoea, cough, ankle oedema and abdominal distension from ascites may be some symptoms experienced by patients with cardiac failure.

Liver disease

Symptoms of jaundice, pruritus, ankle oedema, abdominal distension, haematemesis and confusion (encephalopathy) should be sought to determine the presence of liver disease.

Renal disease – nephrotic syndrome

Severe generalised oedema is the prominent feature with nephrotic syndrome. Patients may also complain of frothy urine due to proteinuria.

Malabsorption

Weight loss, diarrhoea and steatorrhoea may be some of the features associated with malabsorption.

Venous thrombosis

Unilateral leg swelling and pain are the main symptoms of DVT. Occasionally with iliofemoral vein thrombosis, the entire leg may appear blue (phlegmasia cerulea dolens) or white (phlegmasia alba dolens). Bilateral leg oedema with the onset of dilated superficial collateral veins on the trunk and abdomen is suggestive of IVC obstruction.

EXAMINATION

Inspection

Assessment of the distribution of oedema may narrow the differential diagnosis. Generalised causes tend to present with dependent oedema, with fluid accumulating in the ankles in ambulant patients and the sacrum in recumbent patients.

Cardiovascular system

With cardiac failure, palpation of the pulse may reveal tachycardia with pulsus alternans. The measured blood pressure may be low due to systolic failure. The JVP is elevated and a third heart sound with bilateral coarse pulmonary crepitations may be auscultated. Hepatomegaly due to liver congestion and ascites may also be present.

Abdominal examination

Generalised wasting from malabsorption or malignancy may be appreciated on inspection. Clubbing, palmar erythema, Dupuytren's contracture, jaundice, spider naevi and gynaecomastia are signs of liver disease. Dilated collateral veins on the abdomen may be due to portal hypertension or IVC obstruction; therefore, determine the direction of blood flow. Below the umbilicus the direction of blood flow is inferior with portal hypertension, and superior with IVC obstruction. Organomegaly due to carcinoma may be present and predispose to venous thrombosis. Pelvic malignancy may also result in venous outflow obstruction.

Legs

The legs are examined for the presence of tenderness and swelling. Circumferences of both the thighs and calves are compared. Marked painful erythematous unilateral swelling may be indicative of a DVT.

GENERAL INVESTIGATIONS

- **Urinalysis**
  Heavy proteinuria with nephrotic syndrome.
- **FBC**
  WCC ↑ infection and DVT. Hb ↓ malabsorption.
- **U&Es**
  Urea and creatinine ↑ with renal failure.
- **LFTs**
  Abnormal in liver disease.
- **Serum albumin**
  ↓ with nephrotic syndrome, liver disease, malabsorption and malnutrition.

SPECIFIC INVESTIGATIONS

- **24-hour urine collection**
  >3.5 g of protein with nephrotic syndrome.
- **Renal biopsy**
  To determine the cause of nephrotic syndrome in adults.
- **Echocardiography**
  Ventricular dilatation and impaired function with cardiac failure.
- **Liver biopsy**
  Liver cirrhosis.
- **Faecal fat estimation**
  ↑ malabsorption.
- **Duplex Doppler deep veins of the leg**
  Above-knee DVT.
- **Venography**
  Below-knee DVT, IVC obstruction.
- **Lymphangiography**
  Lymphoedema.

OLIGURIA

Oliguria is the passage of less than 400 ml of urine in 24 hours. Anuria is failure to pass any urine.

CAUSES

Renal circulatory insufficiency
- Shock, e.g. haemorrhage and burns
- Dehydration, e.g. vomiting, diarrhoea

Renal causes
- Acute tubular necrosis
- Acute cortical necrosis
- Acute glomerulonephritis
- Acute interstitial nephritis
- Nephrotoxins
- Vascular lesions

Postrenal (obstructive)
- Calculi
- Pelvic tumours
- Prostatic hypertrophy
- Retroperitoneal fibrosis

Others
- Mismatched transfusion (haemoglobinuria)
- Crush injuries (myoglobinuria)

Anuria
- Blocked catheter
- Ureteric damage (bilateral)
- Stone in solitary functioning kidney

HISTORY

Renal circulatory insufficiency
There will usually be a recent history of a condition which causes renal hypoperfusion. This may include haemorrhage, burns or dehydration, e.g. from vomiting, diarrhoea or acute pancreatitis.

Renal causes
In the absence of adequate resuscitation, shock will proceed to cause damage to the tubules, resulting in acute tubular necrosis.

Acute cortical necrosis may arise as a result of antepartum haemorrhage, eclampsia or septic abortion. It may also follow insults similar to those that cause acute tubular necrosis. Vascular lesions may also lead to acute renal failure; these include renal vein thrombosis, renal artery stenosis and intravascular coagulation occurring in haemolytic uraemic syndrome. Other forms of acute renal failure usually present with swelling of the eyelids, ascites and peripheral oedema. Later there may be vomiting, confusion, bruising, gastrointestinal bleeding and eventually fitting and coma. Volume overload may result in pulmonary oedema. With acute interstitial nephritis there may be a history of drug ingestion, e.g. antibiotics, NSAIDs or diuretics, or there may be a history of infection. Nephrotoxins may cause acute renal failure and among the drugs implicated are the aminoglycosides, amphotericin and radiographic contrast media. Organic solvents, particularly carbon tetrachloride used in carpet cleaning, may be responsible. Paraquat, snake bites and mushrooms may also cause acute renal failure.

Postrenal

Often the patient will present with complete anuria. This may occur if there is ureteric damage following surgery or a stone impacted in the ureter of a solitary functioning kidney. The patient may have a history of calculous disease or may have recently suffered an attack of ureteric colic. There may be a history of pelvic tumour or symptoms of prostatic hypertrophy, e.g. difficulty in starting and a poor stream. Retroperitoneal fibrosis often develops insidiously.

Others

Oliguria may follow a mismatched transfusion, due to haemo-globinuria, or crush injuries, due to myoglobinuria. The history will usually be obvious.

Anuria

Before diagnosing anuria, make sure that the patient does not have a palpable bladder (if he or she is not catheterised) and is not therefore in acute retention, or, if the patient is catheterised, that the catheter is not blocked. As indicated above, anuria is more likely to be a symptom of an obstructive lesion rather than one of renal hypoperfusion or an intrinsic renal lesion.

EXAMINATION

General

If the patient has a catheter *in situ*, make sure that it is not blocked. If the patient does not have a catheter *in situ*, palpate the lower abdomen for a distended bladder associated with acute retention. Palpate the abdomen to exclude swelling of the kidneys and perform a rectal examination to exclude prostatic hypertrophy.

Specific

All causes of oliguria are likely to have some common features on examination. The patient will be dyspnoeic due to pulmonary oedema and will either have sacral oedema (if confined to bed) or ankle oedema (if ambulant). There may be confusion, drowsiness, fitting or coma. Hypertension and arrhythmias may be present. The patient will be nauseated, may be vomiting, have hiccups, and there may be evidence of gastrointestinal haemorrhage. Spontaneous bruising may occur eventually.

GENERAL INVESTIGATIONS

- **FBC, ESR**
  Hb ↓ anaemia, renal failure, haemorrhage. WCC ↑ infection. ESR ↑ some causes of glomerulonephritis.
- **U&Es**
  Urea ↑, creatinine ↑ in renal and postrenal causes. These may rise in renal hypoperfusion if not adequately treated.
- **ECG**
  Arrhythmias. Associated with electrolyte imbalance, e.g. hyperkalaemia.
- **CXR**
  Pulmonary oedema. Cardiomegaly.
- **ABGs**
  Metabolic acidosis.
- **MSU**
  Red cells, casts and protein in intrinsic renal disease. Hb positive but no red blood cells suggests myoglobinuria or haemoglobinuria.
- **Urine electrolytes**
  See table on page 346.
- **Urine osmolarity**
  See table on page 346.

Distinction between physiological oliguria and acute renal failure

Urine	Physiological oliguria	Acute renal failure
Specific gravity	>1020	<1010
Osmolality (mosm/kg)	>500	<350
Sodium (mmol/l)	<15	>40
Urine/serum creatinine	>40	<20
Fractional sodium excretion*	<1	>2
Renal failure index†	<1	>2

*Fractional sodium excretion = (urine sodium × plasma creatinine/plasma sodium × urine creatinine) × 100.

†Renal failure index = (urine sodium × plasma creatinine)/urine creatinine.

SPECIFIC INVESTIGATIONS

- **US**
  Obstructive lesion.
- **Cystoscopy and ureteric catheterisation with retrograde pyelography**
  Cause of obstruction, possible relief of obstruction.
- **Antegrade pyelography**
  Cause of obstruction. Relief of obstruction.
- **DMSA scan**
  Renal function. Infarction. Absent outline of kidney.

PALPITATIONS

Palpitation is an awareness of the heartbeat; although benign in the vast majority, palpitations are occasionally a manifestation of a life-threatening disorder.

CAUSES

Cardiac arrhythmia
- Premature ventricular contractions (ventricular ectopic beats)*
- Premature atrial contractions (atrial ectopic beats)*
- Atrial fibrillation*

Supraventricular tachycardia

Ventricular tachycardia

Sinus tachycardia
- Anxiety/emotional stress
- Caffeine
- Nicotine
- Alcohol

HISTORY

A variety of symptoms is used to describe palpitations and this includes 'fluttering', 'pounding' and 'skipping a beat'. Symptoms may also be experienced in the neck. Important aspects are the frequency, regularity of palpitation (e.g. fast and irregular) and precipitating factors. Asking the patient to tap the rate and rhythm of the palpitation (on a table for example) can be very informative. Arrhythmias associated with irregular palpitations are listed above.

Knowledge of precipitating factors is important. Palpitations can be a normal manifestation of anxiety or panic reactions. However, it is vitally important that an organic cause is excluded as it is common for anxiety disorders to coexist in a patient with supraventricular tachycardia. Exercise is associated with excess catecholamines and also a precipitator of arrhythmia (supraventricular tachycardia, atrial fibrillation and ventricular tachycardia usually originating from the right ventricle). Excessive caffeine, smoking and alcohol intake are also thought to be precipitators of arrhythmia.

*Indicates causes that tend to present as irregular palpitations.

A history of any underlying heart disorder is important, as arrhythmia is associated with ischaemic heart disease (ventricular arrhythmia), hypertensive heart disease (atrial fibrillation), heart failure (ventricular arrhythmia), heart valve disease.

Early age of onset of arrhythmia (childhood or teenage years) suggests the presence of a congenital abnormality such as a bypass tract that can lead to supraventricular tachycardia. The reader should consult a cardiology textbook for further details.

Additional features

Dizziness or syncope (page 414) is usually associated with serious arrhythmia such as ventricular tachycardia and occasionally supraventricular tachycardia.

ON EXAMINATION

Examination during an episode of palpitation is very informative as assessment of the rhythm and rate of the pulse can be determined. Auscultation of rate at the cardiac apex is a more accurate as not all beats are conducted to the pulse (for example in atrial fibrillation).

It is important to measure the blood pressure and screen for any evidence of underlying structural heart disease, especially mitral valve prolapse (systolic murmur and a systolic click), as this condition is associated with supraventricular tachycardia and atrial fibrillation.

INITIAL INVESTIGATIONS

12-lead ECG

All patients should have a resting ECG. It is very unlikely that any arrhythmia can be picked up during this investigation; however, conditions that predispose to arrhythmia may be diagnosed. The presence of an accessory pathway (and hence predisposition to supraventricular arrhythmia) is indicated by a short PR interval (less than 0.12 seconds).

Also, the presence of left ventricular hypertrophy can indicate underlying structural heart disease (hypertensive heart disease, hypertrophic obstructive cardiomyopathy). Ischaemic heart disease can be suggested by Q waves, or ST segment/T wave abnormalities.

Occasionally, atrial or ventricular premature contractions (ectopic beats) may be evident.

FURTHER INVESTIGATIONS

Further investigations are best reserved for those who are at high risk of arrhythmia: patients with evidence of underlying structural heart disease, family history of arrhythmia, regular palpitations (especially during sleep) and dizziness or syncope associated with palpitations.

Ambulatory ECG monitoring

Continuous ambulatory ECG monitoring is an excellent method to detect and identify arrhythmia. Upon further investigation, ventricular and atrial premature contractions (ectopic beats) are the most commonly identified arrhythmia. Sinus rhythm is the usual remaining finding. A serious arrhythmia is detected in approximately 7%. The reader is advised to consult ECG textbooks for a detailed discussion of the numerous configurations of each arrhythmia.

▶ PENILE LESIONS

Penile lesions are common. They interfere with sexual intercourse.
The majority of surgical conditions of the penis relate to problems
with the foreskin and glans and the need for circumcision.
Carcinoma of the penis and Peyronie's disease are rare.

CAUSES

Foreskin and glans

- Phimosis
- Paraphimosis
- Balanoposthitis
- Balanitis xerotica obliterans
- Herpes genitalis
- Condylomata (warts)
- Trauma (bite)
- Erythroplasia of Queyrat
- Carcinoma
- Chancre (syphilis)

Shaft of the penis

- Peyronie's disease
- Priapism

Urethra

- Epispadias
- Hypospadias

HISTORY

Foreskin and glans

Phimosis

In most cases phimosis is congenital. The foreskin has been tight
since birth and the patient complains that it will not retract over the
glans. In children, this may cause ballooning of the foreskin during
micturition, with resulting balanoposthitis. In adults, the complaint
is that it interferes with sexual intercourse.

Paraphimosis

This is a result of a patient having a phimosis. The foreskin is
pulled back over the glans while washing and then is not returned.

It may also occur during sexual intercourse. In hospital practice it may occur while the patient is being catheterised and the foreskin is not returned to its correct place following this procedure. The foreskin forms a tight constriction around the glans, interfering with venous return and causing swelling of the glans and foreskin. The patient presents with considerable pain and a swollen glans penis.

Balanoposthitis
This is inflammation of the glans and foreskin. The patient complains of an attack of inflammation of the foreskin and glans. It may be associated with poor hygiene but in children it is often associated with phimosis and collection of urine under the foreskin. In diabetics it is often due to candida.

Balanitis xerotica obliterans
The patient will complain of thickening and tightening of the foreskin, and the inability to retract it.

Herpes genitalis
The patient will complain of painful vesicles on the foreskin or glans penis. There will usually be a history of sexual contact.

Condylomata (warts)
The patient may present with warts on the glans and contiguous surface of the prepuce. They are usually of venereal origin.

Trauma
There may be a history of trauma, often of an unusual nature. Love bites may be responsible.

Erythroplasia of Queyrat
The patient will present having noticed a dark, velvety, red, flat patch on the skin of the glans.

Carcinoma
This usually presents in old age. It is virtually unknown in those that are circumcised. Most patients present with a lump or an ulcer which may be painful. In uncircumcised patients who cannot retract the foreskin there may be a bloodstained purulent discharge from under the foreskin.

Syphilitic chancre
A chancre presents as a painless, hard ulcer on the penis.

Shaft

Peyronie's disease

The patient may have noticed a subcutaneous lump along the penis. He may complain that when he has an erection the penis appears bent.

Priapism

The patient will present with a persistent painful erection. This is unassociated with sexual desire. There may be a history of leukaemia, sickle cell disease, disseminated pelvic malignancy, or the patient may be on haemodialysis. Priapism may also result from alprostadil overdose for erectile dysfunction.

Urethra

Epispadias

This is rare. The patient, a baby or child, usually presents with the urethra opening on the dorsal surface of the glans penis.

Hypospadias

This is more common than epispadias, the patient presenting with the urethral opening on the ventral or undersurface of the penis. In both epispadias and hypospadias, the patient will complain of a problem with micturition.

EXAMINATION

Foreskin and glans

Phimosis

The foreskin is tight and has a pinhole orifice. It will be impossible to retract it over the glans penis. There may be associated balanoposthitis.

Paraphimosis

The diagnosis is usually obvious. The glans penis is swollen and oedematous and there is a deep groove just proximal to the corona glandis, where there is tight constricting ring of skin. The patient is obviously in pain.

Balanoposthitis

There is inflammation of the glans (balanitis) and often associated inflammation of the foreskin (posthitis). There may be a discharge from under the foreskin. In the case of candidiasis there are itchy red patches on the glans. There may be evidence of poor personal hygiene.

Balanitis xerotica obliterans

The foreskin is thickened, with loss of elasticity and fibrosis. It is usually not possible to retract it over the glans.

Herpes genitalis

Initially there will be itchy vesicles but these develop into shallow, painful erosions. There may be associated painful inguinal lymphadenopathy.

Condylomata (warts)

There will be a bunch of warts, usually around the junction between the foreskin and the glans and extending on to the glans.

Trauma

Appearance will depend upon the type of trauma. Teeth marks may be apparent.

Erythroplasia of Queyrat

There is a dark-red, flat, velvety, indurated patch on the glans penis. It is a premalignant condition and represents carcinoma in situ.

Carcinoma

The lesion is usually at the junction of the foreskin and glans. There will be a lump or ulcer. If there is an ulcer it will have raised everted edges and a necrotic base. It feels hard. The inguinal lymph nodes may be affected, either by metastases or secondary infection. In patients where the foreskin cannot be retracted, it may be necessary to carry out circumcision to make the diagnosis.

Syphilitic chancre

There will be a painless, hard ulcer with a sloping edge. The inguinal nodes will be enlarged, rubbery, discrete and non-tender.

Shaft

Peyronie's disease

There are plaques of fibrosis in the corpora cavernosa. These may be felt as hard lumps along the corpora cavernosa. The patient will volunteer the information that the penis becomes bent on erection.

Priapism

The diagnosis will be obvious, there being a painful erection.

Urethra

The diagnosis of epispadias and hypospadias will be obvious. In hypospadias the opening of the urethra may be anywhere along the line of the urethra, from a few millimetres from the tip of the penis to the perineum. In epispadias, which is rare, the urethral opening is on the dorsal surface of the glans penis.

GENERAL INVESTIGATIONS

- **FBC, ESR**
  WCC ↑ infection, leukaemia (associated with priapism). ESR ↑ malignancy.
- **Swab**
  C&S. Microscopy. Balanitis – bacterial or fungal.
- **Blood glucose**
  Diabetes – candida balanitis.

SPECIFIC INVESTIGATIONS

- **Sickle cell test**
  Sickle cell disease with priapism.
- **VDRL**
  Syphilitic chancre.
- **Electron microscopy**
  Identification of herpes virus in vesicular fluid.
- **PCR**
  For rapid diagnosis of herpes.
- **Biopsy**
  Erythroplasia of Queyrat. Carcinoma. Condylomata.
- **Circumcision**
  Diagnostic if tight phimosis prevents retraction of foreskin to inspect glans for carcinoma.

POLYURIA

The volume of urine produced per day varies in each individual and is affected by the amount of fluid intake, physiological requirements and insensible losses. Polyuria is arbitrarily defined as urine output of more than 3 litres in 24 hours.

CAUSES

Diuretics

Therapeutic
- Frusemide
- Bendrofluazide
- Amiloride

Osmotic
- Hyperglycaemia
- Hypercalcaemia
- Mannitol
- Urea

Diabetes insipidus

Cranial
- Idiopathic deficiency of ADH production
- Inherited (dominant or recessive)
- Head injuries
- Neurosurgery
- Brain tumours
- Opiates

Nephrogenic
- Inherited (X-linked)
- Drugs
  - Lithium
  - Demeclocycline
- Chronic hypercalcaemia
- Hypokalaemia
- Chronic tubulointerstitial nephritis
- Recovering acute tubular necrosis
- Recovering obstructive uropathy

Excessive fluid intake
- Psychogenic
- Drug-induced thirst – anticholinergics
- Hypothalamic disease

HISTORY

General

Polyuria is often accompanied by polydipsia, and with all water-losing states severe thirst is often a side-effect. Frequency of urination (frequent passing of small amounts of urine) should be differentiated from polyuria (frequent passing of large amounts of urine). Diabetes insipidus may be hereditary and other family members may be affected.

Drug history

A detailed drug history is invaluable, as a significant number of drugs precipitate polyuria by various mechanisms. Therapeutic diuretics are used in a range of disorders, such as hypertension and cardiac failure. Opiates inhibit ADH secretion and may produce cranial diabetes insipidus, whereas drugs such as lithium and demeclocycline may produce nephrogenic diabetes insipidus. A side-effect of anticholinergics is dryness of the mouth; patients may therefore ingest excessive quantities of water, causing polyuria. Nephrotoxic drugs, such as aminoglycosides, cyclosporin, NSAIDs and ACE inhibitors, may precipitate acute tubular necrosis, which can result in severe polyuria in the recovery phase.

Past medical history

Hyperglycaemia causes an osmotic diuresis, therefore polyuria and polydipsia are common presenting features of diabetes mellitus. Malignancy and hyperparathyroidism are common causes of chronic hypercalcaemia, which can cause polyuria by an intrinsic osmotic effect or by precipitation of nephrogenic diabetes insipidus. Cranial diabetes insipidus can result from severe, blunt, head injuries, craniopharyngiomas, pineal gland tumours or as a transient postoperative complication following neurosurgery. Renal ischaemia from conditions such as sepsis and haemorrhage predisposes to acute tubular necrosis. Chronic tubulointerstitial nephritis can result from reflux nephropathy, polycystic kidney disease, gout and multiple myeloma.

GENERAL INVESTIGATIONS

- **Urine dipstick**
  +++ glucose with diabetes mellitus.
- **24-hour urine collection**
  >3 litres confirms polyuria, and helps differentiate from urinary frequency.
- **U&Es**
  Plasma urea and creatinine levels ↑ renal failure. Sodium ↑ with uncompensated polyuria (inadequate water intake). Sodium ↓ with urea/creatinine ↓ indicates polydipsia as the primary cause. Potassium ↓ may cause nephrogenic diabetes insipidus.
- **Serum calcium**
  ↑ calcium causes osmotic diuresis and chronic tubulointerstitial nephritis.
- **Serum glucose**
  ↑ diabetes.

The above tests may be all that is required to differentiate between osmotic diuresis, excess fluid intake and diabetes insipidus. If the differentiation between primary polydipsia and diabetes insipidus cannot be made confidently then proceed with the following two tests. The reader is advised to consult a reference source regarding the precautions and safety measures to be observed in the water deprivation and DDAVP tests.

- **Water deprivation test**
  Do not perform this test in volume-depleted patients nor in the presence of hypernatraemia.
  After overnight water restriction the plasma osmolality is measured.
  Plasma osmolality ↓: primary polydipsia.
  Plasma osmolality ↑: stop test and measure urine osmolality.
  Urine osmolality ↑: no diabetes insipidus.
  Urine osmolality ↓ in three consecutive samples: diabetes insipidus.
- **DDAVP test**
  Arginine vasopressin is then administered.
  Urine osmolality ↑: cranial diabetes insipidus.
  No urine osmolality ↑: nephrogenic diabetes insipidus.

SPECIFIC INVESTIGATIONS

- **CT/MRI head**
  Tumours, hypothalamic disease.
- **Renal biopsy**
  Acute tubular necrosis, chronic tubulointerstitial nephritis.

▶ POPLITEAL SWELLINGS

Popliteal swellings are not uncommon. The majority are easily diagnosed on clinical examination alone.

CAUSES

Superficial
- Sebaceous cyst
- Lipoma
- Varix of the short saphenous vein

Deep
- Lipoma
- Lymphadenopathy
- Semimembranosus bursa
- Baker's cyst
- Popliteal artery aneurysm

Bony
- Exostoses
- Osteogenic sarcoma

HISTORY

Superficial

Sebaceous cyst
A sebaceous cyst will present as a firm swelling in the skin. It may be tender if it becomes inflamed and there may be a discharge from it.

Lipoma
This presents as a soft lobulated swelling in the subcutaneous tissue.

Varix of the short saphenous vein
This presents as a soft swelling behind the knee, usually associated with varicose veins of the short saphenous system.

Deep

Lipoma
Deeper lipomas are difficult to feel because of the tough overlying fascia. They do not always feel soft and lobulated, as superficial ones do.

Lymphadenopathy

There may be several palpable lumps within the popliteal fossa. The patient will usually draw attention to a lesion distally, either on the leg or foot, usually on the lateral margin of the foot or the back of the leg. Other groups of nodes may be enlarged.

Semimembranosus bursa

The patient complains of a swelling behind the knee that interferes with knee movement, particularly flexion.

Baker's cyst

A Baker's cyst is a pulsion diverticulum of the knee joint caused by chronic disease within the joint. The patient will usually give a history of a painful knee joint and may have osteoarthritis or rheumatoid arthritis. Occasionally the cyst ruptures and the patient complains of severe pain in the calf, which has to be carefully distinguished from venous thrombosis.

Popliteal artery aneurysm

These often get quite large before they are noticed. The patient may be aware of a pulsatile swelling behind the knee but often notices it when crossing the legs, the upper of the crossed limbs moving with each pulse.

Bony

Exostoses may grow in the region of the epiphysial cartilage of the femur. There is a well-defined bony swelling in the popliteal fossa.

Osteogenic sarcoma

This may affect either the lower end of the femur or the upper end of the tibia. There is a rather diffuse swelling around the knee joint. Pain may be a presenting symptom. There may also be general malaise and weight loss. Occasionally pulmonary metastases have occurred at presentation, and there may be cough and haemoptysis.

EXAMINATION

Superficial

Sebaceous cyst

There will be a small, well-defined swelling in the skin with a punctum. If it is infected, the surrounding skin will be red and there may be discharge.

Lipoma
There will be a soft, lobulated swelling in the popliteal fossa.

Varix of the short saphenous vein
This is not uncommon. There will be a soft, compressible dilatation at the termination of the short saphenous vein. There may be an expansile cough impulse. A fluid thrill will be palpable when the short saphenous vein lower down the leg is tapped.

Deep

Lipoma
A deep lipoma in the fat of the popliteal fossa may be difficult to define accurately. It does not always have the soft, lobulated appearance of a more superficial lipoma.

Lymphadenopathy
There may be a number of discrete glands palpable or they may be firm and matted together. Check for a lesion distally on the leg or foot, e.g. malignant melanoma. Check for lymphadenopathy elsewhere.

Semimembranosus bursa
The swelling lies above the level of the knee joint line, slightly to the medial side of the popliteal fossa. It tends to be firm in consistency and transilluminates.

Baker's cyst
Baker's cysts occur more often in elderly patients with long-standing arthritis or in younger patients with rheumatoid arthritis. The lump is below the level of the knee joint and deep to gastrocnemius. It may transilluminate. Pressure over the lump may reduce it into the knee joint. Examination of the knee joint reveals changes consistent with arthritis, i.e. limited movements, crepitus and occasionally an effusion.

Popliteal artery aneurysm
An expansile, pulsatile mass will be palpable in the popliteal fossa. They are often bilateral. Check the distal circulation. Popliteal aneurysms may thrombose with distal ischaemia, or may throw off small emboli causing ischaemic toes or ischaemic ulcers on the tips of the toes. Palpate the abdomen: there is an association between popliteal aneurysms and abdominal aortic aneurysms.

Bony

Exostoses
A bony mass may be felt in the popliteal fossa.

Osteogenic sarcoma

The overlying skin may be reddened, with dilated subcutaneous veins. There may be tenderness. The swelling is usually smooth until it spreads into the surrounding tissues, when it becomes irregular. The swelling feels firm but is not usually bony hard.

GENERAL INVESTIGATIONS

- **FBC, ESR**

  Hb ↓ lymphadenopathy, e.g. part of generalised lymphadenopathy associated with reticulosis. WCC ↑ reticulosis. ESR ↑ reticulosis, osteogenic sarcoma with secondaries.

- **US**

  Lipoma. Semimembranosus bursa. Baker's cyst. Popliteal artery aneurysm.

- **Knee X-ray**

  Exostoses. Osteoarthritis (Baker's cyst). Rheumatoid arthritis (Baker's cyst). Osteogenic sarcoma – bone destruction, grows out of cortex, elevating periosteum with reposition of subperiosteal bone (Codman's triangle), radiating spicules of bone ('sunray' spicules).

- **CXR**

  Secondary deposits from osteogenic sarcoma. Hilar lymph nodes with generalised lymphadenopathy.

SPECIFIC INVESTIGATIONS

- **Duplex Doppler**

  Varix of short saphenous vein. Popliteal artery aneurysm.

- **CT**

  Shows invasion of osteogenic sarcoma. Lung secondaries.

- **MRI**

  Baker's cyst. Bone tumour.

- **Arteriography**

  Popliteal aneurysm. Distal circulation.

▶ PRURITUS

Pruritus is itching of the skin. There are a vast number of
dermatological causes of pruritus which are usually visible on
inspection. The following are causes of generalised pruritus in
the absence of dermatological disease.

CAUSES

Obstructive jaundice

Chronic renal failure

Haematological disease
- Iron deficiency
- Polycythaemia

Internal malignancy
- Bronchial carcinoma
- Hodgkin's disease

Endocrine disease
- Hyperthyroidism
- Hypothyroidism
- Diabetes mellitus

Drugs
- Oral contraceptive pill (cholestasis)
- Opiates (histamine release)
- Alcohol and drug withdrawal

HISTORY

When approaching a patient with generalised pruritus, enquiries are
made regarding the site and duration of symptoms. Occasionally
the onset of pruritus will correlate with the initiation of drug
treatment, allowing you to exclude the offending medication. It may
also occur as a side-effect of alcohol or drug withdrawal. Pruritus
after a hot bath classically occurs with polycythaemia. Iron
deficiency, even in the absence of anaemia, can cause pruritus;
therefore symptoms of blood loss in each system should be
carefully elicited.

Haemoptysis, chronic cough and weight loss in smokers may be
due to underlying bronchial carcinoma, which is an important

subgroup of internal malignancies that present with pruritus. The presence of localised lymphadenopathy, fever, night sweats and weight loss should lead to the consideration of Hodgkin's disease. Patients with obstructive jaundice (page 240) may present with pruritus (due to the accumulation of bile salts), even while the jaundice is not clinically apparent. With complete obstruction, patients may notice pale stools and dark urine.

Lethargy, anorexia, nocturia, oliguria, polyuria, haematuria, frothy urine from proteinuria, skin fragility, oedema and bone pains are some of the multisystemic features suggestive of chronic renal disease. Interestingly, pruritus seldom occurs with acute renal failure.

As pruritus may be due to thyroid disease, clinical assessment of the thyroid status is an important aspect of the history. Features of hyperthyroidism are tremor, heat intolerance, palpitations, increased appetite with weight loss, anxiety and diarrhoea. Features of hypothyroidism are cold intolerance, mental slowing, weight gain, constipation and menorrhagia.

EXAMINATION

Inspection

Wide, staring eyes with lid lag and tremor may be present with thyrotoxicosis. Pallor of the conjunctivae may be evident in severe anaemia, whereas with polycythaemia, conjunctival insufflation and facial plethora occur. The sclera should also be examined for the presence of jaundice. Sallow skin with easy bruising and uraemic frost may be seen with chronic renal failure. Spoon-shaped nails of iron deficiency may be accompanied by angular cheilitis. Clubbing may be due to bronchial carcinoma.

GENERAL EXAMINATION

Asymmetrical, non-tender, localised lymphadenopathy in the absence of infection is suggestive of Hodgkin's disease. The thyroid gland is palpated for abnormalities, such as enlargement, nodularity and asymmetry. A respiratory examination is performed; features of bronchial carcinoma include monophonic inspiratory wheeze (partial endoluminal bronchial obstruction), lobar collapse of the lung, pleural effusion, and Horner's syndrome with apical lung tumours. Chest wall tenderness may also occur as a result of tumour infiltration. Splenomegaly may occur with Hodgkin's disease and polycythaemia rubra vera.

GENERAL INVESTIGATIONS

- **Urine dipstick**
  Protein and blood with renal disease.
- **FBC and blood film**
  Microcytic hypochromic anaemia with iron deficiency, normochromic normocytic anaemia with Hodgkin's, ↑ Hb with polycythaemia.
- **U&Es**
  Urea and creatinine ↑ renal failure.
- **Glucose**
  ↑ with diabetes mellitus.
- **LFTs**
  Bilirubin ↑, alkaline phosphatase ↑ with obstructive jaundice.
- **TFTs**
  TSH ↓ and T_4 ↑ thyrotoxicosis; TSH ↑ and T_4 ↓ hypothyroidism.
- **CXR**
  Bronchial carcinoma, hilar lymphadenopathy with Hodgkin's disease.

SPECIFIC INVESTIGATIONS

- **Excisional biopsy of lymph node**
  Hodgkin's disease – Reed–Sternberg cells.
- **US abdomen**
  Dilated bile ducts with obstructive jaundice, the site and cause of obstruction may be visualised. The size of the kidneys may be decreased with chronic renal disease, and multiple cysts visible with polycystic kidney disease.
- **Serum iron, serum ferritin, protoporphyrin**
  Serum iron ↓, serum ferritin ↓, free erythrocyte protoporphyrin ↑ iron deficiency.

PRURITUS ANI

Pruritus ani is itching around the anal canal. It is a common symptom and in approximately half the cases no cause can be found.

CAUSES

Anal discharge
- Skin tags
- Fistula-in-ano
- Warts
- Haemorrhoids
- Carcinoma
- Polyps
- Gonococcal proctitis

Faecal soiling
- Incontinence
- Poor hygiene
- Diarrhoea

Skin diseases
- Candidiasis
- Tinea cruris
- Lichen sclerosus
- Contact dermatitis
- Scabies
- Psoriasis
- Eczema

Parasites
- Threadworms

Psychogenic
- Anxiety

HISTORY

Anal discharge
Any cause within the anus or lower rectum that produces moisture and sogginess of the anal skin may cause pruritus ani. Patients may volunteer the information that they have haemorrhoids or

perianal warts. They may have noticed an anal discharge, which soils the underwear. Check for a history of anal sexual exposure.

Faecal soiling

The patient may complain of incontinence. This may be associated with poor hygiene. Chronic diarrhoea may be responsible. There may be an underlying cause for the chronic diarrhoea, e.g. colitis or Crohn's disease. Excessive sweating in hot weather may be associated with pruritus ani.

Skin diseases

If the patient is diabetic or immunosuppressed, candidiasis may be responsible. Recent oral antibiotic therapy may result in candidiasis. Check whether the patient has an itchy rash anywhere else. This may be particularly so with scabies or eczema. Contact dermatitis may result from the use of deodorants or a change in washing powder for the underwear. Psoriasis is usually not itchy but sometimes considerable itching occurs, especially if the area becomes infected. Lichen sclerosus is uncommon, occurring chiefly in women, when it may involve both vulva and perineum. In men this may be associated with balanitis xerotica obliterans, so enquire if there is any abnormality of the foreskin.

Parasites

Threadworms usually occur in children. The parents may have noticed them.

Pyschogenic

Idiopathic pruritus may occur in people with anxiety states. An itch–scratch cycle may occur, which is difficult to break.

EXAMINATION

Anal discharge

Inspection of the anus may show skin tags, the external opening of a fistula-in-ano, perianal warts or haemorrhoids. Digital rectal examination may reveal a carcinoma of the anal canal or fibrous anal polyps. Proctoscopy and sigmoidoscopy will confirm any associated anal or rectal lesion. Take a swab if purulent discharge.

Faecal soiling

Soiling of the underwear may be apparent. General poor hygiene may be apparent also in the patient. Carry out a digital rectal examination to check for sphincteric tone.

Skin diseases

Candidiasis may occur in those on long-term antibiotics, diabetics and the immunosuppressed. Tinea cruris is more common in men. The infection often involves the groin and perineum in addition to the perianal areas. The patient may also have coexisting tinea pedis. With lichen sclerosus there are well-defined plaques of superficial atrophy of the epidermis with a whitish colour. In the male, check the penis for balanitis xerotica obliterans. With contact dermatitis there may be changes in the skin in other areas apart from the perianal area. With scabies there are usually lesions on other parts of the body. Burrows 5–10 mm deep appear as long ridges, which may be 'S' shaped. Isolation of the organism with a pin and examination under the microscope will confirm the diagnosis. With psoriasis there will usually be lesions on other areas of the body, and this will also be so with eczema.

Parasites

Threadworms may be visible around the anus.

Psychogenic

There may be an obvious history of psychiatric illness or the patient may appear anxious or depressed.

GENERAL INVESTIGATIONS

- **FBC, ESR**
  These are usually normal.
- **Urinalysis**
  Positive for sugar – diabetic.
- **Blood glucose**
  Diabetic.
- **Stool culture**
  Ova, parasites and cysts, cause of diarrhoea.
- **Anal swab**
  Gram stain – Gram negative intracellular diplococci in gonorrhoea.
- **Skin scrapings**
  For mycotic infection, microscopy and culture.
- **Nocturnal 'Sellotape swab'**
  Threadworms.
- **Biopsy**
  Anal carcinoma. Lichen sclerosus.

▶ PYREXIA OF UNKNOWN ORIGIN

Most pyrexias result from a clearly defined illness, e.g. acute
pyelonephritis or acute appendicitis, or from self-limiting viral
infections, e.g. common cold. Pyrexia of unknown origin is a fever,
the cause of which is undetermined after taking a history and
performing a clinical examination. The fever is often prolonged.

CAUSES

Bacterial
- Subacute bacterial endocarditis
- TB
- Brucellosis
- Typhoid
- Leptospirosis
- Abscess, e.g. subphrenic, pelvic
- Q fever
- Cat scratch disease

Viral
- Influenza
- Glandular fever
- HIV
- CMV

Fungal
- Candidiasis
- Aspergillosis
- *Pneumocystis carinii*

Protozoal
- Malaria
- Amoebiasis
- Toxoplasmosis

Neoplasia
- Hypernephroma
- Lymphoma
- Hepatoma
- Acute leukaemia

Connective tissue disease
- SLE
- Polyarteritis nodosa
- Rheumatoid arthritis
- Temporal arteritis

Granulomatous disease
- Sarcoidosis
- Crohn's disease

Drug-induced

Others
- Myocardial infarction
- Pulmonary embolism
- Familial Mediterranean fever
- Munchausen's disease (factitious)
- Postimmunisation

HISTORY

A full and extensive history should be taken, noting especially travel abroad, contact with infection, contact with animals, bites, abrasions, rashes, diarrhoea. Check the drug history, including non-prescription drugs and drug abuse. Check for any recent history of surgery, particularly abdominal surgery. Is there any history of recent immunisations? Has the patient experienced night sweats, weight loss and general malaise?

EXAMINATION

A full physical examination should be carried out. This should be directed at every system of the body, checking particularly for lymphadenopathy and hepatosplenomegaly. Rectal and vaginal examination should be carried out.

INVESTIGATIONS

It may be necessary to carry out numerous and repeated investigations. It may also be necessary to withhold any drugs one at a time to see if a temperature settles.

GENERAL INVESTIGATIONS

- **FBC, ESR**
  Hb ↓ malignancy, anaemia of chronic disease, e.g. rheumatoid arthritis. WCC ↑ infection, leukaemia. Lymphocytes ↑ viral infection. Platelets ↓ leukaemia. ESR ↑ malignancy, connective tissue disease, TB.
- **U&Es**
  Connective tissue disease affecting the kidneys.
- **LFTs**
  Biliary tract or liver disease, e.g. cholangitis, hepatitis.
- **Blood glucose**
  Diabetes – infections are more common in diabetics.
- **Blood culture**
  Streptococcus viridans suggests infective endocarditis. Isolation of coliforms suggests the possibility of intra-abdominal sepsis.
- **Viral antibodies**
  Hepatitis B, hepatitis C, infectious mononucleosis, HIV, CMV.
- **Sputum culture**
  Microscopy for tubercle bacilli and C&S.
- **Urine microscopy and culture**
  Microscopic haematuria in endocarditis. Haematuria in hypernephroma and blood dyscrasias. White cells – infection. Granular or red cell casts – renal inflammation, e.g. connective tissue disease. Proteinuria suggests renal disease.
- **Stool culture and microscopy**
  C&S. Ova, parasites and cysts on microscopy.
- **CXR**
  Tuberculosis. Atypical pneumonia. Pneumonitis associated with HIV and *Pneumocystis carinii*. Secondary deposits. Hilar glands associated with sarcoidosis, TB and lymphoma.
- **ECG**
  Cardiac disease.

SPECIFIC INVESTIGATIONS

- **Rheumatoid factor**
  Rheumatoid arthritis.
- **Serological tests**
  Q fever, brucellosis, leptospirosis.
- **Autoantibodies**
  Connective tissue disease.

- **Mantoux test**
  TB.
- **Antistreptolysin O titre**
  Rheumatic fever.
- **Bone marrow aspirate**
  Leukaemia. Myeloma.
- **Lumbar puncture**
  White cells and organisms – meningitis. Blood – subarachnoid haemorrhage. Protein – Guillain–Barré syndrome.
- **US abdomen**
  Intraperitoneal abscesses.
- **Gallium scan**
  Localised infection.
- **Labelled white cell scan**
  Localised infection/abscess.
- **Liver biopsy**
  Hepatitis.
- **Renal biopsy**
  Glomerular disease. Malignancy.
- **Muscle biopsy**
  Myositis.
- **CT**
  Infection. Malignancy.
- **Exploratory laparotomy**
  This may be necessary to exclude intra-abdominal sepsis.

▶ RECTAL BLEEDING

Rectal bleeding is a common symptom. The majority of patients
with rectal bleeding have a simple condition such as haemorrhoids
but the symptoms should always be taken seriously and
investigated. Rectal bleeding with change in bowel habit and
colicky abdominal pain should be regarded as due to colorectal
cancer until proved otherwise.

CAUSES

Anus
- Haemorrhoids
- Fissure-in-ano
- Carcinoma
- Trauma

Colon and rectum
- Carcinoma
- Polyps
- Diverticular disease
- Inflammatory bowel disease
  - Ulcerative colitis
  - Crohn's disease
- Ischaemic colitis
- Angiodysplasia
- Irradiation colitis or proctitis
- Rectal prolapse
- Solitary rectal ulcer

Small bowel
- Meckel's diverticulum
- Intussusception
- Mesenteric infarction
- Aortoenteric fistula

Upper gastrointestinal tract
- Massive haemorrhage, e.g. duodenal ulcer

Others
- Anticoagulants
- Bleeding diatheses
- Uraemia

HISTORY

Anus

Haemorrhoids

Piles occur at any age. Bleeding from piles is either noted on the toilet paper or splashes in the toilet after defecation. Uncomplicated piles are not painful.

Fissure-in-ano

Fissure-in-ano is most common under the age of 40 years. It is quite common in children. The patient experiences pain on defecation, which may persist for minutes or hours afterwards. Constipation is usually a precipitating cause, the constipation being made worse by the fissure as the patient avoids defecation because of pain. Blood is noticed on the toilet paper or streaked on the stool.

Carcinoma of the anal canal

Carcinoma of the anal canal usually occurs in the elderly. It presents with pain on defecation and streaking of blood on the stools and blood on the toilet paper. Initially, in the early stages, it may be mistaken for a fissure-in-ano.

Trauma

There may be a history of a penetrating injury to the anal canal. Sexual abuse or homosexual practices may be relevant.

Colorectal

Carcinoma

With colonic carcinoma the blood may be mixed with the stool. There is usually a history of accompanying change in bowel habit and colicky abdominal pain. With rectal cancer the blood is usually streaked on the stool and there may be a history of tenesmus, i.e. a sense of incomplete evacuation of the rectum.

Polyps

The history may be similar to that of carcinoma.

Diverticular disease

Bleeding associated with diverticular disease is typically acute, massive and fresh. There may be a past history of diverticular disease.

Inflammatory bowel disease

With ulcerative colitis and Crohn's disease there is often sudden onset of diarrhoea with watery, brown motions containing mucus and fresh blood. There is usually colicky abdominal pain. With ulcerative proctitis the patient may complain of tenesmus.

Ischaemic colitis

This usually occurs in the elderly. There is colicky abdominal pain associated with the passage of dark-red venous blood PR.

Angiodysplasia

The patient is usually elderly. There is bleeding PR, which may be torrential but is more often repeated small bleeds.

Irradiation proctitis or colitis

There will be a history of irradiation, often for carcinoma of the cervix. The patient passes blood and mucus PR and complains of tenesmus.

Rectal prolapse

The patient will be aware of something hanging out of the back passage that comes down on defecation. Bleeding is due to trauma.

Solitary rectal ulcer

Bleeding occurs after defecation, usually in small volumes. This may be associated with mucus discharge and a feeling of a lump in the anus.

Small bowel

Meckel's diverticulum

This usually results in painless bleeding in young adults. The blood tends to be dark red and may on occasions have the characteristics of melaena.

Intussusception

This usually occurs in infants, but may rarely occur at any age. The child has colicky abdominal pain and draws the legs up, screams and passes a stool consisting of mixed blood and mucus ('redcurrant jelly' stool).

Mesenteric infarction

The patient is usually elderly, or a younger patient who has a history of heart disease (embolism). The patient develops severe central abdominal, colicky pain associated with diffuse tenderness and later collapse and shock.

Aortoenteric fistula

This usually occurs following repair of an infrarenal aortic aneurysm with a Dacron graft. The Dacron graft becomes infected, the fistula forms between the aorta and duodenum. Depending on the speed of the bleed, there may be either melaena or profuse red rectal haemorrhage with shock.

Upper gastrointestinal tract

Massive haemorrhage from the upper gastrointestinal tract, e.g. bleeding oesophageal varices, duodenal ulcer, may present with bright-red bleeding PR. This is due to extremely fast intestinal transit and the patient will always be shocked.

Others

Check for a history of anticoagulants. The patient may have a bleeding disorder. Check for bleeding from other sites or spontaneous bruising.

Uraemia

Rectal bleeding may occur in uraemia and this may be related to a platelet defect.

Rarely, rectal bleeding may occur with collagen diseases, particularly polyarteritis nodosa.

EXAMINATION

Anus

Haemorrhoids

There may be obvious prolapsed haemorrhoids; however, sigmoidoscopy and proctoscopy are usually required to make the diagnosis.

Fissure-in-ano

Separate the buttocks. A chronic fissure-in-ano with a sentinel pile may be seen in the midline posteriorly, or more rarely in the midline anteriorly. Digital rectal examination, if attempted, will be extremely painful.

Carcinoma

This may show a hard ulcer in the anal canal with everted edges; however, in the early stages, carcinoma of the anal canal may be difficult to distinguish from a chronic fissure-in-ano. Biopsy should be undertaken.

Trauma

Bruising may be apparent around the anal canal. There may be a split in the skin or mucosa. Digital rectal examination will be painful.

Colon and rectum

Carcinoma
An abdominal mass may be palpable. There may be signs of intestinal obstruction. Digital rectal examination may reveal a hard, irregular, ulcerating mass.

Polyps
A polyp may be palpable in the rectum. There may be no findings on physical examination.

Diverticular disease
The patient may be tender in the left iliac fossa. Often there are no abdominal findings.

Inflammatory bowel disease
There may be a palpable abdominal mass with Crohn's disease. There may be localised abdominal tenderness. If toxic dilatation has occurred, the abdomen will be distended and tender, and there may be signs of peritonitis if perforation has occurred.

Ischaemic colitis
Physical examination may show left-sided abdominal tenderness and the patient may be shocked.

Angiodysplasia
There may be little to find other than rectal bleeding. There are usually no abdominal signs.

Irradiation colitis or proctitis
There may be some abdominal tenderness. Digital rectal examination will reveal a granular mucosa and blood on the glove.

Rectal prolapse
There will be obvious prolapse of the rectum with ulcerated, bleeding rectal mucosa.

Solitary rectal ulcer
There are no abdominal findings. Digital rectal examination may give the impression of a polypoid swelling just inside the rectum, which may be mistaken for carcinoma. Proctoscopy will reveal redness and oedema of the mucosa and, in about 50% of patients, frank ulceration will be noted.

Small bowel

Meckel's diverticulum
There will usually be nothing to find on abdominal examination.

Intussusception

A mass may be palpable in the right iliac fossa. Eventually, as the intussusception proceeds, the right iliac fossa becomes 'empty'.

Mesenteric infarction

The patient may be in atrial fibrillation and this suggests embolism. There will be diffuse abdominal tenderness, later accompanied by collapse and shock.

Aortoenteric fistula

There will usually be the long midline scar of a recent aortic aneurysm repair. Otherwise there will be little to find on abdominal examination.

Upper gastrointestinal tract

Massive haemorrhage

There may be signs of liver failure associated with a massive bleed from varices. There may be epigastric tenderness associated with duodenal ulceration.

Others

With anticoagulants there may be bleeding from other orifices, as may occur also with bleeding diatheses. Look for signs of bruising. Uraemic bleeding is often seen in patients with established uraemia and they may already be on dialysis and have an arteriovenous fistula or a CAPD tube *in situ*. Rectal bleeding from collagen diseases is rare. Polyarteritis nodosa is probably the most common. Bleeding is due to necrotising vasculitis and there may be signs of vasculitis elsewhere, e.g. skin.

GENERAL INVESTIGATIONS

- **FBC, ESR**
  Hb ↓ may occur in almost any type of rectal bleeding. WCC ↑ inflammatory bowel disease, ischaemic colitis, aortoenteric fistula. Platelets ↓ in bleeding diatheses. ESR ↑ carcinoma, collagen disease.
- **U&Es**
  Urea and creatinine raised with uraemic bleeding. The urea may be raised due to absorption of blood from the bowel. Usually in this case the creatinine is normal.
- **LFTs**
  Liver failure associated with oesophageal varices.

- **Sigmoidoscopy/proctoscopy**
  Anorectal tumours. Haemorrhoids. Distal colitis. Solitary rectal ulcer. Biopsy.
- **AXR**
  Obstruction associated with carcinoma. Inflammatory bowel disease (toxic dilatation of the colon).

SPECIFIC INVESTIGATIONS

- **Barium enema**
  Carcinoma. Diverticular disease. Polyps. Inflammatory bowel disease. Ischaemic colitis.
- **Colonoscopy**
  Diverticular disease. Colonic tumours. Angiodyplasia. Colitis.
- **Angiography (in the acute bleeding phase)**
  Angiodysplasia. Bleeding Meckel's diverticulum.
- **Labelled red cell scan**
  Angiodysplasia. Meckel's diverticulum.
- **Technetium scan**
  Meckel's diverticulum.

SCALP LESIONS

Lesions on the scalp are common; the most common are sebaceous cysts, which are often multiple.

CAUSES

Traumatic
- Haematoma
- Cephalhaematoma

Sebaceous cysts

Neoplastic

Benign
- Ivory osteoma

Malignant
Primary
- Basal cell carcinoma
- Squamous cell carcinoma
- Malignant melanoma
- Leukaemia
- Myeloma
Secondary
- Breast
- Bronchus
- Thyroid
- Prostate
- Kidney

Infective
- Cock's peculiar tumour
- Tinea capitis

Other
- Psoriasis
- Seborrhoeic dermatitis

HISTORY

Traumatic
Check for a history of trauma. A boggy haematoma may overlie a skull fracture. A cephalhaematoma is seen in a newborn baby. It

follows a traumatic delivery. The haematoma is below the periosteum of the skull.

Sebaceous cyst

These may be multiple. The patient usually notices them when combing the hair.

Neoplastic

With an ivory osteoma the patient may notice a rock-hard swelling on the scalp. The patient is usually a young adult and is asymptomatic. Malignant ulcers may occur on the scalp. The patient will notice a lesion when combing the hair and bleeding may occur. These lesions present earlier in bald patients. Bony tenderness and swelling may be a presenting symptom of secondary deposits. There may be a history of a primary or a careful history must be taken to establish the site of a primary.

Infective

With Cock's peculiar tumour the patient may notice a sore, bleeding lesion on the scalp. Cock's peculiar tumour is due to a sebaceous cyst suppurating and granulation tissue appearing on its surface. It may be mistaken for a squamous cell carcinoma. Tinea capitis usually occurs in childhood. There is an itchy, red, scaly patch on the scalp and the hairs break easily, leaving patches of stubble.

Other

Psoriasis may affect the scalp. There is usually a history of lesions elsewhere on the body. Seborrhoeic dermatitis presents with a fine, scaly rash on the scalp. Hair growth is usually normal with both these lesions.

EXAMINATION

Traumatic

A knock on the head may cause a boggy haematoma. X-ray is required to exclude an underlying fracture. Cephalhaematoma occurs in the newborn; the haematoma spreads beneath the periosteum of the skull and is therefore limited by the skull suture lines.

Sebaceous cyst

Sebaceous cysts are spherical, tender, firm swellings in the scalp. They may be multiple. Rarely is a punctum visible with sebaceous cysts on the scalp.

Neoplastic

An ivory osteoma is a bony, hard, smooth swelling arising from the outer table of the skull. The skin is freely mobile over it. A squamous cell carcinoma presents as an ulcer with a hard, everted edge. A malignant melanoma is usually pigmented, ulcerated and bleeds. In both these conditions cervical lymphadenopathy may be present. A basal cell carcinoma is a raised ulcer with a rolled edge with a pearly appearance, often with superficial telangiectasia. Lesions in the skull may be secondaries from lung, breast, thyroid, prostate and kidney. Each of these areas should be examined for a possible primary. Myeloma may present with painful lesions in the skull. There may be areas of localised tenderness.

Infective

Cock's peculiar tumour presents as an open, granulating sebaceous cyst. It appears angry and swollen and may be mistaken for a squamous cell carcinoma. In tinea capitis there are red, scaly patches on the scalp, with broken hairs giving a stubbled appearance.

Other

With psoriasis there are well-demarcated areas of scales heaped up over red plaque. The hair grows normally through the plaques. Check for psoriatic lesions elsewhere. Seborrhoeic dermatitis shows fine scales but the hairs remain intact.

GENERAL INVESTIGATIONS

The diagnosis of most of these lesions is made on clinical examination alone.

- **FBC, ESR**
  Hb ↓ malignancy. WCC ↑ leukaemia. ESR ↑ myeloma and other malignancies.
- **CXR**
  Primary tumour. Secondary malignancy, e.g. secondaries from malignant melanoma.
- **Skull X-ray**
  Fracture. Ivory osteoma. Pepper-pot skull – myeloma. Secondary deposits – osteolytic from lung, breast and thyroid.
  Osteosclerotic from prostate and occasionally kidney.

SPECIFIC INVESTIGATIONS

- **Serum protein electrophoresis**
  Monoclonal gammopathy with myeloma.
- **Bone scan**
  Bony secondaries.
- **Scalp scrapings**
  Fungal infection, e.g. tinea capitis.
- **Biopsy**
  Malignant lesions. Cock's peculiar tumour.

SCROTAL PAIN

This may be due to lesions on the scrotal skin, within the scrotum, or may rarely be due to referred pain.

CAUSES

- Skin
- Dermatitis
- Irritation (urine/faeces in the incontinent)
- Infected sebaceous cyst
- Herpes simplex
- Behçet's disease (rare)
- Fournier's gangrene (rare)

Internal scrotal swellings

- Strangulated hernia
- Testicular torsion
- Torsion of testicular appendage
- Epididymo-orchitis
- Haematocele
- Varicocele

Referred

- Ilioinguinal nerve entrapment after hernia repair
- Groin strain
- Idiopathic cord neuralgia
- Spinal nerve irritation (rare)

HISTORY

Skin

The patient may have noticed a skin lesion, which is itchy, sore or painful. In the elderly, confused and incontinent, pain and soreness may be due to the irritant effect of faeces and urine with superadded infection. Previous history of a superficial swelling may suggest an infected sebaceous cyst. There may be a history to suggest contact dermatitis. Painful vesicular lesions may suggest herpes. Behçet's syndrome may cause painful ulcerative lesions of the scrotum and the patient may also have similar lesions on the penis. Fournier's gangrene usually has acute onset in a young, healthy male with rapid progression to gangrene of the skin. There is often absence of a discernible cause.

Internal scrotal swellings

There may be a previous history of an inguinal hernia descending into the scrotum. Sudden onset of colicky abdominal pain and irreducibility may suggest the development of a strangulated inguinal hernia. Sudden onset of pain, redness, and swelling in a teenager or young male suggests a diagnosis of testicular torsion. This may come on during vigorous exercise. This is a surgical emergency and needs urgent surgery. Gradual onset of pain, redness and tenderness will suggest epididymo-orchitis. Check for symptoms of urinary tract infection, e.g. dysuria or frequency, which may accompany epididymo-orchitis. Orchitis may be associated with mumps and this may be apparent, the patient complaining of bilateral painful parotid and submandibular glands together with painful cervical lymphadenopathy and constitutional illness. A history of trauma will suggest haematocele. A dull ache, often poorly localised, may be associated with a varicocele.

Referred pain

Rarely, the patient may complain of pain in the scrotum with no visible or palpable abnormality. Check for a history of previous inguinal hernia repair, which may have resulted in ilioinguinal nerve entrapment. Idiopathic cord neuralgia may occur but is rare. Occasionally 'groin strain' may cause scrotal pain. Referred pain from spinal lesions may rarely cause scrotal pain.

EXAMINATION

Skin

A red, scaly lesion will suggest dermatitis. There may be superadded infection. In the elderly and incontinent, the diagnosis of irritation from urine or faeces will usually be apparent. An infected sebaceous cyst will present as a localised, tender, red swelling on the scrotum. There may be purulent discharge. Herpes simplex will present with vesicular lesions. They may be present elsewhere, e.g. on the penis. Behçet's disease will present with painful ulcerative lesions on the scrotum as well as on the penis. There may be other signs of Behçet's disease, e.g. arthritis, keratitis, iritis, mouth ulcers. With Fournier's gangrene there is usually a tense, glossy oedema developing over the scrotum. Crepitations develop later before subcutaneous gangrene occurs. The gangrene may spread over the inguinal area and the lower abdominal wall. In the advanced case, the skin will have completely disappeared, leaving the testes hanging naked in the scrotum.

Internal scrotal swellings

There may be a tense, tender scrotal mass, which it is impossible to 'get above'. This would suggest a strangulated hernia. The presence of an enlarged tender testicle drawn up towards the groin suggests testicular torsion. An enlarged tender testis with redness and scrotal oedema suggests epididymo-orchitis. The parotid and submandibular glands should be checked to exclude mumps. Occasionally, torsion of a testicular appendage may occur and cause pain and scrotal swelling out of all proportion to the size of the lesion, which may be less than a few millimetres in diameter. A tender swelling with scrotal bruising and oedema following trauma will suggest a haematocele (a collection of blood between the layers of the tunica vaginalis). A varicocele may not be obvious until the patient has been standing up for 10–15 seconds. Classically it feels like a 'bag of worms' with the warm blood filling dilated veins, which are palpable through the scrotal skin. It is more common on the left-hand side. Rapid onset of a left-sided varicocele may be associated with carcinoma of the left kidney, the tumour growing down the left renal vein and obstructing the left testicular vein. Examine the abdomen for a left renal mass.

Referred pain

Check for the scar of an inguinal hernia repair. In ilioinguinal nerve entrapment there will be anaesthesia/paraesthesia below the scar and on the anterior aspect of the scrotal skin. In the rare case where scrotal pain may be referred from a spinal lesion, a full neurological examination should be carried out. Examine the lumbosacral spine for localised tenderness.

GENERAL INVESTIGATIONS

- **FBC, ESR**
  WCC ↑ infection. ESR ↑ infection, tumour.
- **US**
  Testicular lesion. Haematocele.
- **MSU**
  Urinary tract infection associated with epididymo-orchitis.
- **Swab**
  Ulcer, C&S.

SPECIFIC INVESTIGATIONS

- **Lumbosacral spine X-ray**
  Referred pain due to degenerative disease or metastases.
- **Laser Doppler**
  Check for testicular blood flow. Absent in testicular torsion.
- **Technetium scan**
  Testicular torsion (no outline of testis) versus epididymo-orchitis (good testicular blood flow).
- **US abdomen**
  Left renal carcinoma (varicocele).
- **MRI**
  Spinal lesion.
- **Surgery**
  Diagnostic between torsion and infection. There is rarely time or equipment to carry out laser Doppler or a technetium scan. If a testicular torsion is not dealt with within 6 hours of onset there is likely to be permanent damage to the testis. If there is any doubt in the diagnosis, assume that it is torsion and explore the scrotum surgically.

SCROTAL SWELLINGS

Scrotal swellings are a common presenting complaint in the outpatient clinic. They are also therefore common in clinical examinations. It is important to be able to make a rapid diagnosis of testicular torsion and take appropriate action, i.e. surgery. It is also important to distinguish between those swellings that have underlying serious pathology (testicular tumour) and those that are simple and benign (epididymal cysts).

CAUSES

- Sebaceous cyst
- Indirect inguinal hernia
- Hydrocele
- Epididymal cyst (spermatocele)
- Epididymo-orchitis
- Testicular torsion
- Testicular tumour
- Varicocele
- Haematocele
- Sperm granuloma
- Tuberculosis (rare)
- Gumma (rare)

HISTORY

Sebaceous cyst
The patient may complain of several painful lumps on the scrotal skin. There may be a history of one or more of them becoming red, inflamed and tender with discharge.

Indirect inguinal hernia
The patient will be often aware of what the lump is. He may be able to reduce it. The hernia may present with a painful, irreducible swelling and signs of intestinal obstruction.

Hydrocele
An idiopathic hydrocele presents usually as a painless scrotal swelling which may become quite large. They usually occur over the age of 50 years. Occasionally there may be pain and discomfort if there is underlying testicular disease. A younger

patient presenting with a hydrocele should raise the suspicion of an underlying malignancy.

Epididymal cyst

This presents as a painless scrotal swelling. Epididymal cysts may slowly enlarge over many years. They may be bilateral.

Epididymo-orchitis

The patient complains of pain and swelling, usually unilaterally. There are usually constitutional symptoms of malaise and fever. It may be accompanied by urinary tract infection with dysuria and frequency.

Testicular torsion

This usually occurs around puberty. It is rare over 25 years of age. There is sudden onset of pain in the scrotum and groin, which may radiate into the lower abdomen. This may be accompanied by nausea and vomiting. There may be a history of violent exercise, e.g. straining in the gymnasium, lifting or even masturbation. Always ascertain the exact time of onset of symptoms. To be sure of testicular salvage, surgery should be carried out within 6–8 hours of onset of symptoms.

Testicular tumour

Teratomas occur between 18 and 30 years, seminomas between 30 and 45 years. The common presentation is a feeling of heaviness in the scrotum accompanied by a painless swelling. Occasionally, symptoms are due to secondary deposits, e.g. abdominal pain from enlarged retroperitoneal lymph nodes. Occasionally, distant lymphadenopathy, e.g. cervical, may be a presenting symptom.

Varicocele

The patient (or partner) may notice varicose veins in the scrotum. Often the only symptom is a dragging ache in the scrotum and groin. Subfertility may be a presentation and is associated with bilateral varicoceles. A varicocele is more common on the left.

Haematocele

There will be a clear history of trauma.

Sperm granuloma

This may develop 2–4 months after vasectomy. The patient will complain of a small tender nodule at the site of vasectomy.

Tuberculosis

This is now rare in the UK. A scrotal lump with associated dull, aching pain is the usual presentation. There may be a history of pulmonary or renal TB. There may be malaise, weight loss, haemoptysis or haematuria.

Gumma

This is extremely rare. There is a painless swelling of the testis. It needs to be distinguished from a testicular tumour. Other signs of syphilis may be present.

EXAMINATION

Sebaceous cyst

A small swelling or multiple small swellings occur in the scrotal skin. They are tense and spherical. Because of the thinness of the scrotal skin stretched over the swelling, the cheesy yellow material contained within them can be seen. There may be a small punctum surmounting the cyst.

Indirect inguinal hernia

Hernias that descend in the scrotum are invariably indirect. They may be reducible. It is impossible to get above the swelling. There is an expansile cough impulse and bowel sounds may be heard over the hernia.

Hydrocele

A hydrocele is usually unilateral. It may become very large.
A hydrocele is fluctuant, transilluminates and is dull to percussion. If large enough there may be a fluid thrill. The testis cannot be palpated separately from the hydrocele. It is possible to get above the swelling except with infantile hydroceles, when the fluid extends up to the deep inguinal ring.

Epididymal cyst

An epididymal cyst usually occurs above and behind the testis. The testis can be palpated separately from it. An epididymal cyst frequently feels lobulated because often the fluid is in locules. They are fluctuant. Those containing clear fluid transilluminate. Those containing a milky opalescent fluid are called spermatoceles and do not transilluminate.

Epididymo-orchitis

The scrotal skin is hot, red and oedematous. The tenderness is initially confined to the epididymis but eventually spreads to involve the testis.

Testicular torsion

The scrotal skin is usually hot, red and oedematous. The testis is extremely tender and is often drawn up towards the groin.

Testicular tumour

There is a firm, irregular swelling in the scrotum. Often the patient notices the lump when it is very small but in other cases it may become very large before the patient presents. Rarely the tumour has been allowed to advance so far that it is attached to the scrotal skin. Check for palpable para-aortic nodes. Examine the cervical nodes, especially in the left supraclavicular fossa. Testicular tumours metastasise to the para-aortic nodes, to the mediastinal nodes, and occasionally into the cervical nodes. Inguinal nodes are not involved unless the tumour has invaded the scrotal skin, which is rare.

Varicocele

This can only be palpated with the patient standing up. The dilated veins then become visible and palpable. They are said to feel like 'a bag of worms' but actually feel more like lukewarm spaghetti. The left side is more commonly affected.

Haematocele

There is a tense, tender, fluctuant swelling. There may be obvious scrotal bruising. The testis cannot be felt separately as the blood surrounds it within the layers of the tunica vaginalis.

Sperm granuloma

There is a small, tender, painful nodule at the site of previous vasectomy.

Tuberculosis

The swelling is usually confined to the epididymis, where there is a hard lump. The spermatic cord and vas are thickened. Occasionally a sinus may have formed. Check the chest for signs of pulmonary TB. Check the neck for scars (lymph node drainage for cold abscess) or lymphadenopathy.

Gumma

A gumma is a painless swelling of the whole testis. Other signs of syphilis may be present.

GENERAL INVESTIGATIONS

- **FBC, ESR**
  Hb ↓ chronic disease, e.g. TB. WCC ↑ inflammation, e.g. epididymo-orchitis, torsion. ESR ↑ TB, syphilis, tumour.

- **CXR**
  TB. Secondary deposits from testicular tumour.
- **MSU**
  UTI associated with epididymo-orchitis.
- **US**
  Solid versus cystic. Hydrocele versus epididymal cyst. Always arrange an ultrasound of the underlying testis in the young patient with a lax hydrocele as there may be an underlying tumour.

SPECIFIC INVESTIGATIONS

- **Tumour markers**
  AFP, βHCG, LDH.
- **EMSU**
  TB.
- **VDRL**
  Gumma.
- **US abdomen**
  Carcinoma of left kidney invading the left renal vein, associated with left varicocele.
- **Laser Doppler***
  Torsion versus epididymo-orchitis.
- **Technetium scan***
  Torsion versus epididymo-orchitis.
- **Surgery**
  Distinction between torsion and epididymo-orchitis.
- **MRI**
  Abdominal and chest MRI scan may confirm lymphadenopathy associated with secondary deposits from testicular tumours.

---

*There is rarely time or equipment to carry out these investigations. If there is any doubt about the diagnosis, assume that it is torsion and explore the scrotum surgically.

▶ SHOCK

Shock is an abnormality of the circulation that results in inadequate organ perfusion and tissue oxygenation.

CAUSES

Hypovolaemic
- Haemorrhage
- Burns
- Gastrointestinal losses

Cardiogenic
- Myocardial infarction
- Acute valvular damage
- Arrhythmia

Distributive
- Sepsis
- Anaphylaxis
- Neurogenic shock (spinal injury)

Obstructive
- Cardiac tamponade
- Massive pulmonary embolism
- Tension pneumothorax

HISTORY

Trauma
Trauma is a pertinent feature in the history as haemorrhage invariably accompanies penetrating trauma. The site and approximate amount of blood loss should be assessed. Blunt trauma to the chest is associated with tension pneumothorax, myocardial contusion and cardiac tamponade. Trauma to the pelvis and long bones can result in closed fractures, causing significant haemorrhage that may not always be apparent to the observer. Thermal injury can occur with patients involved in fires, water-heater explosions and gas explosions. Acute onset of paralysis following trauma may be due to spinal or peripheral nerve injury. Disruption to the descending sympathetic pathways with spinal injuries results in loss of vasomotor tone and consequently hypotension.

Dyspnoea

Although tachypnoea is a physiological accompaniment to blood loss, when dyspnoea is the predominant symptom you should consider pulmonary oedema from the causes of cardiogenic shock. In addition, dyspnoea is also a prominent feature of all the causes of obstructive shock.

Chest pain

The consequences of blunt trauma to the chest have been described above. In the absence of trauma, the presence of chest pain should lead you to consider myocardial infarction (central crushing) and pulmonary embolism (pleuritic).

Precipitating factors

Occasionally patients may be aware of allergens that provoke anaphylaxis. In the community, food products (shellfish, eggs, peanuts) and insect venom (bees, wasps) are common causes. In hospital, penicillin, anaesthetic agents and intravenous contrast media are the major provoking factors. Detailed systemic enquiry for presence of infection may elucidate the offending focus for patients in septic shock. A history of profuse vomiting, diarrhoea or intestinal obstruction (vomiting, constipation, colicky abdominal pain and distension) would indicate gastrointestinal losses as the cause for hypovolaemia.

EXAMINATION

Inspection

A thorough systematic inspection should be undertaken; burns and sites of bleeding from penetrating trauma may be obvious. Cyanosis is a feature of large pulmonary emboli and tension pneumothoraces. Patients with anaphylaxis often exhibit angio-oedema and urticaria.

Temperature

Patients in shock are generally cold and clammy. With septic shock, however, the skin is warm to the touch and the patient is usually pyrexial.

Pulse

A tachycardia is the earliest measurable indicator of shock; however, it may not be elevated in cases of neurogenic shock. The character of the pulse is usually weak. The rhythm may suggest an arrhythmia as the precipitating factor in cardiogenic shock. Pulsus paradoxus (decrease in amplitude of the pulse on inspiration) is consistent with cardiac tamponade.

JVP

A low JVP is a useful discriminator for hypovolaemic shock as it will usually be elevated with all causes of cardiogenic and obstructive shock.

Auscultation

Bronchospasm, and consequently wheezing, may be prominent in anaphylactic shock. Unilateral absent breath sounds indicate a pneumothorax, while muffled heart sounds are features of cardiac tamponade. The presence of a new murmur can be due to acute valvular insufficiency as a cause for cardiogenic shock.

GENERAL INVESTIGATIONS

- **Pulse oximetry**
  Although low saturation *per se* is not very discriminatory, severe impairment of oxygen saturation is associated with pulmonary embolus and pneumothorax. This may be confirmed with ABGs.
- **FBC**
  With blood loss a low Hb may be noted, although this will not be evident immediately. A raised WCC occurs with infection. Unfortunately, it will also be raised in most causes of acute physiological stress.
- **U&Es**
  With significant gastrointestinal losses, low serum sodium and potassium accompanied with raised urea and creatinine are the usual abnormalities.
- **ECG**
  The ECG may reveal myocardial infarction or the presence of an arrhythmia as the precipitating aetiology. Electrical alternans (alternating large and small QRS complexes) is a specific indicator of pericardial tamponade. Widespread low-amplitude complexes are common in significant pericardial effusion.
- **CXR**
  May reveal a pneumothorax with deviation of the trachea (although the diagnosis of a tension pneumothorax should be clinical and relieved before a chest X-ray is performed!). The cardiac silhouette may be globular in the presence of a pericardial effusion; however, tamponade is still possible with a normal-appearing chest film.

SPECIFIC INVESTIGATIONS

- **Blood cultures**
  Blood and site-specific cultures are essential in suspected septic shock. The underlying organism may be isolated.
- **Echocardiography**
  An echocardiogram will be able to demonstrate valvular dysfunction, the presence of tamponade and massive pulmonary embolism (when right heart failure is present).
- **Pulmonary angiography**
  Is preferable to V/Q scanning for the diagnosis of pulmonary embolism in the presence of shock, as emergency therapeutic measures (such as thrombolysis) can be performed.
- **CT/MRI spine**
  May be required to assess the extent and confirm the level of injury.

▶ SPLENOMEGALY

The spleen must be enlarged to about three times its normal size before it becomes clinically palpable. The lower margin may feel notched on palpation. The spleen may become so massive in size that it is palpable in the right iliac fossa. Massive splenomegaly in the UK is likely to be due to chronic myeloid leukaemia, myelofibrosis or lymphoma. Splenomegaly may lead to hypersplenism, i.e. pancytopenia as cells become trapped and destroyed in an overactive spleen.

CAUSES

Infective

Bacterial
- Typhoid
- Typhus
- TB
- Syphilis
- Leptospirosis
- Septicaemia
- Abscess

Viral
- Glandular fever

Protozoal
- Malaria

Parasitic
- Hydatid cyst

Inflammatory
- Rheumatoid arthritis
- Sarcoidosis
- Lupus
- Amyloid

Neoplastic
- Leukaemia
- Lymphoma
- Polycythaemia vera
- Myelofibrosis

- Primary tumours
- Metastases

Haemolytic disease
- Hereditary spherocytosis
- Acquired haemolytic anaemia
- Thrombocytopenic purpura

Storage diseases
- Gaucher's disease

Deficiency diseases
- Pernicious anaemia
- Severe iron-deficiency anaemia

Splenic vein hypertension
- Cirrhosis
- Splenic vein thrombosis
- Portal vein thrombosis

Non-parasitic cysts

HISTORY

Infective

Most infective causes present with fever, malaise and anorexia. With typhus there will be a history of foreign travel. Typhus is conveyed between hosts by arthropods. The patient complains of severe constitutional symptoms with headache, vomiting, photophobia and toxaemia. With typhoid there will usually be a history of foreign travel or it will occur in the immigrant population. There will be a history of malaise, headache, fever, cough, constipation initially and then diarrhoea. Epistaxis and abdominal pain may occur. TB usually presents with weight loss, night sweats and a cough. If septicaemia is responsible there will usually be an obvious cause, and the patient may already be hospitalised. With splenic abscess there may be a history of endocarditis, lung abscess, drug abuse, or it may occur in an immunocompromised host. Syphilis is rare and there may be a history of contact. With leptospirosis there is often a history of contact with rats, particularly when swimming in rivers where there are rats by the riverside. Fever, jaundice, headache, haemoptysis and haematuria are presenting symptoms. With malaria there is usually a history of travel to an area where it is endemic. The patient usually presents within 2 months of travel abroad with malaise, myalgia, sweating, coldness, followed by rigors, high fever and drenching sweats. Hydatid disease occurs most frequently in rural sheep-farming regions, e.g. Wales. The commonest presentation is with a cyst in the lung causing dyspnoea, haemoptysis or anaphylaxis.

Inflammatory

Rheumatoid arthritis may be apparent. Sarcoidosis may present with lymphadenopathy, fever and malaise, as well as hepatosplenomegaly. Lupus may present with protean manifestations with cutaneous, musculoskeletal, renal, pulmonary and haematological problems. Amyloid may be primary or secondary. There may be cutaneous, cerebral, cardiac or endocrine manifestations. With secondary amyloidosis there may be a history of chronic infection, e.g. TB; inflammatory disease, e.g. rheumatoid arthritis; or neoplasia. It usually affects the kidney and liver as well as the spleen.

Neoplastic

There will often be generalised signs of malignancy. Often there will be general malaise with weight loss, and with lymphoma there will be a history of night sweats. There may also be a tendency to spontaneous bruising. Primary tumours of the spleen and splenic metastases are rare.

Haemolytic disease

Haemolytic disease usually presents with the symptoms of anaemia, namely tiredness and malaise. Jaundice may be present, although is often not very deep, merely giving a lemonish tinge to the skin. With excessive breakdown of red blood cells, pigment stones may form in the gall bladder and the disease may present with acute cholecystitis.

Storage diseases

Apart from variable hepatosplenomegaly, these may present with neurological problems, skeletal deformities or mental deterioration.

Deficiency diseases

There may be a history of pernicious anaemia. Splenomegaly is usually mild. With iron-deficiency anaemia there may be dietary deficiency, malabsorption or blood loss. Check for a history of blood loss.

Splenic vein hypertension

There may be an obvious history, with cirrhosis and signs of liver failure. Isolated splenic vein thrombosis is rare.

Non-parasitic cysts

These are rare but may arise from organised haematomas, infarcts or inflammation. They are usually isolated findings when the patient is being investigated for other conditions.

EXAMINATION

General

The spleen appears from below the tip of the left tenth rib and enlarges towards the umbilicus. It is firm and smooth and usually has a notch on its upper edge. It moves with respiration, is dull to percussion, and it is impossible to get above it.

Infective

With typhus there is only moderate splenomegaly. The patient will often be toxic with a generalised maculopapular rash. With typhoid there is moderate splenomegaly, the patient being pyrexial with a tender abdomen and with rose spots on the trunk. Again with TB the splenomegaly is only moderate. There may be chest signs. With septicaemia there is usually an obvious cause and again there is only moderate splenomegaly. With splenic abscess, again there is only moderate splenomegaly and the spleen may be tender and feel irregular. With glandular fever the patient will be pyrexial with lymphadenopathy, and occasionally there is a rash, especially if the patient has been given ampicillin. Splenomegaly is moderate. With syphilis there may be fever, malaise, lymphadenopathy, and a rash on the trunk, palms and soles. Rarely there may be hepatitis, meningism and uveitis. With leptospirosis ictohaemorrhagica the patient is usually ill with pyrexia, jaundice and purpuric rash. There may be signs of meningitis. There also may be tender muscles (myositis). There may be signs of acute renal failure. With malaria there is often anaemia, jaundice and hepatosplenomegaly. With hydatid disease the liver is usually more affected than the spleen. There may be hepatomegaly in addition to splenomegaly.

Inflammatory

With inflammatory disease the spleen is rarely grossly enlarged. Changes of rheumatoid arthritis may be apparent elsewhere in the body. With sarcoidosis there may be lymphadenopathy as well as hepatosplenomegaly. With lupus there may be cutaneous manifestations as well as musculoskeletal, renal and pulmonary manifestations. With amyloid, in addition to hepatosplenomegaly, there may be signs of carpal tunnel syndrome, peripheral neuropathy, purpura and a large tongue.

Neoplastic

There may be massive splenomegaly associated with chronic myeloid leukaemia, myelofibrosis and lymphoma. Other signs such as lymphadenopathy and spontaneous bruising may be present.

Haemolytic disease

The patient may have a mild jaundice together with moderate splenomegaly. A purpuric rash may be apparent with thrombocytopenic purpura.

Storage diseases

These are rare. There may be signs of cardiac failure, skeletal deformity or neurological deficits.

Splenic vein hypertension

Signs of liver failure, e.g. spider naevi, liver palms, caput medusae and jaundice may be present.

Non-parasitic cysts

The only finding may be splenomegaly.

GENERAL INVESTIGATIONS

- **FBC, ESR, blood film**
  Hb ↓ anaemias. Hb ↑ polycythaemia. WCC ↑ infection, leukaemia, abscess. ESR ↑ infection, malignancy. WCC ↓, platelets ↓ hypersplenism. PCV ↑ polycythaemia. MCV ↑ pernicious anaemia. Blood film – spherocytosis, malaria.
- **U&Es**
  Urea ↑, creatinine ↑ renal failure, e.g. with leptospirosis, amyloid, septicaemia.
- **LFTs**
  Cirrhosis.

SPECIFIC INVESTIGATIONS

- **Rheumatoid factor**
  Rheumatoid arthritis.
- **Paul–Bunnell test**
  Glandular fever.
- **VDRL**
  Syphilis.
- **Serum iron and serum ferritin**
  ↓ iron-deficiency anaemia.

- **Parietal cell antibodies**
  Pernicious anaemia.
- **Serum vitamin B$_{12}$**
  Pernicious anaemia.
- **Blood culture**
  Septicaemia. Leptospirosis. Typhoid.
- **Stool culture**
  Typhoid.
- **Urine culture**
  Typhoid. Leptospirosis.
- **CSF culture**
  Leptospirosis.
- **Complement fixation test**
  Leptospirosis.
- **ELISA/immunofluorescence**
  Typhus.
- **Bone marrow aspirate**
  Myelofibrosis. Polycythaemia. Leukaemia. Gaucher's disease.
- **US**
  Cause of splenomegaly, e.g. cyst, tumour, diffuse enlargement.
  Cirrhosis of the liver.
- **CT**
  Causes of splenomegaly, e.g. cyst, tumour, diffuse enlargement,
  cirrhosis.

▶ STEATORRHOEA

Steatorrhoea refers to the passing of excessive amounts of fat in the faeces. The causes are listed below, according to pathogenesis.

CAUSES

Lipase deficiency
- Impaired secretion – chronic pancreatitis
- Inactivation – excess gastric acid

Bile deficiency
- Underproduction – liver disease
- Obstruction – obstructive jaundice
- Increased degradation – bacterial overgrowth

Mucosal disease
- Ileal resection
- Coeliac disease
- Crohn's disease

Impaired fat transport
- Abetalipoproteinaemia

Lymphatic deficiency
- Lymphoma
- Whipple's disease

HISTORY

Patients with steatorrhoea often experience bulky, sticky and greasy stool that floats and is often difficult to flush away. Diarrhoea is the usual accompanying symptom (page 103) for most of the causes. Jaundice with pale stools and dark urine implies obstruction to the flow of bile, which is essential for the absorption of fat and fat-soluble vitamins. The causes and diagnostic approach to jaundice are found on page 240.

Abdominal pain

Vague epigastric abdominal pain experienced by patients with chronic pancreatitis may radiate to the back and is usually worse with food. Epigastric pain exacerbated by food may be a symptom of Zollinger–Ellison syndrome, which results in excessive gastric acid production (lowering the pH of gastric chyme) inactivating lipase. It usually presents with symptoms of peptic ulceration refractory to medical treatment. Abdominal pains associated with Crohn's disease are often felt in the right iliac fossa due to regional ileitis.

Associated symptoms

Patients with coeliac disease may also suffer with growth retardation, nutritional deficiencies causing anaemia and muscle wasting. Other symptoms include bone pain due to demineralisation, cerebellar ataxia and peripheral neuropathy. Joint pains, pyrexia, skin pigmentation and peripheral lymphadenopathy are among the varied symptoms of Whipple's disease resulting from infection with the bacterium *Tropheryma whipplei*. Steatorrhoea is the primary manifestation of intestinal lymphoma. It may be accompanied by abdominal pains and pyrexia and occasionally present with intestinal obstruction. Mouth ulcers, perianal abscesses, right iliac fossa pains and blood PR are some of the symptoms experienced by patients with Crohn's disease. Ataxia and night blindness from retinitis pigmentosa may result from abetalipoproteinaemia, which is caused by the absence of apolipoprotein B and therefore this results in defective chylomicron formation.

Past medical history

Previous surgical resection involving the terminal ileum will predispose an individual to malabsorption of fat due to decreased enterohepatic circulation of bile salts. Moreover, with decreased length of absorptive intestine, intestinal transit time decreases and there is a decrease in concomitant fat absorption. Conditions associated with intestinal stasis, hypomotility and decreased gastric acid secretion predispose to intestinal bacterial overgrowth and increased degradation of bile salts.

EXAMINATION

Steatorrhoea is often associated with malabsorption and therefore patients may appear emaciated. Mouth ulcers may be due to Crohn's or coeliac disease. Clubbing is associated with Crohn's, liver cirrhosis, coeliac disease and cystic fibrosis, which is associated with pancreatic exocrine insufficiency. Jaundice may be present with bile duct obstruction and liver disease. Bruising may result from impaired clotting due to vitamin K deficiency, and bone pains on examination may be secondary to osteomalacia from vitamin D deficiency. The classical rash of dermatitis herpetiformis may be seen with coeliac disease. Erythema nodosum is a feature of Crohn's disease and may be accompanied by right iliac fossa tenderness, perianal abscesses and fistulae. Hepatomegaly may be found in liver disease, and splenomegaly with intestinal lymphoma.

GENERAL INVESTIGATIONS

- **Faecal fat estimation**
  Stool collections over a period of 3 days are performed with a diet consisting of 50 g or more of fat per day. The normal value of faecal fat is less than 7 g per day.
- **FBC and blood film**
  WCC $\uparrow$ with active inflammation. Acanthocytes are present on the blood film with abetalipoproteinaemia.
- **ESR**
  $\uparrow$ with acute Crohn's disease.
- **LFTs**
  Bilirubin and alkaline phosphatase $\uparrow$ obstructive jaundice. Transaminases $\uparrow$ liver parenchymal disease. Albumin $\downarrow$ malabsorption syndromes.
- **Blood glucose**
  $\uparrow$ with diabetes, a complication of chronic pancreatitis.
- **Serum amylase**
  Usually normal with chronic pancreatitis, but may be elevated if associated with recurrent acute attacks of pancreatitis.
- **Antigliadin, antiendomysial and antireticulin antibodies**
  To detect coeliac disease.
- **AXR**
  Calcification with chronic pancreatitis.
- **Jejunal biopsy**
  Subtotal villous atrophy and crypt hyperplasia with coeliac disease, which are reversible on a gluten-free diet. Dilated lymphatics and PAS-positive macrophages in Whipple's disease. Absent villi with lymphocytic infiltration of the lamina propria and histological evidence of malignancy with intestinal lymphoma.

SPECIFIC INVESTIGATIONS

- **^{14}C-labelled bile acid breath tests**
  Screening test for bacterial overgrowth.

- **Serum gastrin assay**
  Zollinger–Ellison syndrome.
- **Small bowel enema**
  Strictures, skip lesions, fissures and fistulae with Crohn's disease.
- **Colonoscopy**
  Mucosal hyperaemia, friability, ulceration and contact bleeding with Crohn's disease.
- **CT abdomen**
  Abdominal lymphadenopathy with lymphoma.

▶ STRIDOR

Stridor is a high pitched inspiratory sound produced by upper airway obstruction.

CAUSES

Congenital
- Laryngomalacia (congenital flaccid larynx)

Acquired
- Foreign body
- Laryngeal oedema
  - Anaphylaxis
  - Inhalational injury
- Infection
  - Epiglottitis
  - Retropharyngeal abscess
- Iatrogenic
  - Post-tracheostomy stenosis
  - Postintubation stenosis
  - Post-thyroid surgery
- Cricoarytenoid rheumatoid arthritis
- Goitre

Malignancy
- Intraluminal obstruction
  - Larynx
  - Trachea
  - Bronchus
- External compression
  - Malignant nodes
- Bilateral vocal cord palsy
  - Brainstem stroke
  - Thyroid carcinoma
  - Oesophageal carcinoma

HISTORY

Onset
Instantaneous onset of stridor usually implies an inhaled foreign body. This is accompanied by violent bouts of coughing, and a

clear history may be obtained from a witness. Stridor indicates partial obstruction, as complete occlusion of the upper airway is silent. Stridor that develops over a period of a few seconds to minutes may be due to laryngeal oedema from an anaphylactic reaction. This may be accompanied by urticaria and facial oedema. Enquiries should immediately determine known allergens and treatment can be initiated without delay. The most common cause of infantile stridor is laryngomalacia. During inspiration there is extreme infolding of the epiglottis and aryepiglottic folds due to inadequate cartilagenous support. Head flexion aggravates the stridor, whereas patency of the airway is improved by the prone position and head extension. The stridor gradually resolves in most infants within 2–3 months.

Precipitating factors

Iatrogenic causes of stridor may have clear precipitating factors. Tracheal stenosis may complicate a long period of intubation or tracheostomy. Upper airway obstruction occurring immediately after thyroid surgery may be due to laryngeal oedema, haematoma and bilateral recurrent nerve injury. Patients who have been rescued from fires may suffer inhalation injuries due to the high temperature of inhaled gases.

Associated symptoms

Respiratory obstruction may occur with massive enlargement of the tonsils, e.g. in glandular fever, or when complicated by a retropharyngeal abscess. Patients may notice swelling of the neck in the presence of a goitre and may be either euthyroid or complain of symptoms of abnormal thyroid function (page 173). Symptoms of joint pains, stiffness and deformities occur with rheumatoid arthritis. Associated stridor can result from cricoarytenoid involvement. Weight loss can be an accompanying feature of malignancy. Hoarseness of the voice is an early symptom of laryngeal carcinoma; stridor occurs as a late feature. Chronic cough with haemoptysis in a chronic smoker usually heralds the onset of bronchial carcinoma. The location of the carcinoma may alter the quality of the wheeze. Partial intraluminal upper airway obstruction from bronchial carcinoma produces stridor, whereas partial lower airways obstruction produces the inspiratory monophonic wheeze. Rapid progressive painless dysphagia occurs with oesophageal carcinoma.

EXAMINATION

Inspection

With acute partial upper airway obstruction, patients will often appear very distressed. Immediate assessment for generalised urticaria, facial oedema, hypotension and widespread wheezing will allow the diagnosis of anaphylaxis to be made and appropriate treatment initiated. Soot on the face and singed nasal hair from thermal exposure may be present with inhalational injuries. A large goitre will be visible on inspection. Bilateral symmetrical deforming arthropathy involving the small joints of the hands (MCP, PIP) is suggestive of rheumatoid disease. Clubbing may be present in the fingers with bronchial carcinoma.

The cause of stridor may be visible on inspection of the throat. Further information is obtained on inspection using indirect laryngoscopy. With bilateral vocal cord palsy, the cords lie in a cadaveric position. A small glottic aperture is seen and does not widen on attempted inspiration. Supraglottic and glottic carcinomas may be readily visible.

Palpation and auscultation

The presence of cervical lymphadenopathy may be due to infection or carcinoma of the larynx, pharynx, bronchus or oesophagus. A goitre may also be palpable in the neck, skewing the trachea to one side due to compression effects. The chest is examined for monophonic wheezing, collapse of a segment, pleural effusion and rib tenderness, which are the thoracic manifestations of bronchial carcinoma.

GENERAL INVESTIGATIONS

General investigations should be tailored to the clinical findings.
- **FBC**
  WCC ↑ infection.
- **ESR**
  ↑ with infection and malignancy.
- **TFTs**
  ↑, ↓ or normal with goitres.
- **Lateral soft-tissue neck X-ray**
  Radio-opaque foreign bodies.

- **CXR**
  Both frontal and lateral views are required to identify radio-opaque foreign bodies. Bronchial carcinoma may present as a central mass, peripheral mass, collapse of a segment, consolidation of a lobe or as a pleural effusion. Hilar lymphadenopathy may be apparent, causing external compression of trachea or bronchus.

SPECIFIC INVESTIGATIONS

- **Fibreoptic laryngoscopy**
  Visualisation of the vocal cords, tumour masses, tracheal stenosis and allows biopsies to be taken.
- **Upper GI endoscopy**
  To determine the presence of carcinoma, which may be infiltrating both recurrent laryngeal nerves when associated symptoms of dysphagia are present.
- **FNAC of a goitre**
  To determine the underlying aetiology of a goitre.
- **CT neck and thorax**
  Define the extent and assist in staging of laryngeal carcinoma, thyroid carcinoma, oesophageal carcinoma and bronchial carcinoma.

▶ SWEATING ABNORMALITIES

Excessive sweating is often brought to the attention of the physician when it becomes socially unacceptable, the underlying cause ranging from trivial to serious.

CAUSES

Excessive sweating
- Hypoglycaemia

Systemic infections

Malignancy
- Brain tumours
- Hodgkin's lymphoma

Endocrine
- Phaeochromocytoma
- Thyrotoxicosis
- Carcinoid syndrome
- Diabetic autonomic neuropathy
- Menopause

Psychiatric
- Substance dependency/withdrawal
- Anxiety states

Deficient sweating
- Heat stroke
- Hypohidrotic ectodermal dysplasia
- Miliaria
- Sympathetic tract lesions

HISTORY

Apart from heat stroke, the causes of deficient sweating are rare and usually arise from congenital disorders of the sweat glands, such as hypohidrotic ectodermal dysplasia, a condition associated with poor hair and teeth formation. Absent sweating can also be caused by miliaria, which is caused by plugging or rupture of the sweat ducts.

Excessive sweating is commonly encountered as it is a physiological accompaniment to pain, nausea, vomiting (page 452) and shock (page 392). The causes in the absence of these symptoms have been listed above. Excessive sweating may be episodic or constant. Episodic bouts of sweating may be due to hypogylcaemia, phaeochromocytoma, carcinoid syndrome and menopause. Patients with hypogylcaemia often complain of associated tremor, dizziness, anxiety and hunger. Paroxysmal release of catecholamines by phaeochromocytomas may produce attacks of sweating, hypertension, palpitations, headaches and anxiety. It usually comes to medical attention presenting as a result of hypertension. Carcinoid syndrome is produced by a variety of hormones secreted by enterochromaffin tumours, originating from the small bowel in the presence of hepatic metastasis.

Episodic sweating is associated with brick-red flushing, diarrhoea, wheezing and occasionally right-sided heart lesions. Hot flushes and sweating may also be prominent symptoms experienced by women reaching the menopause; the aetiology has often been attributed to alterations in the concentrations of female reproductive hormones.

Patients with night sweats may complain of waking up with their clothes and bed sheets drenched in perspiration. Classically, these features are reported with TB and Hodgkin's disease. The accompanying symptoms of pulmonary TB include weight loss, cough and haemoptysis. With Hodgkin's disease, patients may complain of localised lymphadenopathy, weight loss, pruritus, fever and malaise.

Constant sweating and heat intolerance are features of thyrotoxicosis. This may result from increased metabolic rate and may be accompanied by symptoms of increased appetite with weight loss, emotional lability, diarrhoea and palpitations. Rarely excessive sweating may result from tumours encroaching on the hypothalamus.

Enquiries should be undertaken regarding substance dependency, as withdrawal states can produce severe sweating and hallucinations.

EXAMINATION

A complete examination is required for each system in turn to exclude the possibility of underlying infection. A mental state examination is required if an anxiety disorder is suspected. The following are specific features in the examination that may suggest an underlying cause.

Temperature

The presence of pyrexia (page 368) would suggest infection as the underlying cause for sweating. However, it can also occur with Hodgkin's disease.

Inspection

Wide, staring eyes with lid lag may result from thyrotoxicosis causing sweating; in addition, the presence of exophthalmos or ophthalmoplegia specifically indicates Graves' disease as the underlying cause. Episodic brick-red flushing of the face may be experienced with carcinoid syndrome.

Palpation and auscultation

The thyroid is palpated to exclude enlargement of the gland. Regional lymph nodes are examined for enlargement, which may be due to infection or malignancy. A tachycardia is present with thyrotoxicosis and systemic infection. A rapid pulse may also be palpated during paroxysmal attacks with phaeochromocytoma, and the blood pressure will be markedly elevated. With primary pulmonary TB, pleural effusion or segmental collapse may be the only features found on examination. Detection of a new or changing heart murmur may imply endocarditis. However, either stenosis or regurgitation of the tricuspid or pulmonary valve have been reported with carcinoid syndrome. The presence of splenomegaly on abdominal examination may be due to Hodgkin's disease.

GENERAL INVESTIGATIONS

- **BM stix**
  Rapid assessment of blood sugar and may be confirmed by blood glucose estimation. Glucose may be $\uparrow$ with phaeochromocytoma.
- **FBC and blood film**
  WCC $\uparrow$ infection.
- **ESR**
  $\uparrow$ with infection, malignancy and lymphoma.
- **TSH and free T$_4$**
  TSH $\downarrow$ and T$_4$ $\uparrow$ with thyrotoxicosis.
- **CXR**
  TB, bronchial carcinoid, chest infection.

SPECIFIC INVESTIGATIONS

- **Mantoux test**
  Diluted Mantoux test if no previous BCG immunisation has been performed to screen for TB.
- **Urinary 5HIAA**
  ↑ with carcinoid tumours.
- **Urinary catecholamines and metanephrines**
  ↑ with phaeochromocytoma.
- **Lymph node excision biopsy**
  Reed–Sternberg cells with Hodgkin's disease.
- **MRI head**
  Hypothalamic tumours.

▶ SYNCOPE

Syncope is the transient loss of consciousness due to impaired cerebral blood flow.

CAUSES

Cardiovascular
- Vasovagal syncope
  - Situational syncope
  - Micturition syncope
  - Cough syncope
- Orthostatic hypotension
  - Prolonged bedrest
  - Drug-induced
  - Hypovolaemic
  - Autonomic failure
- Arrhythmia
  - Sick sinus syndrome
  - Stokes–Adams attack
  - Supraventricular tachycardia
  - Ventricular tachycardia
- Myocardial infarction
- Cardiac outflow obstruction
- Carotid sinus syndrome
- Pulmonary embolism

Neurological
- Seizure
- Hysterical syncope

Metabolic
- Hypoxia
- Hypoglycaemia

HISTORY

Vasovagal syncope (the common faint), is the most common cause of syncope. It is associated with peripheral vasodilatation and a vagally-mediated slowing of the heart rate. It may be precipitated by situations such as fear, emotion, prolonged standing or pain. The patient may complain of nausea, weakness and blurred vision, and appear pale with bradycardia on examination. Palpitations (page 347) preceding collapse may suggest an arrhythmia. Situational syncope are faints classified according to the precipitating factors and are often due to an excessive vagal response to the offending stimuli.

Orthostatic hypotension is a drop in blood pressure on standing. This causes a transient decrease in cerebral perfusion and therefore loss of consciousness. Prolonged bedrest can result in the deconditioning of the baroreceptors in the body, resulting in a postural drop of blood pressure. A drug history may exclude offending medication such as antihypertensives and opiates. Hypovolaemia is also a cause of postural hypotension (see shock, page 392); it is associated with a pallor, tachycardia and a low urine output. Disease states such as diabetes mellitus and Guillain–Barré syndrome can result in autonomic failure and inability of the body to maintain an appropriate blood pressure.

Cardiac outflow obstruction, which occurs with aortic stenosis and hypertrophic obstructive cardiomyopathy, will result in syncope on effort as the cardiac output cannot be increased on demand.

In carotid sinus syndrome, the receptors of the carotid sinus are more sensitive than normal, thus minor stimulation, such as turning the head or pressure from a tight collar, may elicit the carotid sinus reflex and precipitate syncope.

Seizures are paroxysmal discharges in the cortex which are sufficient to produce clinically detectable events, e.g. convulsions, loss of consciousness or behavioural symptoms. Although it is not strictly syncope, atonic seizures may present in a similar fashion, with a sudden loss of muscle tone and collapse. Patients may be incontinent during a seizure and drowsy or confused during the postictal phase.

Hysterical syncope tends to be very dramatic with normal examination findings during the attack.

Hypoglycaemia causes faintness and even results in loss of consciousness. It tends to be more common with insulin-treated diabetics but may also occur in normal individuals after an alcohol binge. Symptoms usually occur when the glucose is below 2.5 mmol/l.

EXAMINATION

Appearance

Vasovagal syncope often results in pallor of the complexion and clamminess. Convulsions may occur with seizures.

Blood pressure

Should be taken supine and standing, only then will a postural drop be noted.

Pulse

During the attack of syncope, taking the pulse is a good way to detect an arrhythmia. Bradycardia is the usual finding in vasovagal syncope. Stokes–Adams attacks result from complete heart block causing a transient period of asystole, with full recovery. The sick sinus syndrome is associated with alternating episodes of bradycardia and tachycardia. Shock, supraventricular and ventricular tachycardias may result in very rapid heart rates.

Pressure on the carotid sinus, located at the bifurcation of the carotid arteries, will cause syncope in patients with carotid sinus syndrome.

Auscultation

The soft second heart sound and an ejection systolic murmur radiating to the carotids characterises aortic valvular stenosis. An ejection systolic murmur can also be auscultated in hypertrophic obstructive cardiomyopathy, where the outflow of blood from the left ventricle is obstructed owing to hypertrophy of the cardiac muscle.

GENERAL INVESTIGATIONS

- **BM stix**
  Testing the blood for glucose with BM stix is a simple and very fast way of obtaining a blood glucose level. More accurate readings can be confirmed with a serum sample.
- **FBC**
  Will indicate anaemia when haemorrhage is the underlying cause of hypovolaemia. Septic shock with peripheral vasodilatation may be associated with an elevated white cell count.
- **U&Es and serum glucose**
  Electrolyte abnormalities will predispose to seizures.
- **Blood glucose**
  Hypoglycaemia.
- **ECG**
  When obtained during an attack may reveal an arrhythmia. Pulseless ventricular tachycardia should be treated as ventricular fibrillation and cardiac resuscitation should commence. Q waves and ST elevations may be seen with myocardial infarction.

SPECIFIC INVESTIGATIONS

- **EEG**
  Although epilepsy is essentially a clinical diagnosis, seizures associated with specific electrical changes in the cortex can be used to confirm the diagnosis. A negative EEG does not, however, exclude epilepsy.
- **24-hour ECG**
  Will be able to document any arrhythmia associated with episodes of syncope.
- **Echocardiography**
  Allows assessment of the aortic valve and diagnosis of hypertrophic obstructive cardiomyopathy.
- **V/Q scan**
  Allows diagnosis of the majority of acute pulmonary emboli.
- **Tilt table testing**
  This is usually reserved for patients with recurrent syncope of indeterminate cause. In patients with vasovagal syncope, a 60° tilt will produce hypotension, bradycardia and syncope within 30 minutes.

▶ THROAT CONDITIONS

A sore throat is an extremely common symptom, especially in children and young adults. Prolonged sore throat in an elderly patient is a cause for concern as it may indicate the presence of neoplasia.

CAUSES

Infective
- Tonsillitis
  - Bacterial, e.g. streptococcus, gonococcus
  - Viral, e.g. glandular fever
- Pharyngitis
  - Viral
  - Fungal
- Quinsy

Inflammatory
- Thyroiditis (rare)

Neoplastic
- Carcinoma
  - Tonsil
  - Posterior third of the tongue
  - Larynx
- Lymphoma
- Blood dyscrasias

Neurological
- Glossopharyngeal neuralgia

Referred pain
- Angina
- Oesophageal spasm

Other
- AIDS
- Reflux oesophagitis

HISTORY

Infective
Sore throat, dysphagia, referred pain to ear, headache, malaise. A history of oral sex may suggest oropharyngeal gonorrhoea.

Quinsy is a peritonsillar abscess. There is usually a history of acute tonsillitis but the patient becomes more ill with a high temperature, dysphagia and referred pain to the ear. In glandular fever the patient can present with a severe membranous tonsillitis but usually has malaise and lymphadenopathy elsewhere.

Inflammatory
Subacute thyroiditis presents with a swelling of the thyroid, with neck pain, fever, weakness and malaise. It is a rare condition.

Neoplastic
Carcinoma of a tonsil presents with painful ulceration with induration. There is often referred pain to the ear and the patient may spit blood. Occasionally, the presenting symptom is a lump in the neck representing metastatic cervical lymphadenopathy. Carcinoma of the posterior third of the tongue may present with a feeling of soreness in the throat with difficulty in swallowing. The patient may spit blood and pain may be referred to the ear. Supraglottic carcinoma may present with a feeling of a lump in the throat but there is usually a change in voice and early cervical lymphadenopathy. Lymphoma of the tonsil rarely causes pain, the patient presenting with enlargement of one tonsil. Patients with a blood dyscrasia may present with a sore throat resulting from infection consequent upon neutropenia.

Neurological
Glossopharyngeal neuralgia presents as a sharp stabbing pain at the root of the tongue, radiating into the throat and ear, triggered by swallowing or touching the pharynx.

Referred pain
Angina may cause pain in the throat. It is usually associated with exercise. There may also be pain in the chest, radiating into the jaw and down the left arm. Occasionally, diffuse oesophageal spasm gives rise to chest pain radiating into the throat and jaw.

Other
Sore throat may occur in AIDS. It may be due to a variety of infective organisms, e.g. viral or fungal. Reflux oesophagitis may cause a burning pain in the throat or a sensation of a lump in the throat.

EXAMINATION

Infective

With tonsillitis there is usually pyrexia, foetor and pus exuding from the tonsillar crypts. The pharyngeal mucosa is often inflamed. Cervical lymphadenopathy. Check for lymphadenopathy elsewhere, and splenomegaly, which may be associated with glandular fever. Quinsy is associated with trismus and the tonsil is pushed downwards and medially by the quinsy. The uvula is usually oedematous.

Inflammatory

Thyroiditis presents with a tender, diffuse swelling in the thyroid gland, which moves on swallowing. It is rare.

Neoplastic

Carcinoma of the tonsil presents as a hard, ulcerated swelling on the tonsil. Cervical lymphadenopathy may be present. In carcinoma of the posterior third of the tongue and supraglottic larynx there is usually an indurated ulcer. Laryngoscopy is required as part of the examination. Check for cervical nodes and other sites for metastases, e.g. lung, liver. Lymphoma usually presents as painless enlargement of the tonsil. Blood dyscrasias may present with lymphadenopathy and hepatosplenomegaly. Agranulocytosis results in ulceration and membrane formation on the tonsils and oral mucosa.

Neurological

The diagnosis of glossopharyngeal neuralgia is usually made from the history. Touching the palate may trigger the symptoms.

Referred pain

Angina and oesophageal spasms are usually diagnosed from the history.

Others

Pharyngitis and tonsillitis may occur as part of AIDS, due to either viral or fungal infections. Other signs of AIDS, e.g. malaise, fever, weight loss, chest infections, Kaposi's sarcoma. Diagnosis of reflux oesophagitis is usually made on a history. There is little to find on examination.

GENERAL INVESTIGATIONS

- **FBC, ESR**

  Hb ↓ malignancy. WCC ↑ infection. Blood dyscrasia. Lymphocytosis in glandular fever. ESR ↑ malignancy. Infection. Thyroiditis.

- **Swab**
  Culture and sensitivity – streptococcus and gonococcus.
- **Viral antibodies**
  Glandular fever.
- **ECG**
  Cardiac ischaemia.
- **CXR**
  Metastases.

SPECIFIC INVESTIGATIONS

- **Indirect laryngoscopy**
  Infection. Malignancy.
- **OGD**
  Oesophagitis. Hiatus hernia.
- **HIV testing**
  AIDS.
- **Biopsy**
  Benign versus malignant.
- **CT**
  Tumour. Spread of tumour.

▶ TOE LESIONS

Lesions of the toes are extremely common. They are caused by a variety of conditions ranging from simple ingrowing toenail to severe pain caused by ischaemia. Deformities of the toes are also exceptionally common, particularly in the elderly.

CAUSES

Toenails
- Ingrowing toenail
- Subungual haematoma
- Subungual melanoma
- Subungual exostosis
- Onychogryphosis

Deformities
- Hallux valgus
- Hallux rigidus
- Hammer toe
- Claw toes

Ulcers

Ischaemic
Large vessel disease
- Arteriosclerosis
- Embolism
Small vessel disease
- Diabetes
- Raynaud's
- Buerger's
- Embolism
- Vasculitis, e.g. scleroderma, SLE, rheumatoid

Neuropathic
Peripheral nerve lesions
- Diabetes
- Nerve injuries
- Leprosy
Spinal cord lesions
- Spina bifida
- Spinal injuries
- Syringomyelia

Neoplastic
- Discoloration
- Chilblains
- Ischaemia

HISTORY

Nails

Ingrowing toenail usually presents with pain at the sides of the nail and often with infection and local inflammation. With infection the toe is painful and throbs, especially in bed at night. With subungual haematoma there is a history of injury to the nail. Bleeding occurs beneath the nail, which is extremely painful, and occasionally the patient may faint with the pain. Subungual melanoma presents with pigmentation under the nail. With subungual exostosis there is lifting of the nail with deformity. Onychogryphosis is a 'ram's horn' deformity of the nail. The nail thickens and curves over the end. It is common in the elderly but may occur in young people after injury to the nailbed.

Deformities

A patient with hallux valgus normally presents with a 'bunion'. The first metatarsal deviates medially. It is more common in females. The patient may complain that the great toe overrides the second toe. Unsuitable, tight footwear may be a precipitating cause. Hallux rigidus is osteoarthritis of the first MTP joint. It occurs in young adults. The patient complains of pain on walking, especially when 'pushing off', and stiffness in the joint. Hammer toe usually affects the second toe. There is a fixed flexion deformity of the PIP joint and compensatory hyperextension of adjacent joints. The patient merely complains of a deformed toe, and may also complain of painful callosities that have developed where the deformed toe presses against the footwear. With clawed toes both IP joints are flexed. The tips of the toes may develop painful callosities.

Ulcers

Ulcers are usually ischaemic (painful) or neuropathic (painless). Check for a history of intermittent claudication, smoking, Raynaud's disease, cardiac disease, diabetes. With neuropathic ulcers there may be a history of diabetes, nerve injuries, spinal cord lesions. Ulcers usually occur on the pressure points over the tips of the toes. Neoplastic ulcers on the toes are extremely rare. Melanoma may occur on the toes but is usually subungual.

Discoloration

Painful discoloration, either red or shiny, white, blue or black (gangrene), suggests ischaemia. Chilblains occur in childhood and early adult life, usually in females. They are more likely in those with outdoor occupations. Painful swelling occurs on the toes, which may become itchy. They are often multiple and may develop into shallow ulcers.

EXAMINATION

Nails

With ingrowing toenails there is often a serous discharge or purulent discharge from the nailfold. The toe becomes red and swollen. Granulation tissue may be apparent at the nailfold. Subungual haematoma is usually obvious. Occasionally, however, the patient forgets the injury and presents with a brownish discoloration under the nail and this has to be distinguished from a melanoma. Haematoma is usually reddish–brown with sharp edges, the melanoma being brownish–grey with an indistinct edge. A haematoma grows out with the nail. A melanoma does not. With suspected melanoma, examine the regional lymph nodes and liver for secondaries. Subungal exostosis results in deformity of the nail, which is pushed up and deformed. The swelling between the toe and the end of the nail eventually becomes obvious. Onychogryphosis is obvious with a thick discoloured nail, which curves over at the end (ram's horn deformity).

Deformities

With hallux valgus the first metatarsal bone deviates medially, the great toe laterally. There may be a thickened bursa over the medial aspect of the joint (bunion). The great toe may override the second toe. In hallux rigidus there is a stiff, painful, enlarged, first MTP joint. With hammer toe the second toe is usually affected. There is a fixed flexed deformity of the PIP joint and compensatory hyperextension of the adjacent joint. Check for the presence of corns and callosities. In claw toes both IP joints are flexed (see foot deformities, page 157).

Ulcers

Punched out, painful ulcers over pressure points suggest ischaemic ulcers. Check for discoloration of the toe, capillary return and absence of foot pulses. Neuropathic ulcers are painless; the circulation is usually good, but sensation is absent or blunted locally. Carry out a full neurological examination.

Discoloration

With ischaemic toe it may be shiny red, blue, white or black with gangrene. Examine the pulses. Chilblains are usually reddish–blue, the skin being oedematous, and blistering may occur, which bursts leaving superficial ulcers.

GENERAL INVESTIGATIONS

- **FBC, ESR**
  Hb ↓ anaemia of chronic disease, e.g. rheumatoid arthritis, SLE. WCC ↑ infection, e.g. with diabetes. ESR ↑ vasculitis, e.g. rheumatoid arthritis, SLE.
- **U&Es**
  Chronic renal failure with connective tissues diseases.
- **Blood glucose**
  Ischaemia with small vessel disease in diabetes.
- **X-rays**
  Subungual exostosis. Hallux rigidus.

SPECIFIC INVESTIGATIONS

- **Antibody screen**
  Connective tissue disease.
- **Doppler studies**
  Ischaemia.
- **Arteriography**
  Arterial disease.
- **MRI**
  Spinal cord lesions with neuropathy.
- **Nerve conduction studies**
  Peripheral neuropathy.
- **Excision biopsy**
  Malignant lesions, e.g. subungual melanoma.

▶ TONGUE DISORDERS

Tongue disorders are extremely common, ranging from minor furring of the tongue to extensive infection and malignancy. Tongue disorders are often a manifestation of systemic disease.

CAUSES

Furring
- Gastrointestinal disease
- Dehydration
- Mouth breathers
- Smokers
- Antibiotics

Colour change
- White patches, e.g. leukoplakia, thrush
- Pallor (anaemia)
- Blue (central cyanosis)
- Red
  - Pernicious anaemia
  - Vitamin B deficiency
- Pigmented
  - Addison's disease

Swelling (macroglossia)
- Cretinism
- Myxoedema
- Down's syndrome
- Acromegaly
- Trauma, e.g. hot liquids, corrosive substances
- Allergy

Chronic superficial glossitis
- Syphilis
- Smoking
- Spices
- Spirits
- Sepsis
- Sharp teeth

Ulceration
- Aphthous ulcer
- Dental trauma

- Chancre
- Gumma
- Carcinoma

Wasting
- Hypoglossal nerve palsy

HISTORY

Furring
A history of gastrointestinal disease, dehydration, mouth breathing, smoking or antibiotics.

Colour change
White patches on the tongue are suggestive of leukoplakia or candidiasis, the latter being associated with antibiotic therapy, chemotherapy or immunosuppression. Hairy leukoplakia is associated with Epstein–Barr virus and is found almost exclusively in patients with HIV. A pale tongue may indicate anaemia, a blue tongue central cyanosis. The patient may present with a red, painful tongue which may occur in pernicious anaemia or other forms of vitamin B deficiency. Pigmentation may be a sign of Addison's disease.

Swelling
The patient may present with a swollen tongue, which may or may not be painful. Difficulty in articulation or swallowing may be apparent. Cretinism will be obvious (extremely rare nowadays), as will Down's syndrome. A swollen tongue may be a presentation of myxoedema. Other symptoms of myxoedema may be present, e.g. slowness, weight gain, dry skin, hoarse voice, constipation, lethargy, dislike of cold weather. Acromegaly may be obvious, the patient having noticed an increase in shoe size, change in voice and jaw changes. Infection (see below) may present with swelling, as may allergies or trauma, especially burns with hot fluids or caustic substances. Infection will result in a painful tongue, the classical predispositions to chronic superficial glossitis being the six Ss: syphilis, smoking, spices, spirits, sepsis, sharp teeth.

Chronic superficial glossitis
There is a sequence of chronic inflammatory, degenerative and hypertrophic changes in the tongue which terminate in the development of a carcinoma. There may be a history of the six Ss – syphillis, smoking, sharp tooth, spirits, spices and sepsis. The

patient is usually over the age of 50 and presents with a tongue that has become shiny or white, or has developed a lump on the tongue. There is usually no pain and no interference with eating.

Ulceration

Ulceration is common. Aphthous ulcers are painful and are often associated with chronic debilitating disease. Dental trauma from a sharp tooth or ill-fitting dentures may cause ulcers. Chancre and gumma associated with syphilis are rare. Carcinoma has a peak incidence at 60–70 years and presents with a painless ulcer on the tongue, often at the margins on the dorsal surface. Carcinoma of the posterior third of the tongue may present with referred pain to the ear, the pain being referred from the lingual branch of the trigeminal nerve, which supplies the tongue, to the ear via the auriculotemporal nerve.

Wasting

Wasting of the tongue is caused by paralysis of the hypoglossal nerve. Check for a history of recent trauma or surgery to the neck, which may have damaged the hypoglossal nerve. Atrophy of the tongue occurs on the same side as the lesion.

EXAMINATION

Furring

Examination will reveal uniformed furring of the tongue. Note its colour. Look for signs of gastrointestinal disease.

Colour change

This will usually be obvious. White patches on the tongue may be due to leukoplakia. The white plaques may fissure with time. This is a premalignant condition. Other white patches may be due to candidal infection (thrush). Unlike leukoplakia, these white plaques may be rubbed off, revealing ulcerated buccal mucosa underneath. Colour changes may be uniform (pallor and cyanosis) or patchy (the pigmentation of Addison's disease). In pernicious anaemia the tongue is red, bald and painful.

Swelling

The tongue is large and tends to protrude in Down's syndrome. Other signs of Down's syndrome will be apparent, e.g. epicanthic folds, mental retardation. Look for signs of cretinism, e.g. stunted growth, relatively large head, thick eyelids, thick broad nose, thick lips, widely spaced eyes. With myxoedema there will be dry skin, dry hair, goitre, slow relaxing reflexes, congestive cardiac failure and non-pitting oedema. With acromegaly there will be large feet, prognathism, thick spade-like hands, deep voice and possibly cardiac failure. In generalised infections the tongue will be red and swollen. Allergies may present with a swollen tongue, lips, larynx, bronchospasm and rash. There will usually be a history of exposure to an allergen. The ingestion of corrosive or hot fluids will result not only in inflammation to the tongue but also to the rest of the mouth and the pharynx.

Chronic superficial glossitis

Examination reveals a thin, grey transparent film on the tongue in the early stages. Leukoplakia occurs next and eventually overt carcinoma develops.

Ulceration

Aphthous ulcers start as tender vesicular lesions with a hyperaemic base, which ulcerate leaving a small, white, circular, deep, painful ulcer. Dental trauma will usually result in ulcers at the lateral margins of the tongue adjacent to a sharp tooth. Chancres and gummas are rare, as is tuberculous ulcer of the tongue. A carcinomatous ulcer usually occurs on the upper surface of the tongue, usually at the lateral margins. It feels hard, has an everted edge and is friable and bleeds. Local lymph nodes may be palpable, either due to secondary infection or metastases.

Wasting

Ask the patient to protrude the tongue. Wasting will be noted on the affected side and the tongue deviates to the side of the lesion. Check for scars on the neck to suggest hypoglossal nerve damage.

GENERAL INVESTIGATIONS

- **FBC, ESR**
  Hb ↓ anaemia (microcytic, macrocytic). WCC ↑ infection. ESR ↑ infection, malignancy.
- **Serum vitamin B$_{12}$**
  Reduced in pernicious anaemia.
- **TFTs**
  T$_4$ ↓, TSH ↑ in myxoedema.
- **Swab**
  Culture and sensitivity. Infection. Vincent's angina. Syphilis. Bacterial, viral and fungal infections.

SPECIFIC INVESTIGATIONS

- **VDRL**
  Syphilis.
- **HIV test**
  Hairy leukoplakia
- **CT**
  Pituitary tumour in acromegaly.
- **Oral glucose tolerance test with growth hormone measurement**
  Acromegaly.
- **ACTH stimulation tests**
  Addison's disease.
  Biopsy
  Carcinoma.

TREMOR

A tremor is a rhythmic oscillation of a body part and usually refers to the movements around the small joints of the hands.

CAUSES

Resting tremor
- Parkinson's disease

Action tremor
- Idiopathic
- Benign essential tremor
- Physiological
- Anxiety
- Exercise
- Pathological
- Thyrotoxicosis
- Drugs
  - Beta agonists
  - Caffeine
  - Alcohol
  - Lithium
  - Phenytoin
  - Cyclosporin

Intention tremor
- Cerebellar disease

HISTORY

Tremor is divided into three groups: (1) resting tremor; (2) an action tremor, which is evident when the hand is held in a sustained position or against gravity; and (3) an intention tremor, which is present during movement. Physiological causes of tremor usually have clear precipitating factors, such as anger and exercise.

An action tremor that resolves when the limb is fully supported against gravity is characteristic of benign essential tremor; in addition it may also be relieved by alcohol and is attenuated during movement. Up to a third of patients with benign essential tremor have a family history. In addition to tremor, patients with thyrotoxicosis may also complain of heat intolerance, palpitations, increased appetite with weight loss, anxiety and diarrhoea.

A detailed drug history will easily allow you to identify any drug that may potentially cause tremor. Enquiries should also include the amount of coffee and alcohol intake.

Associated symptoms of slowness, difficulty initiating and stopping walking, muscle rigidity and muscle fatigue (especially with writing) may be present with Parkinson's disease. With cerebellar disease, difficulties may be experienced with balance and coordination.

EXAMINATION

Tremor

Observe the patient at rest: the presence of a pill-rolling tremor is suggestive of Parkinson's disease. In addition, there may be expressionless facies, titubation and drooling of saliva. Thyrotoxic patients will be thin with wide, staring eyes, lid lag, a goitre and exophthalmos with Graves' disease.

The arms are then held outstretched; all other causes of tremor will now be visible. Fine tremors can be accentuated by placing a piece of paper on the outstretched hands. The arm should be fully supported and this will cause resolution of benign essential tremor.

An intention tremor is demonstrated by the finger–nose test; a tremor is markedly increased when the finger approaches the target. In addition, there may also be past-pointing where the finger overshoots the target.

General

Following this evaluation, further examination may be required to determine the underlying cause. The gait is assessed (page 169) and differences between the parkinsonian and ataxic gait of cerebellar disease will be obvious. Further features of cerebellar dysfunction are scanning speech, dysdiadochokinesia, nystagmus and pendular reflexes. When thyrotoxicosis is suspected, the thyroid gland is palpated, ocular movements assessed and the thyroid gland auscultated for a bruit associated with Graves' disease.

GENERAL INVESTIGATIONS

- **TSH and free T$_4$**
  $\uparrow$ TSH and $\downarrow$ T$_4$ with thyrotoxicosis.

SPECIFIC INVESTIGATIONS

- **CT head**

  For the evaluation of patients with impaired coordination
  suggestive of cerebellar disease.

▶ URETHRAL DISCHARGE

Any inflammatory condition within the urethra may cause a discharge. It is important to diagnose venereal conditions so that appropriate treatment is given, not only to the patient but also to sexual contacts.

CAUSES

- Gonorrhoea
- Non-gonococcal urethritis
- Other bacterial
  - Coliforms
  - *Haemophilus ducreyi* (chancroid)
  - TB
  - Syphilis (chancre)
- Reiter's disease
- Prostatitis
- Traumatic
  - Instrumental
  - Accidental
  - Foreign body
- Chemical
- Neoplastic

HISTORY

General

For any sexually transmitted disease check for a history of sexual contact, time of last sexual intercourse, contraceptive methods, number and duration of relationships, sexual practices and unusual sexual practices.

Gonorrhoea

The patient will complain of a thickish, purulent urethral discharge and dysuria. Prostatitis and epididymitis may occur, the patient complaining of deep perineal pain or scrotal swelling.

Non-gonococcal urethritis

The patient complains of urethral discharge, which may be thinner than with gonorrhoea. The presentation may be less acute than with gonorrhoea.

Other bacterial

Urethritis may occur with urinary tract infections. Infection with *Haemophilus ducreyi* causes chancroid or soft sore. It is a tropical infection causing painful genital ulcers and swelling of the inguinal glands. The soft sores may affect the terminal urethra, resulting in dysuria and a profuse, thin, watery discharge. TB of the urethra is very rare. It is usually secondary to TB elsewhere in the genitourinary tract. A syphilitic chancre is now rare but presents as a painful swelling involving the terminal urethra.

Reiter's disease

The patient is usually a young male with recent non-specific urethritis, or it may follow an attack of dysentery. Apart from a urethral discharge, there may be a history of conjunctivitis and joint pains.

Prostatitis

Urethral discharge is rare with acute prostatitis. With chronic prostatitis there may be a clear white urethral discharge. The patient may also complain of suprapubic pain, low back pain, perineal discomfort and pain referred to the testicles.

Trauma

Urethral instrumentation or prolonged catheterisation may cause urethritis. There will be a clear history of this. Foreign bodies may be introduced by the patient. The variety of these defies description! Other foreign bodies include stones passing from the bladder or fragments of urethral catheters. The patient may be too embarrassed to confess that he has introduced a foreign body into the urethra.

Chemical

Chemical urethritis is more common in females. There may be a history of change of soap or bath oils.

Neoplastic

Urethral carcinoma is rare. The patient will complain of dysuria and bloodstained urethral discharge.

EXAMINATION

Gonorrhoea

Often a bead of pus may be seen at the external urethral meatus. It is appropriate to check for evidence of proctitis or anal discharge (homosexuals). There may be evidence of prostatitis, there being a tender, boggy prostate on digital rectal examination. Palpation of the scrotum may reveal epididymitis.

Non-gonococcal urethritis

Pus may again be seen at the external urethral meatus. Check for prostatitis and epididymitis.

Other bacterial

Other forms of urethritis may show a discharge at the external urethral meatus. With chancroid there may be sores on the genitals with sores around the meatus. Check for inguinal lymphadenopathy. Urethral TB is very rare. Check for evidence of TB elsewhere, e.g. lungs, kidneys, epididymis. With a syphilitic chancre the meatus is oedematous and swollen. There may be inguinal lymphadenopathy.

Reiter's disease

Examine for conjunctivitis and arthritis. There may be coexistent plantar fasciitis and Achilles tendonitis. Examine for abscesses on the soles of the feet and palms of the hands (keratoderma blenorrhagica).

Prostatitis

There may be a tender, occasionally boggy prostate on digital rectal examination.

Traumatic

Feel along the course of the urethra for tenderness or palpable stone or foreign body.

Neoplastic

A hard lump may be felt along the course of the urethra. Pressure on it may cause a bloodstained urethral discharge.

GENERAL INVESTIGATIONS

- **FBC, ESR**
  WCC ↑ in infection, e.g. gonorrhoea. ESR ↑ inflammation, e.g. syphilis.
- **Swab**
  Microscopy and culture and sensitivity of urethral discharge. This may grow gonococcus, *Chlamydia trachomatis*, *Trichomonas* sp., *Ureaplasma urealyticum*. Secondary infection, e.g. with candida or coliforms, may occur. *Haemophilus ducreyi* may be grown in chancroid. Dark-ground microscopy may reveal treponemes in syphilis.

SPECIFIC INVESTIGATIONS

- **EMSU**
  TB.
- **Prostatic massage**
  C&S of discharge in chronic prostatitis.
- **VDRL**
  Syphilitic chancre.
- **Cystourethroscopy**
  Foreign body. Urethral carcinoma.

► URINARY INCONTINENCE

Urinary incontinence is the involuntary loss of urine from the
bladder. Loss of urine occurs at times and places which
are inconvenient, inappropriate and socially embarrassing.
Stress incontinence is loss of urine during coughing or straining.
Urge incontinence is the inability to maintain urinary continence in
the presence of frequent and persistent urges to void. Overflow
incontinence occurs when the detrusor muscle becomes flaccid and
often insensitive to stretch and the bladder distends. Weakness of
the sphincter mechanism eventually leads to overflow, when urine
leaks out through the urethra.

CAUSES

Stress incontinence

Pelvic floor injury
- Childbirth
- Prostatectomy

Urge incontinence

Detrusor instability
- Prostatectomy
- Cystitis
- Postradiotherapy
- Tuberculo-cystitis
- Interstitial nephritis
- Stones
- Tumour

Overflow incontinence

Lower motor neurone lesions
- Sacral centre injury
- Cauda equina injury
- Sacral nerve damage, e.g. pelvic surgery
- Diabetes

Chronic outflow obstruction
- Prostatic enlargement

Neurological

Upper motor neurone lesion
- Spinal cord injury above sacral centre
- Disc lesions
- Spinal tumours
- Head injury
- Cerebrovascular accident
- Multiple sclerosis
- Syringomyelia

Anatomical
- Ectopia vesicae
- Ectopic ureter
- Vesicovaginal fistula

Other
- Nocturnal enuresis

HISTORY

Stress incontinence
History of multiple childbirth. Difficult delivery. Recent prostatectomy. History of loss of urine during coughing and straining.

Urge incontinence
The patient is unable to maintain urinary continence in the presence of frequent and persistent urges to void. Recent prostatectomy. Recurrent attacks of cystitis with dysuria and frequency. Past history of pelvic radiotherapy. History of TB. History of ureteric colic. Persistent suprapubic discomfort and haematuria associated with stone. Haematuria associated with tumour.

Overflow incontinence
History of spinal injury involving lumbar vertebra (sacral centre, cauda equina). History of pelvic surgery, e.g. abdominoperineal resection of rectum with damage to pelvic nerves. History of diabetes. History of prostatism with chronic retention with overflow. The patient may still be able to void reasonably normally but feels the bladder is not emptying and leakage continues.

Neurological
With upper motor neurone lesions there may be a history of spinal trauma affecting the cord above the sacral centre. History of head injury, CVA, multiple sclerosis or syringomyelia.

Anatomical

Ectopia vesicae will be obvious at birth with an abdominal wall defect and the ureter opening into exposed bladder mucosa on the lower abdominal wall. Duplex ureter may be associated with an ectopic opening of the ureter into the vagina. Vesicovaginal fistula may follow pelvic surgery or pelvic radiotherapy. It may occasionally be the presenting symptom of pelvic malignancy. Rarely ureterovaginal fistula may occur from an erosion of a ureteric calculus into a vaginal fornix. With duplex ureter, vesicovaginal fistula or ureterovaginal fistula, urine dribbles from the vagina continuously.

Other

Nocturnal enuresis occurs in up to 5% of 10-year-old children. Bed-wetting after puberty usually indicates the presence of an unstable bladder or other pathology.

EXAMINATION

Stress incontinence

Observe leakage when patient coughs. A cystocele or complete prolapse may be seen.

Urge incontinence

There may be little to find on examination.

Overflow incontinence

There may be a palpable bladder. Carry out a full neurological examination. Digital rectal examination may reveal prostatic hypertrophy.

Neurological

Reflex emptying of the bladder occurs. Carry out a full neurological examination.

Anatomical

Ectopia vesicae – ureters opening into bladder mucosa on abdominal wall. With vesicovaginal fistula, examination with a vaginal speculum may indicate the site of the fistula.

GENERAL INVESTIGATIONS

- **FBC**
  WCC $\uparrow$ in infection.
- **MSU**
  C&S for infection.
- **IVU**
  Assess upper tracts, obstruction, bladder lesions, fistula.

SPECIFIC INVESTIGATIONS

- **Cystoscopy**
  Bladder stone. Neoplasia.
- **Cystography**
  Vesicovaginal fistula.
- **Urodynamics**
  Uroflowmetry – measures flow rate. Cystometry – detrusor contractions. Videocystometry – leakage of urine on straining in stress incontinence – urethral pressure profiles – sphincter function and outlet obstruction.
- **CT**
  Cord lesion. Spinal tumour.
- **MRI**
  Cord lesion. Disc lesion. Spinal tumour. Syringomyelia.

▶ URINARY RETENTION

Retention of urine may be acute, chronic or acute-on-chronic. Patients with acute retention present as surgical emergencies. Acute retention is the sudden inability to pass urine, with the presence of painful bladder. Chronic retention is the presence of an enlarged, painless bladder with or without difficulty in micturition.

CAUSES

Local

Urethral lumen or bladder neck
- Urethral valves
- Tumours
- Stones
- Blood clot
- Meatal ulcer

Urethral or bladder wall
- Urethral trauma
- Urethral stricture
- Urethral tumour

Outside the wall
- Prostatic enlargement
- Faecal impaction
- Pregnant uterus
- Pelvic tumour

General

Postoperative

Neurogenic
- Spinal cord injuries
- Spinal cord disease
  - Tabes dorsalis
  - Spinal tumour
  - Multiple sclerosis
  - Diabetic autonomic neuropathy

Drugs
- Anticholinergic drugs
- Antidepressants
- Alcohol

HISTORY

Local

Check for a history of problems with micturition, e.g. difficulty in starting, poor stream, nocturia, frequency, dysuria. Is there any history of urinary tract infection, urethritis, ureteric colic (to suggest a stone which may have passed into the bladder and then impacted into the bladder neck or urethra) or haematuria? Is there a past history of prolonged catheterisation to suggest a urethral stricture? A history of trauma will be apparent. Has the patient fallen astride an object? Has trauma caused a pelvic fracture? Is the patient constipated, to suggest faecal impaction? A pregnant uterus will be obvious.

General

Postoperative acute retention is common, especially in elderly males. This may be due to anxiety, embarrassment, supine posture, pain, drugs, fluid overload or previous unrecognised prostatism with minimal symptoms. After urological procedures it may be due to blood clot in the bladder. Check for a history of neurological disease. Has the patient suffered spinal cord injury? Check the drug history.

EXAMINATION

Local

The patient may have a tender, palpable, painful bladder with sudden onset of retention. In acute retention the bladder rarely extends far above the pubic symphysis. In chronic retention the distended bladder is often painless and more markedly distended than in acute retention, often reaching to the umbilicus. With chronic retention there may be overflow incontinence. Feel along the course of the urethra for stone or stricture. Perform a digital rectal examination to check for prostatic hypertrophy or pelvic tumour. Following pelvic trauma with urethral injury there will be a high 'floating' prostate on rectal examination. Check the urethral meatus for ulcer or stone. Examine the patient for signs of uraemia, which may be present with chronic retention.

General

Postoperative retention will be obvious. Occasionally it is difficult to palpate the bladder because of pain and guarding related to a surgical incision. Neurological causes of acute retention or those

related to spinal trauma are often obvious. Carry out a full
neurological examination.

GENERAL INVESTIGATIONS

- **FBC, ESR**
  Hb ↓ in chronic renal failure, tumours, haematuria. WCC ↑
  infection. ESR ↑ malignancy and infection.
- **MSU**
  Microscopy. C&S for UTI. Cytology to confirm malignancy.
- **U&Es**
  Renal failure. Obstructive uropathy.
- **CXR**
  Pulmonary oedema (chronic renal failure). Possible tumour
  metastases.
- **US**
  Bladder size confirms diagnosis. Dilated upper urinary tract due
  to back pressure. Pregnant uterus.

SPECIFIC INVESTIGATIONS

- **Urethrography**
  Urethral valves. Stricture. Urethral trauma.
- **PSA**
  Carcinoma of the prostate.
- **Cystoscopy**
  Stone, tumour, stricture.
- **Urodynamics**
  Identification and assessment of neurological or bladder neck
  problems.

VISUAL PROBLEMS

Sight is a very important sense, and patients who present with a visual problem are often very distressed. Below is a list of common conditions that may give rise to visual problems, grouped according to symptoms.

CAUSES

Visual disturbances (flashing lights or floaters)
- Migraine
- Retinal detachment
- Vitreous haemorrhage
- Vitreous detachment

Blurring of vision
- Refractive errors
- Head injuries
- Blunt trauma to the eye
- Acute angle-closure glaucoma

Loss of vision

Partial loss
- Homonymous hemianopia – stroke, tumour
- Bitemporal hemianopia – pituitary tumour
- Horizontal field loss – retinal vascular occlusion
- Peripheral field loss – glaucoma, papilloedema
- Central field loss – macular degeneration

Total loss
Acute
- Amaurosis fugax
- Temporal arteritis
- Optic neuritis
- Central retinal vein occlusion
- Central retinal artery occlusion
- Papilloedema
  - Raised intracranial pressure
  - Malignant hypertension

Gradual
- Cataract
- Glaucoma
- Diabetic retinopathy
- Age-related macular degeneration

HISTORY

First establish if visual loss is monocular or binocular. Ocular or optic nerve pathology generally causes monocular visual loss, whereas lesions at the optic chiasma or more posteriorly cause binocular loss that will respect the vertical meridian. Loss of central vision may be due to macular or optic nerve pathology. Retinal lesions cause a 'positive' scotoma (the patient is aware that the part of the field is obstructed), whereas damage posterior to the retina cause a 'negative' scotoma (the patient does not see that a segment of the visual field is missing).

Visual disturbances

Bilateral flashing lights and zigzag lines are often reported by patients suffering with attacks of migraine. This is accompanied by throbbing headache, nausea, vomiting and photophobia. Posterior vitreous detachment, vitreous haemorrhage and retinal detachment are all associated with floaters and flashing lights. Visual acuity and visual fields are normal at first but may be impaired with a large vitreous haemorrhage or advanced retinal detachment.

Blurring of vision

Errors of refraction (long- or short-sighted) are the most common cause of blurring of vision. This is a common problem and is usually corrected with glasses by optometrists. Head and eye injuries may also give rise to transient blurring of the vision. With acute angle-closure glaucoma, corneal oedema will give rise to the appearances of haloes around lights and is associated with a red and painful eye.

Loss of vision

Visual loss may be partial or total. The description of the area of partial visual field loss is very informative. Complaints of vertical visual field losses are due to lesions posterior to the optic chiasma and most commonly caused by strokes, although similar effects can be produced by space-occupying lesions such as cerebral tumours. Horizontal visual field losses imply that the cause lies within the retina and is usually due to retinal vascular occlusions. Patients with glaucoma may complain of tunnel vision, and patients with macular degeneration may experience sudden central visual field loss.

Sudden total visual loss is usually due to a vascular aetiology. Amaurosis fugax is sudden transient monocular blindness due to artheroembolism of the ophthalmic artery. Patients classically complain of a 'curtain descending across the field of vision'. With giant cell arteritis affecting the ophthalmic artery, sudden onset of blindness can occur in conjunction with the symptoms of temporal headache and jaw claudication. It is often associated with polymyalgia rheumatica. Papilloedema may cause transient visual loss, lasting seconds, related to posture.

Monocular blindness due to optic neuritis may occur with multiple sclerosis; it is often associated with retro-orbital pain that worsens with eye movements and starts with a progressive dimming of vision over a few days.

Diabetic retinopathy is the most common cause of blindness in western society. In addition, diabetics are also more prone to develop cataracts and glaucoma. In the elderly, gradual onset of visual loss may be due to cataracts, glaucoma or age-related macular degeneration. Due to the gradual onset of symptoms, these groups of patients may present very late. A cataract may be visible on examination of the eye.

EXAMINATION

Visual acuity unaided and corrected with a pinhole should be assessed with a Snellen chart. If visualisation of the largest letter is not possible then assess vision by counting fingers. Further tests to use are those of movement and, finally, the ability to discriminate between light and dark. With refractive errors, vision can be corrected by viewing the Snellen chart through a pinhole. Visual fields are examined by confrontational testing, and the extent of visual field loss can be assessed approximately.

Pupillary response to light (direct and consensual) allows the assessment of the visual pathway. Direct light reflex may be lost in lesions involving the unilateral optic nerve and with central retinal artery occlusion.

Colour vision will be reduced disproportionately compared to visual acuity in optic nerve diseases. This may be assessed with the use of Ishihara plates.

Fundoscopy

A wealth of information is obtained on fundoscopy. The red reflex is lost with cataracts. Examination of the retina may reveal background retinopathy with diabetes, consisting of dot and blot haemorrhages with cotton-wool spots. With hypertensive retinopathy, silver wiring, arteriovenous nipping, retinal haemorrhages and eventually papilloedema may be appreciated. Growth of new vessels on the retina indicates proliferative retinopathy. An infarcted retina appears oedematous and pale; the macula appears prominent and red (cherry-red spot). Detached retinal folds may be seen, and clots of blood are visible with vitreous haemorrhage. The margins of the optic disc becomes blurred with papilloedema and optic neuritis but later may appear pale. A cupped optic disc appearance occurs with chronic glaucoma.

Upon completion of the examination of the eye, a neurological examination should be performed, followed by a cardiovascular examination to exclude sources of emboli. The rhythm of the pulse is assessed for atrial fibrillation and the heart and carotids are auscultated for murmurs. The blood pressure is measured to exclude hypertension.

GENERAL INVESTIGATIONS

- **ESR**
  Giant cell arteritis.
- **Blood glucose**
  Glucose ↑ diabetes.
- **Intraocular pressure measurements**
  ↑ with glaucoma.
- **Perimetery**
  Formal charting of visual fields. Arcuate scotomas are found with glaucoma. Central scotomas may be seen with optic neuritis. Bitemporal hemianopias/homonymous hemianopias and quadrantanopias in neurological pathology.

SPECIFIC INVESTIGATIONS

- **CT/MRI head**
  Tumours, stroke, multiple sclerosis.
- **Carotid Dopplers**
  Atherosclerotic plaques with amaurosis fugax.
- **Temporal artery biopsy**
  Temporal arteritis.
- **US**
  To assess retina if no visualisation of fundus behind cataract or vitreous haemorrhage.

VOICE DISORDERS

Voice disorders can be caused by a number of conditions. The changes in the quality of the voice ranges from mild hoarseness to aphonia. It is extremely important to exclude laryngeal carcinoma, which is easily treated in the early stages but has a poor prognosis once metastatic spread has occurred.

CAUSES

Infective
- Laryngitis

Traumatic
- Blunt trauma
- Excessive vocal use

Neoplastic
- Laryngeal papilloma
- Laryngeal carcinoma

Recurrent laryngeal nerve palsy
- Goitre
- Oesophageal carcinoma
- Bronchial carcinoma
- Thoracic aortic aneurysm
- Postoperative – thoracic, parathyroid and thyroid surgery

Psychogenic
- Myasthenia gravis

HISTORY

Onset
The temporal profile of deterioration in quality of the voice is useful in discriminating between the causes. Infection and excessive vocal use may result in transient deterioration. Progressive deterioration may be due to tumours, and sustained hoarseness due to recurrent laryngeal nerve palsy.

Precipitating factors
Viral infections usually precede and cause acute laryngitis. It is most commonly due to the influenza virus. Smoking and vocal cord trauma from excessive use by singers, or simply excessive

shouting, are often enough to precipitate hoarseness. A history of blunt trauma to the larynx may be evident and hoarseness from resulting laryngeal fractures may be the first indication of a precarious airway.

Past medical history

Recurrent laryngeal nerve palsy associated with a goitre is usually due to thyroid malignancy. Tumour infiltration of the recurrent nerve may also result from malignancy occurring in oesophagus and lung. Hoarseness of the voice may be the first complaint of patients with a thoracic aneurysm. Previous thyroid or thoracic surgery may have resulted in vagus or recurrent laryngeal nerve injuries.

Associated symptoms

Sore throat from pharyngitis may accompany acute laryngitis. Pain referred to the ear or dysphagia can be late presenting features of laryngeal carcinomas. Rapidly progressive dysphagia is also a symptom of oesophageal carcinoma. Nasal voice may be accompanied by ptosis, diplopia and muscle fatigue with myasthenia gravis. Bizarre associated symptoms with impaired voice intensity but normal coughing ability should lead to the consideration of a functional cause; however, this should be a diagnosis of exclusion.

EXAMINATION

Indirect laryngoscopy is performed with a mirror and headlamp. If unsuccessful, the larynx can easily be examined with a flexible fibreoptic laryngoscope under local anaesthetic. A dry erythematous larynx is seen with acute laryngitis. Vocal cord papillomas and supraglottic carcinomas may be readily visible. Recurrent laryngeal nerve injury will result in paralysis of the unilateral vocal cord. Upon observing this, a detailed examination is undertaken to determine the underlying cause. The neck should be examined for the presence of a goitre. Palpable supraclavicular lymphadenopathy may arise from oesophageal carcinoma.
The chest is carefully examined for signs of collapse and effusion, which may be secondary to bronchial carcinoma.

GENERAL INVESTIGATIONS

- **FBC**
  ↑ White count with laryngitis.
- **ESR**
  ↑ with laryngitis, carcinoma.
- **CXR**
  Bronchial carcinoma, widened mediastinum with thoracic aneurysm.

SPECIFIC INVESTIGATIONS

- **Tensilon test**
  Myasthenia gravis.
- **Endoscopy**
  Oesophageal carcinoma.
- **CT neck**
  Diagnosis and staging for laryngeal and thyroid carcinoma.
- **CT thorax**
  Lung tumours, thoracic aneurysms.
- **Arch aortography**
  Thoracic aneurysm.
- **FNAC**
  Thyroid carcinoma.

▶ VOMITING

Vomiting is the forceful ejection of gastric contents through the mouth. It occurs when the vomiting centre in the medulla oblongata is stimulated. This may be due to direct stimulation of the vomiting centre (central vomiting) or via afferent fibres (reflex vomiting).

CAUSES

Central vomiting

- Drugs, e.g. narcotic analgesics, chemotherapeutic agents
- Acute infections, especially in children
- Endocrine/metabolic
  - Pregnancy
  - Uraemia
  - Hypercalcaemia
  - Diabetic ketoacidosis
  - Addison's disease

Reflex vomiting

Gastrointestinal disease
Inflammation
- Appendicitis
- Cholecystitis
- Pancreatitis
- Peptic ulceration
- Peritonitis
- Biliary colic

Obstruction
- Pyloric stenosis
- Small bowel obstruction
- Large bowel obstruction

Gastrointestinal irritants
- Bacteria, e.g. *Campylobacter* spp, *Salmonella* spp
- Drugs, e.g. aspirin, NSAIDs, alcohol, iron, antibiotics
- Poisons, e.g. arsenic
- Emetics, e.g. sodium chloride, ipecacuanha

CNS causes
- Raised intracranial pressure
- Labyrinthine disorders

- Ménière's disease
- Head injury
- Migraine
- Motion sickness

Psychogenic
- Psychiatric disorders, e.g. hysterical, bulimia, anorexia nervosa
- Offensive sights and smells

Others
- Myocardial infarction
- Severe pain, e.g. testicular torsion, fractures
- Irradiation
- Widespread malignant disease
- Severe coughing, e.g. chronic bronchitis

HISTORY

General

Nature of the vomiting
Bright-red blood, e.g. bleeding peptic ulcer. Altered blood (coffee grounds). Bile (high small bowel obstruction), faeculent (low small bowel obstruction). Recently eaten food. Food several days old (pyloric stenosis), projectile vomiting (infantile pyloric stenosis).

Time of vomit
Soon after meal (gastric ulcer, gastric carcinoma). Early morning (pregnancy). Chronic chest infection (after bout of coughing).

Relief of pain by vomiting
Peptic ulcer disease.

Central vomiting
Take a careful drug history. It will be obvious if the patient is having chemotherapy. Acute infections in children will usually be obvious. Check for pregnancy. Endocrine and metabolic disorders will largely be determined by the result of blood tests.

Reflex vomiting

Gastrointestinal
There will usually be a clear history of a gastrointestinal problem, e.g. localised tenderness of peritonitis or colicky abdominal pain associated with obstruction. Take a careful drug history for irritant drugs, e.g. aspirin. Check for abuse of emetics, e.g. bulimia.

CNS

With raised intracranial pressure there will usually be headache, drowsiness, fits in addition to vomiting. With labyrinthitis there will be nausea, vomiting, vertigo and invariably a hearing defect. Ménière's disease presents with vertigo, tinnitus and deafness. The tinnitus is usually constant but more severe before an attack. Tinnitus may precede other symptoms by many months. Attacks of Ménière's disease may last from minutes to hours. Migraine will present with a visual aura with unilateral throbbing headaches and sometimes photophobia. With motion sickness the history is usually obvious.

Psychogenic

Bulimia is eating followed by self-induced vomiting. Vomiting may also occur in anorexia nervosa but failure to eat is usually the prominent feature. Hysteria may be responsible for vomiting. Full psychiatric assessment is recommended.

Others

For other causes the history will usually be obvious. There will usually be severe chest pain in myocardial infarction, and severe pain associated with testicular torsion or trauma. A history of a fracture will be obvious. There may be a history of severe chest infection, e.g. bronchitis or bronchiectasis, associated with coughing bouts followed by vomiting. There may be a recent history of radiotherapy for malignant disease. Widespread malignant disease may cause vomiting.

EXAMINATION

Gastrointestinal

A full gastrointestinal examination should be carried out. Look for signs of localised tenderness or signs of intestinal obstruction.

CNS

With raised intracranial pressure there will be listlessness, irritability, drowsiness, and the pulse rate will be low with a rising blood pressure. Check for papilloedema. Ultimately coma and irregular breathing will occur. With acute labyrinthitis there may be nystagmus to the opposite side from the lesion. The fistula test will be positive (pressure on the tragus causes vertigo or eye deviation by reducing movement of the perilymph). Sensorineural deafness may occur in purulent labyrinthitis. With Ménière's there will be rotatory nystagmus and unsteadiness of stance and gait during an attack, together with past-pointing.

Psychogenic

In anorexia nervosa, a wasted hirsute female will present, often with anxious parents.

Others

With myocardial infarction there may be signs of acute congestive cardiac failure. With causes of severe pain, attention will normally be drawn to the appropriate area, e.g. scrotum with testicular trauma or torsion. With irradiation there may be skin signs of recent radiotherapy. With widespread malignant disease the patient is often cachectic. A site of the primary may be obvious. With severe coughing, chest signs may be obvious.

GENERAL INVESTIGATIONS

- **FBC, ESR**
  Hb ↑ gastrointestinal disease. Malignancy. Anorexia nervosa.
  WCC ↓ abdominal inflammation. ESR ↓ inflammation. Tumour.
- **U&Es**
  Dehydration. Uraemia. Hyperkalaemia occurs in Addison's disease.
- **LFTs**
  Biliary tract disease.
- **Serum amylase**
  Pancreatitis.
- **CXR**
  Congestive cardiac failure – pulmonary oedema. Malignancy. Pneumonia. Bronchiectasis.
- **ECG**
  Myocardial infarction.
- **AXR**
  Obstruction.

SPECIFIC INVESTIGATIONS

- **Blood glucose**
  Raised in diabetes. Low in Addison's disease.
- **Serum calcium**
  Hyperparathyroidism and other causes of hypercalcaemia.

- **ABGs**
  Diabetic ketoacidosis.
- **βHCG**
  Pregnancy.
- **Toxicology screen**
  Drug causes of vomiting.
- **Barium enema**
  Malignancy. Diverticular disease.
- **Small bowel enema**
  Gastrointestinal disease, e.g. Crohn's disease.
- **OGD**
  Peptic ulcer disease. Malignancy.
- **US**
  Gastrointestinal disease, e.g. gallstones.
- **CT**
  Abdominal malignancy. Intracranial lesion associated with raised intracranial pressure.
- **Rinne's test**
  Ménière's disease, labyrinthitis.
- **Caloric tests**
  Labyrinthitis, Ménière's disease.
- **Audiometry**
  Ménière's disease, labyrinthitis.

WEIGHT GAIN

In most cases, weight gain is not pathological. With the exception of pregnancy the conditions listed below account for less than 1% of patients presenting with weight gain.

CAUSES

Pregnancy

Increased fat
- Cushing's syndrome
- Hypothyroidism
- Polycystic ovarian syndrome
- Hypothalamic disease

Increased fluid
- Cardiac failure
- Renal failure – nephrotic syndrome
- Ascites
- Lymphatic obstruction

Increased muscle
- Growth hormone
- Androgenic steroids
- Athletes, e.g. weightlifters

HISTORY

General
Enquire about the possibility of pregnancy and any changes in dietary habits that may result in simple weight gain. Rapid weight gain is often secondary to increased fluid as opposed to an increase in dry weight. A drug history is taken to exclude the use of anabolic steroids and growth hormone, especially in body builders.

Cushing's syndrome
Patients with Cushing's syndrome present with hair growth, acne, abdominal striae, muscle weakness, back pain, amenorrhoea, thin skin, bruising and depression. A drug history should be taken to exclude exogenous corticosteroids as the cause for Cushing's syndrome.

Hypothyroidism

With hypothyroidism, patients may complain of lethargy, anorexia, cold intolerance, goitre, dry hair, dry skin, constipation and menorrhagia.

Polycystic ovarian syndrome

Women with this condition present with hirsutism, obesity and menstrual irregularities. It is also associated with insulin resistance.

Hypothalamic disease

Prior history of neurosurgery, craniopharyngioma or other brain tumours may have resulted in damage to the hypothalamus. As it is the regulatory centre for appetite, uncontrolled excessive eating may result.

Cardiac failure

Fluid retention from cardiac failure may be accompanied by symptoms of exertional dyspnoea, orthopnoea, paroxysmal nocturnal dyspnoea. Ascites and peripheral oedema may also result from congestive heart failure.

Renal failure

Patients with renal failure may present with lethargy, fragile pigmented skin, peripheral oedema, periorbital oedema, thirst and polyuria.

ASCITES

See page 37.

EXAMINATION

Inspection

The distribution of body fat should be noted. Patients with Cushing's syndrome have truncal obesity with proximal muscle wasting. Hirsutism is a feature of both polycystic ovarian syndrome and Cushing's syndrome. With hypothyroidism there may be loss of the outer third of the eyebrows and a 'peaches and cream' complexion.

Inspection of the trunk may reveal thin skin with easy bruising in both Cushing's syndrome and renal failure. In addition, striae and thoracic kyphosis may be present with Cushing's from wedge fractures caused by osteoporosis.

Proximal muscle weakness is found in both Cushing's and hypothyroidism. Check for signs of 'body building'.

Palpation and auscultation

Peripheral oedema may be a feature of fluid overload with renal failure, cardiac failure. Non-pitting oedema is characteristically found with hypothyroidism. The JVP should be examined and will be elevated with congestive cardiac failure and fluid overload with renal failure. The pulse is taken and bradycardia may be noted with hypothyroidism. The blood pressure is measured and hypertension may be due to incorrect cuff size or may occur as a complication of Cushing's disease. A third heart sound may be present with cardiac failure, and widespread pulmonary crepitation suggests pulmonary oedema from cardiac failure or fluid overload in renal failure.

Further examination of the abdominal system may reveal the presence of ascites (page 37), which may result from liver disease, malignancy or cardiac failure. A complete neurological examination is performed to screen for neurological deficits, which will warrant diagnostic imaging to look for lesions involving the hypothalamus. If there is any suspicion that a patient is taking body-building drugs, e.g. anabolic steroids, check for testicular atrophy and prostatic hypertrophy.

GENERAL INVESTIGATIONS

- **Urine dipstick**
  +++ Glucose – diabetes from Cushing's or as a complication of obesity. Protein +++ is present with nephrotic syndrome. Blood may be present with renal diseases.
- **U&Es**
  Potassium ↓ Cushing's. Urea and creatinine ↑ renal failure.
- **TFTs**
  Screen for hypothyroidism.
- **Random cortisol**
  ↑ evening levels may suggest Cushing's syndrome; a normal result does not exclude it. Although commonly performed, has little diagnostic value.

SPECIFIC INVESTIGATIONS

- **24-hour urinary free cortisol**
  ↑ with Cushing's.
- **24-hour urine collection for protein**
  >3.5 g with nephrotic syndrome.
- **Low-dose dexamethasone test**
  Failure of cortisol suppression with Cushing's.
- **US abdomen and pelvis**
  Renal disorders, polycystic ovaries.
- **Echocardiography**
  Cardiac failure.
- **CT/MRI head**
  Hypothalamic disease.
- **Renal biopsy**
  To determine the aetiology of renal parenchymal disease.

WEIGHT LOSS

Unintentional weight loss may be a manifestation of underlying disease. The following are causes of occult weight loss.

CAUSES

Systemic disease
- Malignancy
- Cardiac failure
- Chronic respiratory disease
- Malabsorption
- Renal failure
- Liver failure

Endocrine
- Hyperthyroidism
- Diabetes mellitus
- Addison's disease

Infective
- TB
- HIV
- Helminth (worms) infection

Psychiatric
- Depression
- Anorexia nervosa

HISTORY

General
The time frame and amount of weight loss should be noted. A dietary history is required to determine the amount and type of food ingested. Decreased dietary intake may result from loss of appetite or loss of interest in eating due to depression. On the other hand, patients with thyrotoxicosis lose weight despite a voracious appetite.

Enquiries should be undertaken regarding perception of body image, as patients with anorexia nervosa believe that they are fat despite being severely underweight. Risk factors for HIV should be screened for and a sexual history as well as information regarding intravenous drug use should be obtained. Systemic enquiry is required to identify features suggestive of malignancy or organ failure in each system to account for unintentional weight loss.

Cardiorespiratory system

Dyspnoea, orthopnoea, paroxysmal nocturnal dyspnoea, peripheral oedema are symptoms suggestive of congestive cardiac failure. With long-standing cardiac failure, cardiac cachexia results from loss of total body fat and lean body mass. Currently the most common aetiology is end-stage heart failure. Dyspnoea without accompanying orthopnoea or paroxsysmal nocturnal dyspnoea suggests respiratory disease. With any chronic respiratory disorder, basal metabolic rate is increased as a result of the increased work of breathing. The presence of haemoptysis may be due to malignancy or TB. A long smoking history is a strong predisposing factor for the development of bronchial carcinoma and COPD. Night sweats and weight loss may be accompanying features of both TB and Hodgkin's disease.

Gastrointestinal system

Lethargy, diarrhoea, steatorrhoea (page 402) and abdominal discomfort are various symptoms suggestive of malabsorption. Jaundice, dark urine, pale stools, itching, prolonged bleeding, abdominal swelling from ascites, and confusion are symptoms associated with liver disease. Vague abdominal pains, change in bowel habit, tenesmus, blood or mucus mixed with the stools may be due to gastrointestinal malignancy. Patients with helminth infections, such as ascaris, may complain of perianal itching and notice worms in their faeces. Although this is rare in the UK, it may be encountered in patients returning from foreign travel.

Renal system

Lethargy, anorexia, nocturia, oliguria, polyuria, haematuria, frothy urine from proteinuria, skin fragility, pruritus, oedema and bone pains are some of the multisystemic features suggestive of renal disease.

Haematological system

Localised non-tender lymphadenopathy from Hodgkin's disease may be accompanied by pyrexia and pruritus. Persistent generalised lymphadenopathy, however, is a recognised presenting feature of HIV.

Endocrine system

Polydipsia and polyuria with weight loss may be presenting features of diabetics. Patients with thyrotoxicosis may complain of tremor, staring eyes, heat intolerance, palpitations and diarrhoea.

With Addison's disease, anorexia, malaise, nausea, vomiting, diarrhoea or syncope from postural hypotension may be experienced.

EXAMINATION

The causes of occult weight loss are very varied. The following specific features that may be identified on examination may be useful in determining an underlying cause.

Inspection

Signs suggestive of endocrine disorder may be obvious; a goitre may be visible with thyrotoxicosis, accompanied by exophthalmos and tremor. Pigmentation of the skin creases and buccal mucosa in a cachectic patient with postural hypotension are the usual findings with Addison's disease. Jaundice, caput medusae, spider naevi and gynaecomastia may be seen with liver disease. Tachypnoea and pursed-lip breathing may be evident with COPD. Clubbing may be a feature of bronchial carcinoma, suppurative lung disease, cirrhosis and inflammatory bowel disease. The JVP is elevated with congestive cardiac failure.

Palpation and auscultation

Peripheral oedema may be present with cardiac failure, malabsorption, renal and liver disease. Auscultation of the chest may reveal widespread crepitations with pulmonary oedema from cardiac failure, or uniformly decreased breath sounds with COPD. Palpation of the abdomen may reveal hepatomegaly and ascites with liver disease; ascites may also occur with cardiac failure and gastrointestinal malignancies. Lying and standing blood pressure should be measured, as a postural drop is present with Addison's disease.

GENERAL INVESTIGATIONS

- **Urine dipstick**
  Glucose with diabetes. Protein and blood with renal disorders.
- **FBC**
  Hb ↓ chronic disease, malabsorption, renal and liver failure.
- **ESR**
  ↑ with malignancy.

- **U&Es**
  Urea and creatinine ↑ renal failure. Sodium ↓, potassium ↑ and bicarbonate ↓ Addison's disease.
- **Blood glucose**
  More than 11.1 mmol/l on two separate occasions indicate diabetes mellitus.
- **LFTs**
  Bilirubin ↑, transaminases ↑ and albumin ↓ liver failure.
- **Clotting screen**
  PT ↑ liver failure.
- **TSH and free T$_4$**
  TSH ↓ and T$_4$ ↑ thyrotoxicosis.
- **CXR**
  Malignancy, TB.

SPECIFIC INVESTIGATIONS

- **Faecal fat estimation**
  ↑ with fat malabsorption.
- **Faecal occult blood**
  Colorectal carcinoma
- **AXR**
  Pancreatic calcification with chronic pancreatitis.
- **Colonoscopy**
  Colorectal carcinoma, inflammatory bowel disease.
- **Gastroscopy**
  Gastric carcinoma.
- **US abdomen**
  Malignancy, small kidneys with renal failure.
- **Short synacthen test**
  Failure of plasma cortisol to increase with Addison's disease.
- **Echocardiography**
  Ventricular impairment with cardiac failure.
- **Stool cultures**
  Microscopy for helminths and their ova. Helminths may occasionally be visible with the naked eye.
- **HIV antibodies**
  For the diagnosis of HIV.

INDEX